FUNDAMENTALS
of
ORTHOPAEDICS

Third Edition

John J. Gartland, M.D.

James Edwards Professor of Orthopaedic
Surgery and Chairman of the Department,
Jefferson Medical College of Thomas Jefferson
University, Philadelphia, Pennsylvania

1979

W.B. SAUNDERS COMPANY

Philadelphia • London • Toronto

W. B. Saunders Company: West Washington Square
                          Philadelphia, PA 19105

                          1 St. Anne's Road
                          Eastbourne, East Sussex BN21 3UN, England

                          1 Goldthorne Avenue
                          Toronto, Ontario M8Z 5T9, Canada

Fundamentals of Orthopaedics   ISBN   0-7216-4047-8

Last digit is the print number: 9   8   7   6   5   4   3   2   1

To L. M. L.

With the gratitude and affection of the entire Department

Preface to the Third Edition

The call for a third edition of Fundamentals of Orthopaedics since 1965 would seem to signal the establishment of this book as a basic primary text for Orthopaedic Surgery. Each chapter has been carefully reviewed for content, clarity and balance, and appropriate changes have been made. My sole intent, as before, has been to make the book more readable, more logical and more timely. New illustrations have been added, and the references made more complete and current.

The chapter on Neuromuscular Disorders has been written by Dr. John Dowling, a member of the orthopaedic faculty at Jefferson. Dr. Dowling joins Dr. Phillip Marone as Jefferson orthopaedic faculty contributors to the book. As time goes on, it is my intent to involve other orthopaedic faculty members in the writing of chapters.

It is my hope that, eventually, the book will become more of a Departmental effort and less of a solo effort. Regardless of possible future editorial changes, the goal of this and all future editions will remain exactly the same as that expressed for the first edition. That is, and will remain, a basic and introductory book intended principally to acquaint the student with the disorders of the musculoskeletal system and to indicate the scope, the limitations, and the possibilities of this fascinating field of medicine.

My grateful thanks are extended to the entire orthopaedic resident staff at Thomas Jefferson University Hospital for their assistance in selecting timely and current references. Most of the new photographs were made by Larry Kradle of our departmental photographic unit.

The manuscript was typed and retyped in a flawless fashion by Ann Louise Smith.

My thanks are sincerely offered again to the staff of W. B. Saunders Company for their friendly professionalism and skillful expertise.

JOHN J. GARTLAND, M.D.
Philadelphia, Pennsylvania

June 1979

Contents

CHAPTER 1

THE TASK
THE MATERIAL,
AND THE TOOLS

THE TASK

Orthopaedics is that part of medicine directly concerned with the disorders that befall the musculoskeletal system including bone, joints, and muscles and their associated ligaments, tendons, and bursae. This specialty is surgically oriented and has been formally defined as that branch of medicine especially involved in the preservation and restoration of the function of the skeletal system, its articulation, and associated structures.

It can be expected that most practicing physicians will have some contact with the patient with a musculoskeletal complaint. An estimated 20 to 30 per cent of patients seeking medical advice from family practitioners have complaints arising from the musculoskeletal system. The task facing these physicians, as well as the orthopaedic physician, now properly encompasses all of the congenital, traumatic, infectious, hereditary, metabolic, neoplastic, and degenerative processes to which the musculoskeletal system is subject.

The term orthopaedic originally appeared in 1741 in the title of a book, published by Nicholas Andry of the University of Paris, in which certain basic problems of the musculoskeletal development of children were discussed as factors contributing to adult deformity. The word was synthesized by Andry from the Greek roots *orthos*

1

(straight) and *paidios* (child). He submitted the proposition that the prevention of deformed adults lies in the development of straight children. Modern orthopaedics has expanded from this narrow view to apply to patients of all ages and now includes in its scope injuries, diseases, and deformities of bones and joints and their related muscles, tendons, ligaments, and nerves.

The early orthopaedist made extensive use of braces and mechanical appliances to prevent and correct skeletal deformity. The modern orthopaedic surgeon, though equally concerned with mechanical correction, can now operate with safety to obtain earlier and more complete correction of a deformity by direct surgical approach.

In recent years there has been an increased awareness of the importance of engineering principles in explaining the behavior of biological systems. This awareness has stemmed from the combined efforts of orthopaedists and engineers who have applied engineering concepts to the field of orthopaedic surgery, thereby demonstrating the usefulness of biomedical engineering principles for better understanding the musculoskeletal system.

FIGURE 1–1. Fracture of proximal femur after open reduction and nail-plate fixation.

FIGURE 1–2. Lack of appreciation of bio-mechanical principles has led to device failure after one week.

This improved understanding has resulted in more sophisticated approaches to orthopaedic problems. Clinical application of basic research in biomedical engineering has led to new orthopaedic procedures and surgical techniques. Advances in biomedical engineering have also led to the widespread use of joint implants in reconstructive surgery. The emergence of biomechanics as a defined area of knowledge in orthopaedics is relatively new, but has already produced developments that have resulted in improvement in patient care (Figs. 1–1 and 1–2)

The present-day orthopaedic surgeon, in addition to solving clinical problems related to both form and function, has developed a deep interest in the cause of deformity and takes an active part in helping to find answers for unsolved questions. Orthopaedic research laboratories, making use of tools supplied by other areas of scientific investigation, are engaged in basic research applied to musculoskeletal disorders and have already produced new information relative to many problems, including arthritis, genetic disorders, and tumors. It is hoped that an increased knowledge of biophysical processes will provide the orthopaedic physician with a key to both the prevention and the cure of many of the perplexing deformities and diseases that befall the musculoskeletal system. Much that is hopeful and exciting in this direction lies on the orthopaedic horizon.

THE MATERIAL

The essential material with which the orthopaedist must work is bone — a hard, specialized connective tissue with a calcified collagenous intercellular substance. Trapped within this hard connective tissue are small living cells, the osteocytes, in communication by means of a network of thin cellular processes that lie in minute tubules called canaliculi. The most striking and obvious difference between bone and all other forms of connective tissue is that bone is the only tissue to contain inorganic mineral deposits within its intercellular matrix space at almost all stages of its normal development (Fig. 1–3). These mineral salts have a distinct morphologic relationship to the organic elements of the bone matrix, fulfill a definitive mechanical function within this tissue, and are involved in critical metabolic and homeostatic processes that are under stringent physiologic control.

FIGURE 1–3. Radiograph of dried specimen of adult proximal femur. Mineral content maintains the bone architecture in spite of total cellular death.

Chemically, the mineral portion of bone is composed of calcium phosphate salts containing a small but significant amount of carbonate (4 to 6 per cent) and a very small amount of other ions, such as sodium, potassium, magnesium, and chloride. It is believed that a large proportion of the calcium phosphate in bone exists in crystalline form, having a configuration very similar to that of the geologic family of calcium phosphate minerals, the apatites.

Bone mineral, then, is an integral part of bone tissue, having individual physical and chemical properties that directly affect those of the tissue as a whole. It is the mineral portion of the skeleton that is involved in the unique role that bone tissue plays in maintaining mineral metabolism and homeostasis. Bone serves as a storehouse for 99 per cent of the body's calcium, 80 to 90 per cent of its phosphate, and 70 per cent of its magnesium.

The organic matrix of bone consists of collagen, protein, polysaccharides, and lipids. The matrix is a complex substance that provides the general mechanical and morphological architecture of the skeleton. Long considered relatively inert from a biologic viewpoint, recent evidence suggests that the protein and lipid fractions may play some role in the process of ossification and mineralization.

Thus it can be seen that bone has several important functions within the body. It serves a *mechanical* function by forming the skeletal support of the body: protecting vital structures, providing attachments for muscles, and housing the bone mineral. It also serves a *physiologic* function related to its mineral content. Bone acts as a storage depot for calcium and phosphorus and plays a significant role in meeting the needs of the patient for these elements. Abnormal physiologic demands on bone may result in pathologic changes in bone tissue. If the serum calcium falls below its normal value, the body can react in three specific ways to restore it to normal: (1) it may increase intestinal absorption; (2) it may decrease urinary excretion; and (3) it may increase the release of calcium from bone. If calcium is released from bone, the first supply comes from the surfaces of the canaliculi and Howship's lacunae. If this supply is insufficient, parathyroid hormone secretion is increased, which influences the release of calcium successively from the cells and bone surrounding the osteocytes, from the large mass of cancellous bone, and finally from cortical bone. If not corrected, this process could continue indefinitely until the skeleton becomes depleted.

Belying its appearance, normal bone is a living tissue in a constant state of physiologic activity. The sequence of bone formation, bone destruction, and new bone formation is repeated many times in the life cycle of a bone. Resorption of bone in one region and deposition in other regions are responsible for the growth changes in the skeleton. This process of resorption and deposition continues throughout the life of the healthy individual in response to various mechanical and hormonal stimuli.

Bone develops by transformation of pre-existing connective tissue. After vascularization of the condensed connective tissue, the cells begin to actively secrete proteoglycans and collagen to form the bone matrix *(osteoid)* and bone collagen. The deposition of mineral salts in the matrix or osteoid tissue, probably through the mechanism of direct cellular action, begins the process of ossification. Osteoblasts are found on the surfaces where bone is being formed. Mineral crystals developed from the calcium and phosphate in the intercellular matrix and, under the influence of mesenchymal cells, called *osteoblasts,* are deposited in relation to both collagen fibrils and proteoglycans of the matrix. As the calcification progresses, many osteoblasts become trapped and embedded within the calcified matrix. These embedded cells are then called *osteocytes.* Although the structure of bone tissue is complete at this point, the development process continues until mature bone is produced.

Bone resorption begins while bone formation is in progress. The two processes go on simultaneously and their dynamic interaction is responsible for establishing the final shape and architecture of each bone. The cells associated with bone removal are called *osteoclasts.* The osteoclast is a large, multinucleated cell that plays an active role in bone resorption. It is found in notches or indentations of bone surfaces called *Howship's lacunae.*

Bone is also a plastic tissue and is highly sensitive to alteration of its normal mechanical function. Bone responds to change in function and to stress put upon it by *remodeling;* that is, bone being added where it is needed and removed from where it is not needed. The general principle of this remodeling process is known as Wolff's Law (1868), which holds that every change in the form or function of the bone is followed by certain definite changes in its internal architecture and its external shape (Fig. 1–4). Thus increased skeletal use is accompanied by. bone hypertrophy with an increase in bone mass, whereas skeletal disuse results in bone atrophy with a decrease in bone mass.

Biomechanical studies of bone tissue have identified an elastic phase and a plastic phase. Up to a certain point of loading bone deforms under load, but snaps back to normal shape with release of the load. Beyond this point, bone deforms permanently with load, or if the load is sufficiently high, bone breaks or fractures. The strength of a bone is directly related to its density (bone mass per unit volume). When bone density is reduced by disease, the

FIGURE 1-4. Dried specimen of adult proximal femur. Thickened cortical bone on medial aspect of femoral neck and alignment of cancellous trabecular systems illustrates Wolff's law.

stresses necessary to produce fracture are much smaller. It has also been shown that bone becomes less elastic, or stiffer, with age. Putting drill holes or screw holes in bone is also known to weaken its structure.

Because of its ability to undergo internal reconstruction in response to external stimuli, bone may, to some extent, be modified at will by surgical and experimental procedures.

Like other body tissues, bone tissue may react to abnormal stimuli in a variety of ways, but these reactions are modified somewhat by its peculiar structure. Fracture healing, for example, consists of stages of inflammation and repair like any wound healing, but has the additional stage of osteogenesis. Infection has a particular effect on bone tissue and periosteum. Inflammatory granulation tissue may erode bone, with a loss of normal bone rigidity. Vascular phenomena may occur with infection and include vascular occlusion and ischemic or avascular necrosis of bone. When an area of bone is completely deprived of its blood supply, local cell death occurs; this type of response is known as *avascular necrosis* or *osteonecrosis*. The body's attempt to heal the segment of bone by ingrowth of vascular tissue from the live bone is known as "creeping substitution."

Bone that remains alive can respond to abnormal stimuli by an alteration of bone deposition, by an alteration of bone resorption, or by a combination of these two processes. Bone deposition involves two stages, the osteoblastic formation of matrix or osteoid and its subsequent calcification to form bone. Either process can be altered by an abnormal state. As the reader progresses through this book, numerous clinical examples will be noted in which the pathologic bone response is based either on increased or decreased bone deposition or on increased or decreased bone resorption.

BONE DEVELOPMENT

As already noted, bone always develops by the transformation of embryonic or adult connective tissue into calcified connective tissue. When this process occurs in cartilage, it is called *endochondral ossification.* Bone formed without a preceding cartilaginous base is called *membranous bone.* The only difference between the two processes is that the former occurs within a cartilage model that must be removed before ossification can take place, although some of the cartilage matrix may remain as a framework on which bone is deposited. In both instances, actual bone tissue formation is the same.

BONE STRUCTURE

The gross structure of bone is very closely related to its function. Bone is strongest in areas where the greatest stress is applied. It is angulated or presents external prominences where such deviations can best serve muscle function. Bone assumes three general shapes: flat bone such as skull and pelvis; cuboidal bones such as vertebral and tarsal bones; and long bones such as femur and tibia. Generally, the ends of long bones are covered with articular cartilage and are broad in order to distribute weight-bearing loads through the joints. The cartilage is supported by a bony plate, the subchondral bone, which represents the visible margin of the joint seen on a radiograph.

Grossly, bone tissue occurs in two types: *cancellous* (spongy) and *cortical* (compact). Cancellous bone consists of a latticework of interconnecting bony trabeculae surrounding spaces filled with bone marrow. This type of bone is found in abundance beneath the subchondral bone plate and provides an efficient structural means of supporting the articular surface against weight-bearing loads.

Cortical bone is the outer surface of bone and appears as a continuous hard mass giving rigid strength to the bone. Almost every bone contains varying proportions of both types of tissue in separate but merging zones. The cortical surface of bone is covered with periosteum. The inner surface of cortical bone is lined with endosteum, which also lines the marrow spaces.

A long bone is divided into several anatomic zones, the names of which are frequently used in orthopaedic terminology (Fig. 1–5). The zone at either end of the long bone is called the *epiphysis*. This is a mass of cartilage at birth and is joined to the shaft of the bone by a specialized layer of cartilaginous cells known as the *growth plate*. By the time skeletal maturity is reached, the cartilaginous epiphysis

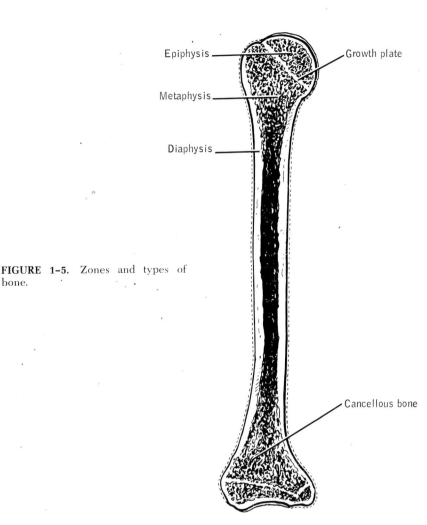

Epiphysis

Growth plate

Metaphysis

Diaphysis

Cancellous bone

FIGURE 1–5. Zones and types of bone.

has become completely ossified except for its covering of articular hyaline cartilage, and the growth plate has become only a line across the bone. The *metaphysis* is that part of the shaft of the bone immediately adjacent to the epiphysis. The *diaphysis* is the shaft of the long bone.

THE TOOLS

Diagnostic Tools

HISTORY

The history is the story of the patient's condition related by the patient with the guidance of the examiner. At its conclusion, the examiner should understand clearly why the patient is seeking medical attention.

The story should be built around specific complaints. Disorders of musculoskeletal origin frequently give rise to specific complaints of pain, deformity, and loss of joint motion, or to symptoms of neurologic involvement. The examiner should guide the patient through an exact description in chronologic sequence by using appropriate questions concerning manner of onset, duration of symptoms, previous symptoms, progress of the complaint, and extent of disability.

It is important to characterize the complaint. Deformity, for example, may be static or progressive, constant or intermittent. Pain may be localized to one area or may radiate to another part of the body. Pain may be described as aching, dull, sharp, or shooting.

Since musculoskeletal complaints are frequently associated with body mechanics, the examiner should determine the effect on the specific complaint of weight-bearing, motion of the part, weather change, and rest. The examiner should ask the patient what aggravates the complaint, what relieves it, whether it has ever been treated and, if so, what the effects of treatment were.

PHYSICAL EXAMINATION

The orthopaedic physical examination includes evaluation of the body as a whole in addition to a more detailed examination of the part in question.

GENERAL ORTHOPAEDIC EXAMINATION

The general posture and alignment of the body, both front and back, are observed. It is important to evaluate the patient's body

attitude when standing and the carriage when the patient is walking. The relationships of the feet to the legs and of the hips to the
pelvis are noted. The relationship of the upper extremities,
shoulder girdle, and neck to the upper trunk is observed. The general contour of the spine is evaluated and its relationship to the
shoulder girdle, thorax, and pelvis is noted.

· The patient is observed while walking and any effect upon
these various relationships should be evaluated. The manner of
walking and the presence of a limp and its type should be observed. Any physical abnormality associated with walking, bending,
sitting, or lying should be noted.

LOCAL ORTHOPAEDIC EXAMINATION

Specific physical findings of orthopaedic significance referable
to each part of the body are discussed in detail in appropriate sections of the text.

Whenever the complaint refers to an area of either the lower or
upper extremity, it is a good plan to examine the opposite side first.
This affords the examiner the chance to establish a normal base line
for that particular patient.

In general, the local physical examination should include:

Inspection. By inspection the examiner should note contour,
appearance, color, or deformity of a part, and its general relationship
to the body as a whole.

Palpation. By palpation the examiner should detect tenderness, swelling, muscle spasm, local temperature changes, or gross
alterations in shape of the part.

Range of Motion. Each joint has characteristic motions that
can be measured passively or actively. Motion is normally limited
by the resistance of other nearby structures or by actual impingement on the joint by muscles, ligaments, or bone. Motion is abnormally limited by pain and muscle spasm, by inflammation or scarring of the muscles, ligaments, or synovial membrane, or by deformity
of the bone or joint.

Joint motion is measured in degrees of a circle (Fig. 1–6). An
extended limb with the bones in a straight line can be said to be
either in 0 degrees of flexion or 180 degrees of extension. This represents the diameter of a circle with the joint at its center. As the
joint is flexed from this position, the angle is increased or reduced
depending upon which style of measurement is chosen, reaching 90
degrees at a right angle.

Passive joint motion is measured manually by the examiner
while the patient is relaxed. The examiner tests the range of motion

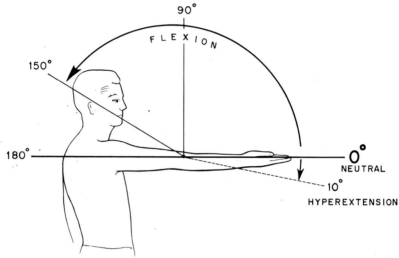

FLEXION and HYPEREXTENSION

FIGURE 1-6. Joint motion is measured in degrees of a circle. (From Joint Motion Manual, American Academy of Orthopaedic Surgeons.)

of which the part is normally capable and compares this range with that obtained on the opposite side.

Active joint motion represents the degree to which the patient can, without assistance, move the affected part.

Except for patients with problems associated with muscular weakness or paralysis, the information related to joint motion obtained by testing passive motion is generally more valuable to the physician than the information obtained by evaluating active motion.

Joint Position. There are two important definitive positions that may be assumed by a joint under particular circumstances. The significance of these positions must be appreciated by the examiner.

The *position of function* for a joint is that position which gives the joint its maximum strength and efficiency. The position of function for the wrist joint, for example, is 30 degrees of dorsiflexion and 10 degrees of ulnar deviation. If injury or disease threatens to result in fusion or stiffness of the joint, disability will be minimized if the fusion occurs in the position of function.

The patient with an injured or diseased joint may assume the *position of comfort.* This is the position in which the joint feels most comfortable to the patient and is usually quite the reverse of the position of function. For example, the position of comfort for the wrist joint is palmar flexion. If the joint remains in this position following injury or disease, the disability that results from fusion or stiffness in this position will be markedly exaggerated.

Patients with damaged or diseased joints will naturally attempt to assume the position of comfort. It is part of the physician's responsibility to make sure that the affected joints are always supported in the position of function.

Measurement. Atrophy or hypertrophy of a part may be determined by comparing circumferential measurements made with a tape measure with those obtained at the same point on the opposite side of the body.

The lengths of the limbs should be measured and compared in order to assess any inequality that may be present. Leg length is usually measured with the patient lying supine on an examining table, with the pelvis level. Using a tape measure, the distance between the anterior superior iliac spine and the base of the medial malleolus is noted on either extremity. Differences in leg length up to one-quarter inch are considered within normal variation.

Neurologic Examination. The strength of muscle power should be assessed whenever the presence of muscular weakness is suspected. The quality of the superficial and deep tendon reflexes and the integrity of cutaneous sensation should be determined when indicated. More detailed information referable to the neurologic examination, particularly as it relates to the upper and lower extremities, is given in appropriate sections of the text.

RADIOGRAPHIC EXAMINATION

Properly exposed and processed radiographs are an important part of the examination of a patient with a musculoskeletal complaint.

Generally, the most useful views are the anteroposterior and lateral, with the films taken as the patient or the extremity lies upon the x-ray table. Visualization of bone should be in both planes whenever possible. It is frequently misleading and often impossible to attempt to evaluate the extent or character of a bone lesion from a single radiographic view. In certain conditions, it is helpful to obtain these views during weight bearing or while traction stress is being applied to the part (Fig. 1–7). In certain instances, oblique radiographic views or films made at other special angles are indicated to obtain special information.

Laminography. Laminography (tomography) or body-section radiography is occasionally helpful in locating overshadowed lesions, small cavities, and foreign bodies. It is also useful in determining whether or not a bone graft is firmly united to the host bone.

FIGURE 1–7. Stress x-ray of ankle, showing marked talar tilting of right ankle.

FIGURE 1–8. Myelogram. The radiopaque dye outlines the subarachnoid space and nerve root sleeves.

Scanography. This is a radiographic technique used to measure accurately the length of the long bone. Scanograms are frequently obtained of children with leg length inequality upon whom epiphyseal surgery is contemplated (see p. 93).

Myelography. Myelography is a radiographic technique that allows visualization of the spinal cord by the use of either air or a radiopaque dye injected into the subarachnoid space (Fig. 1–8). This test may be informative if pressure upon the spinal cord or nerve roots is suspected. Herniated intervertebral discs usually either indent the dye column or interfere with the filling of a nerve root sleeve, or both.

Arthrography. Arthrography is a special type of radiographic examination in which radiopaque dye or air, or both, are injected into a joint cavity to serve as a contrast medium to outline soft tissue components of the joint not usually visualized on an ordinary radiograph. This study is particularly useful in the knee joint as an aid to the diagnosis of meniscal tears or other suspected internal derangements (Fig. 1–9). It is frequently helpful as an aid to diagnosing tears in the rotator cuff of the shoulder joint.

Bone Scanning. Frequently, the use of radioisotopes can aid in demonstrating the presence of treatable disease earlier than con-

FIGURE 1–9. Normal knee arthrogram. Arrow points to triangular-shaped shadow representing a normal medial meniscus.

ventional radiographs. At the present time, radioactive technetium polyphosphate is considered the most useful radioisotope for clinical bone scanning. Any disorder that causes reactive bone formation will also produce scan abnormalities. In new bone formation, hydroxyapatite crystals are deposited in the osteoid matrix laid down by osteoblasts. If sufficient radioactive atoms are available for incorporation into the hydroxyapatite crystals, the new bone can be visualized by scintillation scanning.

Bone scanning is useful in detecting roentgenographically occult bone metastases, bone infection, and fractures, particularly pathologic fractures. The bone scan has proven valuable in the work-up of patients with bone or radicular pain when conventional roentgenograms are normal.

Axial Tomography. Axial tomography and computerized tomography are recently developed techniques designed to aid the physician in assessing the three-dimensional structure of the body and the relationship of the various organ systems. Use of these modalities appears helpful in the evaluation of some bone and soft tissue tumors and certain fractures of the spine.

LABORATORY STUDIES

The laboratory tests that are of greatest value in orthopaedic disorders are those performed on the blood, urine, synovial fluid, and tissue removed from the involved area.

The red and white blood cell count, hemoglobin determination, and erythrocyte sedimentation rate are frequently affected in the presence of anemia, blood dyscrasias, infection, and tissue destruction.

The blood chemical findings that are of most significance in skeletal disorders include serum calcium, serum inorganic phosphorus, serum alkaline phosphatase, serum acid phosphatase, blood nonprotein nitrogen, blood sugar, and blood uric acid levels (Table 1–1).

In certain skeletal conditions, abnormal amounts of calcium and phosphorous may be found in the urine. An abnormal protein (Bence Jones protein) may be detected in the urine of some patients with multiple myeloma. Many of the mucopolysaccharidoses can be diagnosed biochemically by identifying in the urine the specific mucopolysaccharide excreted in excess.

In many pathologic conditions of the musculoskeletal system, confirmation of the diagnosis rests upon the histologic interpretation of tissue removed from the lesion by biopsy.

TABLE 1-1. Laboratory Findings in Bone Disease*

CONDITION	SERUM			URINE	
	Calcium	Inorganic Phos- phorus	Alkaline Phos- phatase	Calcium	Phos- phorus
Hyperparathyroidism, primary	↑	↓	↑	↑	↑
Hyperparathyroidism, secondary	N–↓	↑	R ↑	↑	↓
Hyperthyroidism, marked	N	N	↑	↑	↑
Hypothyroidism	N	N	N	N	N
Senile osteoporosis	N	N–O ↓	N	N	N
Rickets (child)	↓	↓	↑	N	N
Osteomalacia (adult)	N–↓	↓	↑	N	N
Paget's disease	R ↑	R ↓	↑	N	N
Multiple myeloma	↑	N–↑	R ↑	↑	↑

CODE
N–normal
O–occasionally
R–rarely
↑ –increased
↓ –decreased
*Adapted from table of Dr. James L. Quinn, III. *In* Meschan, I.: Synopsis of Roentgen Signs. Philadelphia: W. B. Saunders Co., 1962.

SPECIAL TESTS

On occasion special tests may be required to aid in establishing diagnosis or proper treatment.

Joint Aspiration. A joint may be aspirated to relieve pain, to aid in making a diagnosis, or to instill medication. The aspirant obtained may be blood, pus, or synovial fluid, which may appear normal or abnormal.

This procedure must be performed under aseptic precautions and usually local anesthesia. The needle used for aspiration should be long enough to penetrate the joint capsule successfully and be of sufficient gauge to allow withdrawal of thickened fluid.

The joint most frequently aspirated is the knee. This joint may be aspirated through one of two approaches: (1) with the knee joint extended, a swollen suprapatellar pouch may be entered just medial to the superior pole of the patella; (2) with the knee flexed, the joint proper may be entered through the articular cleft just medial to the patellar tendon. This approach is generally the most useful.

Arthroscopy. Arthroscopy is the insertion of a specially designed endoscope into a joint cavity under anesthesia for the purpose of direct visualization of the joint's structure and contents. The technique has its greatest usefulness in the knee joint.

Ultrasound. Ultrasound, sometimes called sonography, sonics, or ultrasonography, is the technique of using sound waves and their echoes to locate and examine objects and parts of the human body. In the musculoskeletal system it is most useful in helping to define soft tissue masses and cysts.

Electromyography. Electromyography is a technique in which monopolar or coaxial needles are inserted directly into the muscle for the purpose of studying and measuring the electrical potential change associated with skeletal muscle contracture. Both this test and nerve conduction studies are frequently helpful in the differential diagnosis of neuromuscular disorders.

Biopsy. The term biopsy refers to the removal of tissue from a lesion for examination by a clinical pathologist for the purpose of diagnosis. In many instances, an open operation must be performed to obtain the tissue.

On occasion a core of tissue may be removed from a musculoskeletal lesion by a special type of needle or bore introduced through the skin. This type of biopsy is referred to as aspiration, needle, or punch biopsy. In certain areas of the body such as the spine, it is necessary to perform aspiration biopsy under radiographic control.

Treatment Tools

In the treatment program, the orthopaedic physician makes use of general medical measures, such as reassurance and encouragement, rest, attention to diet, and drugs when needed. Special treatment tools are also available for specific tasks. Among these special tools are plaster bandages, traction devices, braces and appliances, special dressings, orthopaedic surgical procedures, and rehabilitative measures. There should be no hesitation on the physician's part about requesting consultation with other physicians if the information obtained will aid in the diagnosis or management of the patient's problem.

PLASTER OF PARIS

One of the most useful tools available to the orthopaedist is plaster of paris, from which splints, circular casts, and molds of body parts can be made (Figs. 1–10 and 1–11).

Plaster is supplied by commercial manufacturers as rolled bandages of varying size wrapped in waxed paper. Plaster of paris bandages are rolls of crinoline-like bandage impregnated with anhydrous calcium sulfate. When these bandages are soaked in lukewarm water, the anhydrous calcium sulfate absorbs water to re-

FIGURE 1–10. A, short leg cast. B, long leg cast.

FIGURE 1–11. Hip spica cast.

crystallize or set as calcium sulfate dihydrate or gypsum. This process of recrystallization is an exothermic reaction that makes the plaster feel warm as it sets and hardens. Before the plaster bandages are applied, the part is usually padded with some type of sheet wadding, cotton bandage, or stockinette. Bony prominences should be protected by extra padding. The types of plaster casts most commonly used include:

Short leg cast, in which the plaster extends from the toes to the level of the tibial tubercle.

Long leg cast, in which the plaster extends from the toes to the upper thigh area.

Short arm cast, in which the plaster extends from the knuckles to just below the elbow.

Long arm cast, in which the plaster extends from the knuckles to just below the axilla.

Hip spica cast, which is used to immobilize the hip joint and pelvis. A double hip spica cast immobilizes both hip joints and allows the patient to be turned completely without moving the affected part. The plaster extends from the nipple line of the chest to the toes on the affected side and to the knee on the opposite side.

Shoulder spica cast, in which the plaster encases the upper extremity, shoulder region and trunk. This type of cast is used to immobilize parts of the upper extremity and shoulder joint.

TRACTION DEVICES

Some details regarding skin and skeletal traction devices are given in Chapter 2 (see p. 38).

In addition to its possible use as maintenance traction in the treatment of some fractures, the form of skin traction to the lower extremity known as Buck's extension may be used for any condition of the knee, femur or hip joint in which partial immobilization with a light traction force is desired. Thus, it may be used for temporary immobilization of a fractured hip or for immobilization following reduction of a dislocated hip joint. It may be used for short periods of time as a treatment of Legg-Calvé-Perthes disease or other causes of painful synovial irritation of the hip joint to help relieve pain caused by muscle spasm.

BRACES AND APPLIANCES

Braces and appliances may be used to rest a part of the body, to limit or encourage its activity, to aid in correcting or preventing deformity, or to provide mechanical support (Fig. 1–12).

FIGURE 1–12.   An ischial weight bearing brace.

Braces and appliances may be purely passive supports or may make use of spring devices to become dynamic splints.

The cast-brace is a device that has recently become popular in the ambulatory treatment of certain fractures of the distal femur and proximal tibia because it allows both knee motion and protected ambulation while the fracture is healing. Made of plaster of paris or molded plastic, the cast-brace must be firmly molded to the part in order to support the soft tissues and bone. Hinges at the knee connect the thigh and leg portions and allow knee motion (Fig. 1–13).

SPECIAL DRESSINGS

The Velpeau bandage and Gibney boot are examples of special dressings that find great usefulness in the treatment of some musculoskeletal problems.

The Velpeau bandage binds the arm and shoulder to the chest and is used mostly for immobilization of certain fractures about the upper end of the humerus and the shoulder joint. It is usually constructed from either wide-meshed gauze bandages or elastic bandages (Fig. 1–14). For the treatment of some conditions, a plaster of paris Velpeau dressing may be made.

FIGURE 1–13. Cast-brace.

The Gibney boot is an adhesive tape support useful in the treatment of sprains and other painful conditions about the ankle joint. The tape is applied by alternate strips in a basket weave fashion (Fig. 1–15).

ORTHOPAEDIC SURGICAL PROCEDURES

When proper indications exist, the orthopaedist may perform a surgical procedure as a method of treatment. The definitions of these surgical terms are given here. The indications for their use are discussed under the appropriate diagnoses in the body of the text. Orthopaedic surgical procedures may be performed on soft tissues or on bone. Surgical procedures that are performed on soft tissue by orthopaedists include:

Arthrotomy — the surgical opening of a joint for the purpose of exploring the joint for evidence of disease or removal of injured or diseased tissue.

Synovectomy — the surgical excision of abnormal synovial membrane from a joint.

FIGURE 1–14. Velpeau dressing.

FIGURE 1–15. Gibney boot.

Tenotomy — the surgical cutting of a tendon.

Capsulotomy — the surgical cutting of a joint capsule.

Tendon lengthening — a surgical technique designed to lengthen a shortened tendon without interrupting its continuity.

Tendon transplantation — the surgical relocation of the tendon of a normal muscle to another site to take over the function of a muscle permanently inactivated by trauma or disease.

Surgical procedures that are performed on bone include:

Osteotomy — the surgical cutting of bone in order to correct deformity in the bone or adjacent joint (see Fig. 2–11).

Arthrodesis — a surgical procedure designed to cause the bones of a joint to grow firmly together, or fuse. Arthrodesis, or fusion, involves surgical removal of articular hyaline cartilage and usually the addition of bone grafts across the joint surface. Metallic and internal fixation devices may or may not be used. Successful arthrodesis usually results in a stiff but stable and painless joint (Fig. 1–16).

Arthroplasty — a surgical procedure designed to restore motion to a joint deformed by injury or disease. Arthroplasty may involve replacement of part of the joint by a metallic prosthesis. Arthroplasty may also involve the surgical reshaping of the bones of the joint and, on occasion, the addition of a soft tissue or metallic interposition device between the reshaped bone ends to aid in establishing motion between the bone (Fig. 1–17).

FIGURE 1–16. AP radiograph of a surgically fused knee joint.

FIGURE 1-17. AP radiograph of hip after arthroplasty utilizing a metallic cup in patient with rheumatoid arthritis of both hips.

Total joint replacement — a special type of arthroplasty in which both sides of the joint are replaced by metal or plastic implants anchored to the bone by methyl methacrylate bone cement (see Fig. 14-26).

Bone grafting — the surgical transplantation of pieces of compact or cancellous bone to another location in the body. Bone grafts or transplants are commonly used to fill gaps and defects in bone, to facilitate the healing of fractures that otherwise would not heal or in which healing would be greatly delayed, and to bring about bony fusion in joints damaged by injury or disease.

The cells in a bone graft die soon after removal from the donor site. The dead bone graft acts as a framework in the host area and is eventually replaced by new bone tissue growing in from the host area. Bone grafts or transplants are classified according to the source of material to be grafted: those cut from the individual who will receive them are called *autografts;* those from another individual of the same species are called *homografts;* those from animals of another species are called *heterografts.* Whenever possible, autografts are used in orthopaedic surgical procedures because they produce no immunologic graft reaction phenomena. Homografts of stored or banked bone are occasionally necessary if large skeletal defects are to be filled. Heterografts are generally unsatisfactory and are seldom used in orthopaedic surgical procedures.

References

Andry, N.: Orthopaedia, Vols. I and II. Facsimile Reproduction of the First Edition in English, London 1743. Philadelphia: J. B. Lippincott Co., 1961.

Bick, E. M. (Ed.): Historical orthopaedics. Clin. Orth. and Rel. Res., No. 44, 1966.

Bourne, G. H. (Ed.): Biochemistry and Physiology of Bone, Vols. I, II, and III, 2nd Edition. New York: Academic Press, 1972.

Boyne, P. J.: Autogenous cancellous bone and marrow transplants. Clin. Orth. and Rel. Res., 73:199, 1970.

Brookes, M.: The Blood Supply of Bone. An Approach to Bone Biology. New York: Appleton-Century-Crofts, 1971.

Capener, N.: Surgical implants. J. Bone and Joint Surg., 47-B:3, 1965.

Chalmers, J.: Transplantation immunity in bone homografting. J Bone and Joint Surg., 41B:160, 1959.

Close, J. R.: Functional Anatomy of the Extremities. Springfield, Illinois: Charles C Thomas, 1973.

Crenshaw, A. H. (Ed.): Campbell's Operative Orthopaedics, Vols. 1 and 2, 5th Edition. St. Louis: C. V. Mosby Co., 1971.

D'Ambrosia, R. D. (Ed.): Musculoskeletal Disorders. Regional Examination and Differential Diagnosis. Philadelphia: J. B. Lippincott Co., 1977.

Duchene, G. B. A.: Physiology of Motion. Translated and Edited by E. B. Kaplan. Philadelphia: J. B. Lippincott Co., 1949.

Forrester, D. M., and Nesson, J. W.: The Radiology of Joint Disease. Philadelphia: W. B. Saunders Co., 1973.

Frankel, V. H., and Burstein, A.: Orthopaedic Biomechanics. Philadelphia: Lea and Febiger, 1970.

Frost, H. M.: Bone Biodynamics. Boston: Little, Brown & Co., 1964.

Hejna, W. F.: Clinical applications of electrodiagnostic studies. Am. Academy of Orthopaedic Surgeons Instructional Course Lectures, Vol. XIX. St. Louis: C. V. Mosby Co., 1970.

Hoppenfeld, S.: Physical Examination of the Spine and Extremities. New York: Appleton-Century-Crofts, 1976.

Howell, D. S.: Current concepts of calcification. J. Bone and Joint Surg., 53-A:250, 1971.

Jaffe, H. L.: Metabolic Degenerative and Inflammatory Diseases of Bone and Joints. Philadelphia: Lea & Febiger, 1972.

McLean, F. C., and Urist, M. R.: Bone: Fundamentals of the Physiology of Skeletal Tissue, 3rd Edition. University of Chicago Press, 1968.

Murray, R. O., and Jacobson, H. G.: The Radiology of Skeletal Disorders. Baltimore: Williams & Wilkins Co., 1971.

Raney, R. B., and Brashear, H. R., Jr.: Shands' Handbook of Orthopaedic Surgery, 8th Edition. St. Louis: C. V. Mosby Co., 1971.

Rang, M.: Anthology of Orthopaedics. London: E. & S. Livingstone, Ltd., 1968.

Rosse, C., and Clawson, D. K.: Introduction to the Musculoskeletal System. New York: Harper & Row, 1970.

Salib, P. I.: Plaster Casting. New York: Appleton-Century-Crofts, 1975.

Salter, R. B.: Textbook of Disorders and Injuries of the Musculoskeletal System. Baltimore: Williams & Wilkins Co., 1970.

Stein, I., Stein, R. O., and Beller, M. L.: Living Bone in Health and Disease. Philadelphia: J. B. Lippincott Co., 1955.

Termine, J. D.: Mineral chemistry and skeletal biology. Clin. Orth. and Rel. Res., 85:207, 1972.

Trueta, J.: Studies of the Development and Decay of the Human Frame. Philadelphia: W. B. Saunders Co., 1968.

Turek, S. L.: Orthopaedics. Principles and Their Application, 3rd Edition. Philadelphia: J. B. Lippincott Co., 1977.

Vaughn, J.: The Physiology of Bone. Oxford: Clarendon Press, 1970.

Wilson, F. C. (Ed.): The Musculoskeletal System. Philadelphia: J. B. Lippincott Co., 1975.

CHAPTER 2

PRINCIPLES OF MANAGEMENT OF FRACTURES AND DISLOCATIONS

THE PROBLEM

The problem facing the physician who is called upon to treat a patient with a broken bone or dislocated joint is that of restoring full function to the part, with the bone or joint solidly healed in a position as near to the normal as possible. These results can be obtained only through knowledge and judgment on the part of the physician and cooperation on the part of the patient.

Only the principles of management will be given in this chapter. Details regarding particular fractures and dislocations will be found in the chapters dealing with the specific regions involved.

FRACTURES

Definition

The standard definition of fracture is a break in the continuity of bone. However, a fracture is a rupture of living connective tissue and, as such, is more than a broken bone. It ultimately involves all the soft tissues in the injured area as well as the bone. Thus, fractures may be accompanied by extensive soft tissue edema, hemorrhage into muscles and joints, dislocation of joints, rupture of tendons, contusions or severance of nerves, and damage to major blood vessels.

As might be expected, fractures are most common in males in the 20 to 40 age group, with the bones of the extremities being most often involved. Although the forces causing fractures are no respecters of age or sex, certain fractures show characteristic predilections. Thus, fractures of the clavicle and through the supracondylar area of the humerus are most common in children. Fracture through the surgical neck of the humerus and Colles fracture at the wrist occur most frequently in middle-aged women. Compression fracture of a vertebra and fracture of the hip show the greatest incidence in the aged.

Normally, the age of the patient is no deterrent to fracture healing. Although it is true that fracture repair is more rapid and certain in children, the notion that fractures heal poorly in the aged is erroneous. Age and ability to repair bone are virtually unrelated in the normal adult. Rather, the rate and certainty of fracture healing are in direct relation to the vascularity of the bone and the surrounding soft tissues and the efficacy of the treatment received. In normal patients, the healing of fractures is not influenced by the use of vitamins, hormones, or extra dietary calcium. However, the coexistence of certain disease states, such as hypoproteinemia and severe anemia may delay fracture healing. The layman's suspicion that once a bone is broken it is forever weak is not true. Provided that normal anatomic alignment of the bone has been obtained, remodeling of the bone tissue after healing has occurred will restore normal strength and structure to the part. However, evidence does exist to indicate that the segment of bone containing the healed fracture does not fully regain its normal tissue elasticity.

Causes of Fractures

Normal bone with an intact blood supply exhibits a degree of elasticity that can withstand, within limits, compression and shearing forces and to a lesser extent, tension forces. Bone fractures, therefore, when its capacity to absorb energy is exceeded.

The most common cause of fracture of normal bone is violence. The violence may be applied directly to a bone, as in a fall on the part or when a person is struck by an automobile. Less violent transmitted forces may be applied indirectly to a bone by means of tension strain. Thus torsion injuries to the foot and ankle while skiing may cause an oblique fracture of the tibial shaft, or a fall on the outstretched hand may cause fracture of the radial head at the elbow.

An angulatory force applied to a long bone in a young child may fracture the cortex on the convex side of the bend, but only bend the cortex on the concave side, owing to the increased elasticity of young bone. This is the so-called "greenstick" fracture frequently seen in young children.

Sudden forceful muscle contraction may deliver a shearing force sufficient to break bone. Certain fractures of the patella and os calcis occur in this manner.

Stress or fatigue fractures occur in certain bones in the absence of documented violence. Bone reacts to repeated loading as do other materials. Occasionally bone fatigues and develops a crack that may go on to become a complete fracture. March fractures, seen in the metatarsals, are examples of stress fractures (see p. 450).

Much less violence is required to break a bone in elderly patients because of accompanying osteoporosis (see p. 118). Evidence indicates that osteoporosis causes quantitative, not qualitative, changes in bone. There is simply less bone present. The bone that remains exhibits no decrease in its strength characteristics or energy-absorbing capacity, but does exhibit decreased bone density.

A *pathologic* fracture is a fracture that occurs through an area of bone previously weakened by disease or tumor. In this instance, the involved bone is weakened both quantitatively and qualitatively by the underlying disease. As a rule, only minimal trauma is required to induce such a fracture. Examples of disease states that might be associated with pathologic fractures are osteomyelitis, metabolic bone disease, and lytic tumors of bone caused by deposits of metastatic carcinoma.

Classification of Fractures

Fractures may be classified according to the types of fracture sustained, the direction of the fracture line, or the type of bone tissue involved. The proper combination of these terms "describes the fracture."

TYPES OF FRACTURE (FIG. 2–1)

Closed fracture — a fracture of a bone not associated with a wound extending from the skin surface to the area of bone injury.

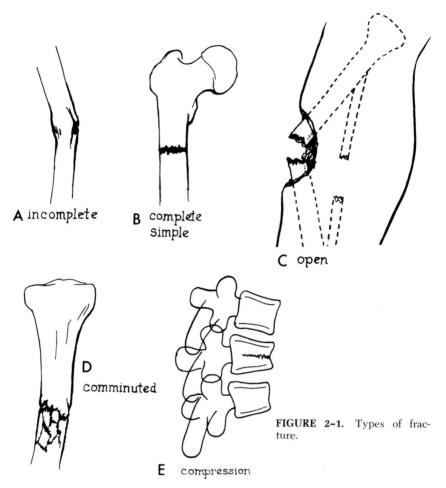

A incomplete   B complete simple   C open

D comminuted

E compression

FIGURE 2-1. Types of fracture.

Open fracture — a fracture of a bone associated with an open wound extending through the skin surface and down to the area of bone injury. Bone fragments may or may not be protruding through the open skin defect. All open fractures are potentially infected and require emergency surgical care.

Incomplete fracture — an incomplete break in the continuity of bone.

Complete fracture — a complete interruption in the continuity of bone.

Comminuted fracture — a fracture consisting of three or more bone fragments.

Impacted fracture — a fracture in which one fragment is imbedded in the substance of the other.

Compression fracture — a type of impacted fracture characterized by crushed bone tissue.

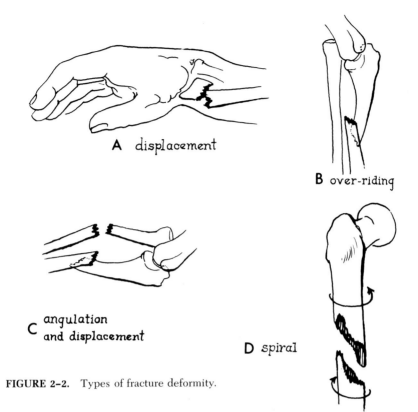

A displacement

B over-riding

C angulation and displacement

D spiral

FIGURE 2-2. Types of fracture deformity.

DIRECTIONS OF FRACTURE LINE (FIG. 2-2)

As seen on a radiograph, the fracture line may be described as *longitudinal, transverse, oblique,* or *spiral.* The fracture is said to be *displaced* when the bone fragments have been moved or changed from their normal position; it is said to exhibit *overriding* when the bone fragments overlap, resulting in shortening of the bone. The fracture is said to show *angulation* when the fragments have been moved out of the linear relationship into an angular relationship, and *rotation* is present when one fragment has rotated on its axis in relation to the other.

TYPES OF BONE TISSUE

Cancellous bone — Owing to the extremely rich blood supply, fractures involving the cancellous bone rarely fail to unite.

Cortical bone — Cortical or compact bone is thick and relatively avascular, enclosing a small vascular medullary canal. Repair of this type of bone tissue is slow.

Healing of Fractures

Most tissues have a common response to injury. This response includes inflammation and repair. Fracture healing is similar to any other type of wound healing except that osteogenesis occurs to re-establish bone continuity. Furthermore, the requirements of bone healing differ from those of soft tissue in that not only is tensile strength needed, but torsional, bending, and compressive strengths are also required to achieve stability.

Once a bone is broken into two or more parts, each part is thereafter called a *fragment*. The new tissue that forms at and around the area of the break to join the fragments together for healing is called *callus* or *callus tissue* (Fig. 2–3). Callus that arises from the periosteum is called external callus. Callus that arises from the endosteum of the marrow cavity and from marrow cells is called internal callus. In successful healing, the callus is first composed of both cartilage and bone but eventually consists only of bone tissue. In unsuccessful repair, the callus may be composed of dense fibrous tissue and fibrocartilage that does not convert to bone. If this occurs, the fragments are said to be joined by a fibrous union.

The events that take place in the healing of the fracture involve a number of tissues including the bone itself, its periosteum, endosteum, marrow and the soft tissues adjacent to the fracture. The following steps in fracture repair have been described:

1. The violence that causes fracture results in a tearing or rupture of haversian, marrow and periosteal blood vessels. Loss of their blood supply leads to the death of bone and periosteal cells in the area adjacent to the fracture line. Bleeding from the ends of a broken bone results in the formation of a blood clot or a fracture hematoma between the bone fragments. The normal inflammatory response of the tissue permits gradual removal of cellular debris and fibrin by macrophages. Within 48 to 72 hours a few connective tissue cells appear in the wound and begin to multiply, having invaded the fracture site from the adjacent vascular connective tissue and marrow. These cells can differentiate into chondroblasts or osteoblasts. The periosteum and endosteum also act as sources of osteoblasts.

2. For the first seven days, the fracture site is similar to any wound except for the presence of fibroblasts and osteoblasts. The fibroblasts and osteoblasts actively engage in the synthesis and se-

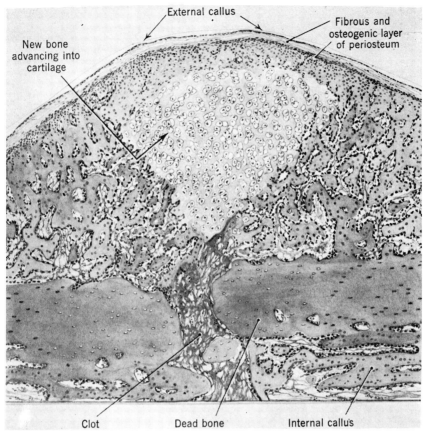

FIGURE 2-3. Drawing of part of a section cut from a rabbit's fractured rib that has healed for 2 weeks. This drawing illustrates the external callus to advantage and shows that the cartilage in it is being replaced by bone along a V-shaped line. Some clot, still unorganized, can still be seen. (Ham, A. W., and Harris, W. R.: *In* Bourne, G. H.: The Biochemistry and Physiology of Bone, 2nd ed. New York: Academic Press, 1972.)

cretion of collagen, which takes the form of fibrils of varying diameter within the wound site. They also synthesize and secrete proteoglycans that form an integral part of the proliferative connective tissue matrix or callus at the repair site. Callus begins to calcify within 14 to 17 days and ultimately bone mineral (hydroxyapatite) is deposited in it.

3. External callus grows and develops from osteogenic cells of the torn periosteum as a collar of cartilage and new bone. This collar encircles the fragments, enlarges, and grows towards the collar associated with the adjacent bone fragment.

4. Internal callus, arising from the endosteum of the marrow cavity and from marrow cells, infiltrates the blood clot. The remain-

ing blood clot aids in the joining process by becoming converted into osteoid tissue. Eventually, bone trabeculae from each fragment meet and join.

5. The fracture fragments become firmly united by an external bridge of trabeculated bone and an internal bridge of trabeculated bone. These newly formed trabeculae are joined to living and dead portions of the original bone fragments.

6. Final remodeling of the healed area is the last step in fracture healing. The dead portions of the original fragments are slowly resorbed and the bone gradually assumes a more normal shape and architecture (Fig. 2–4).

The time required for healing varies with the severity of the fracture, the age of the patient, and the bone that is broken. In general, closed fractures, fractures in children, fractures through small bones, and fractures through cancellous bone heal faster than open fractures, fractures in adults, fractures through long bones, and fractures through cortical bone.

FIGURE 2–4. *A*, supracondylar fracture of humerus treated by skeletal traction. *B*, same area five years later showing final remodeling of bone.

If the healing process is disrupted for any reason — as by loss of fracture hematoma, lack of adequate blood supply to the fragments, poor immobilization, or infection — it may be delayed or stopped completely.

HEALING OF ARTICULAR CARTILAGE

Unlike bone, articular cartilage is very limited in its ability to regenerate. It differs from other tissues in its lack of blood supply. The absence of vessels within cartilage and the low mitotic activity of its cells impose severe limitations on the healing ability of this tissue. The healing of cartilage is slow and usually incomplete. Hyaline articular cartilage heals not by hyaline cartilage, but by fibrous tissue and fibrocartilage, which is a form of scar tissue.

This is of clinical significance when a fracture involves a joint with a splitting of the articular cartilage. If the fracture surfaces of the cartilage are perfectly reduced, the thin band of fibrocartilage is of little clinical significance. If a gap remains between the fragments, however, the fibrocartilage filling the gap will not withstand normal wear and tear stresses and the joint may eventually show degenerative changes.

FRACTURE MANAGEMENT

General Examination

In some patients, fracture of bone may be just one aspect of a multiple injury problem. Under certain circumstances, the accompanying soft tissue injury, particularly if it involves brain, spinal cord, thoracic or abdominal viscera, a major artery, or a peripheral nerve, may assume much greater clinical significance than the fracture itself. In these instances, definitive fracture care will occupy a lower priority on the treatment scale.

The general condition of the patient must be evaluated and any associated hemorrhage immediately controlled. Severe trauma may stimulate a diffuse and widespread series of physiologic reactions, primarily through the neuro-endocrine system that attempts to maintain body homeostasis, which may result in abnormal systemic effects. One such abnormal effect of extreme seriousness is shock. The management of shock is of primary importance in the care of the acutely injured patient. Failure to prevent or control a diffuse, low-flow state will result in death regardless of how expertly the actual injuries are managed. Shock is suspected on the basis of hypotension, tachycardia, oliguria, cool moist skin, and confusion or coma, and it must be treated and stabilized before fracture treatment is begun.

Local Examination

Fracture of a bone may cause physical deformity of the part, resulting in unnatural or impaired motion on careful manipulation. Swelling and local tenderness may characterize the injured area. Exquisite pain is usually produced by active or passive attempts to move the injured part. Protective muscle spasm may be present as a physiologic effort to splint the fracture fragment and to protect against the pain caused by movement (Fig. 2–5).

Visual examination of the part will determine if the patient has sustained an open wound through the skin surface. Such an open wound may indicate the presence of an open fracture.

The presence or absence of any associated muscle, tendon, blood vessel, or nerve damage must be determined. All suspected fractures should be immobilized immediately until adequate radiographic studies have been obtained.

FIGURE 2–5. *A*, normal muscle tension pull on bone. *B*, after fracture, muscle tension pull may displace the bone fragments.

RADIOGRAPHIC EXAMINATION

The presence of a fracture and its type is confirmed by radiographic examination. Radiographs taken for this purpose should always include at least two planes: the anteroposterior and lateral views. Because of the possibility of multiple injuries of the same bone, it is essential to x-ray the joint above and the joint below the bone involved.

Children with suspected joint fractures should also have radiographs of the uninvolved joint on the opposite side for comparison purposes. The normal variations found in the epiphyses of growing children make it essential to have comparison views if the presence of an epiphyseal injury is to be determined.

Treatment of the Closed Fracture

Once the patient has been examined and the radiographs reviewed, the physician is in a position to decide on a course of treatment.

The term *reduction*, as applied to fractures, refers to the means employed to bring the fracture fragments back into close apposition and alignment.

The term *immobilization*, as applied to fractures, refers to the means employed to maintain the reduction until successful repair of the fracture has occurred.

Successful healing of a fracture is determined to a great extent by three factors: (1) the accuracy of the reduction of the displayed fracture fragments, (2) the efficiency of the immbolization by which the fracture fragments are held in the reduced position, and (3) the local blood supply available to the fracture fragments. Whenever bone has lost its normal blood supply or when there is serious soft tissue damage interfering with the surrounding invasion of blood vessels, fracture healing is delayed.

MEANS EMPLOYED TO OBTAIN REDUCTION

The goal of reduction is to bring the fracture fragments into close apposition to each other so that normal position, length, and alignment of the bone are restored. The means employed to obtain reduction are manipulation (closed reduction), use of traction devices, and open operation (open reduction). The choice depends upon the nature of the fracture and the experience and training of the physician.

Closed Reduction (Manipulation). Closed reduction of a fracture means the manual restoration of normal alignment to the bone. Manipulation is carried out under anesthesia, either general, regional or local. In most instances, closed reduction consists of manual traction applied by the physician with manual countertraction supplied by an assistant. The physician attempts to manually bring the broken bone fragments to a straightened position and to lock the ends of the fragments together, thereby restoring normal position, length, and alignment (Fig. 2–6).

Traction Devices (Reduction Traction). Reduction of certain fractures is best obtained by the use of some type of traction device whose purpose is to restore alignment to the broken bone by mechanical means. In practice, traction is exerted on the distal fragment, aligning it with the less manageable proximal fragment. The traction force necessary to attain alignment is called reduction traction and is usually intense in application, but short in duration (See Maintenance Traction, p. 41).

SKIN TRACTION. A light traction force may be delivered to a bone if pull is exerted on adhesive strips attached to the skin of an extremity. The main disadvantage of skin traction is that it cannot provide more than 8 or 10 pounds pull to the part and this limits its usefulness. It is frequently employed with reduction of fractures in younger children. The most common form of skin traction in use is called Buck's extension.

FIGURE 2–6. A, fracture dislocation of ankle joint. B, same patient after closed reduction and application of cast.

FIGURE 2-7. Buck's extension in place. (From Schmeisser, G., Jr.: A Clinical Manual of Orthopedic Traction Techniques. Philadelphia: W. B. Saunders Co., 1963.)

Buck's Extension (Fig. 2-7). Strips of ordinary adhesive tape or moleskin are applied to the leg and attached to a spreader block at the foot. The leg is wrapped with an elastic bandage to improve the purchase of the tape on the skin. A piece of traction cord attaches the spreader block to the weight, which is hung over the foot of the bed. The lower leg is supported on a pillow to reduce friction of the heel against the bed linen. Countertraction is supplied by elevating the foot of the bed on shock blocks.

SKELETAL TRACTION. A heavy traction force may be delivered to a broken bone by pulling on a metal pin or wire inserted directly into or through a bone. Particularly in adults, strong traction and countertraction are usually necessary for the reduction of transverse and oblique fractures of major long bones showing displacement and overriding. A traction force of up to 40 pounds can be delivered to a bone by means of skeletal traction.

In the lower extremity the metal pin may be drilled through the os calcis, the distal tibia and fibula, the proximal tibia, or the supracondylar area of the femur, depending upon the location of the fracture to be treated.

The pin is drilled through the crest of the ulna below the olecranon when skeletal traction is applied to certain fractures of the elbow, humerus, or shoulder joint.

A traction bow or yoke is attached to the metal pin and the traction force is transmitted through a system of ropes and pulleys. The main disadvantages of skeletal traction are the danger of infection developing in or around the pin tract and the possibility that the use of excessive traction may increase the chance of delayed union or nonunion.

A form of skeletal traction currently in use is called skeletal traction with balanced suspension. This consists of a traction system that supplies the skeletal traction and a suspension system that balances or floats the limb in the traction splint apparatus (Fig. 2–8).

Open Reduction. Open reduction of a fracture means the restoration of normal bone alignment under direct vision through an open surgical incision. The decision to employ open reduction should be made only by a physician trained and experienced in fracture management. The main disadvantage of open reduction is the theoretical danger of introducing infection into the bone. In general, open reduction is accompanied by some delay in bone healing time because of loss of fracture hematoma and increased trauma to the fracture fragments by operative manipulation.

FIGURE 2–8. Skeletal traction with balanced suspension. (From Schmeisser, G., Jr.: A Clinical Manual of Orthopedic Traction Techniques. Philadelphia: W. B. Saunders Co., 1963.)

MEANS EMPLOYED TO MAINTAIN REDUCTION

Once the fracture fragments have been brought into close apposition and alignment by reduction, some means must be employed to immobilize the bone fragments in position. The goal of immobilization is to maintain the fracture fragments in contact and alignment until successful repair of the fracture has occurred.

The means employed to maintain reduction are external fixation devices, traction devices, and internal fixation devices. The choice of method depends on the nature of the fracture and the experience and training of the physician.

External Fixation Devices. The most commonly used form of external fixation is a plaster cast encircling the injured part to insure immobilization. Complete fixation of a broken bone with a plaster cast involves immobilizing the joints above and below the fracture site (see Fig. 1–10).

Efficient external fixation for some small bone fractures, such as those of the fingers or metacarpals, may be supplied by plaster splints.

Frequently, a combination of closed reduction and plaster cast fixation is employed in the treatment of fractures.

Over the past decade, several centers have accumulated considerable experience with a new approach to fracture immobilization called *fracture bracing* or *functional bracing* of long bone fractures. Denying both the need for absolute rigid immobilization and the need to immobilize the joints above and below the fracture, proponents of this method have reported success with its use in fractures of the tibia, femur, humerus, and forearm by making use of support afforded the broken bone by the visco-elastic properties of the surrounding soft tissue (see Fig. 1–13).

Following a short initial period of standard fracture treatment using a circular plaster cast or skeletal traction, the patient is placed in a functional cast that allows weight bearing and some joint motion. The functional cast is replaced shortly by a functional brace, usually made of a molded plastic, that also allows weight bearing but, in addition, allows motion of the joints above and below the fracture. The cast brace used for some types of femoral shaft fractures is an example of fracture functional bracing. The technique is demanding and often requires the assistance of an orthotist to apply the functional brace.

Traction Devices (Maintenance Traction). The fracture that has been reduced in some form of traction device is generally maintained in that traction for immobilization until fracture healing has occurred. Once reduction of the fracture has been effected by the traction force, the weight is reduced to the least amount capable of holding the fragments in apposition and alignment. This is called maintenance traction.

Internal Fixation Devices. An internal fixation device is a metallic pin, wire, screw, plate, nail, or rod that is used to hold bone fragments in apposition and alignment mechanically until successful healing occurs (Fig. 2–9). Internal fixation devices must be biologically inert, nontoxic to the body, and absolutely corrosion proof. These devices are made of stainless steel, cobalt, chromium and molybdenum alloys, and titanium and titanium alloys. These devices may be fixed to the sides of the bone, placed through bone fragments, or in the case of rods, inserted directly into the medullary cavity of the bone. Although some pins and wires may be inserted percutaneously, most of these devices must be applied to bone by means of an operation. Thus, the use of internal fixation is most frequently combined with open reduction of the fracture.

A very effective recent innovation in the internal fixation of fractures has been the development of compression plating. Compression plating involves the use of heavy rigid plates and the enhancement of fixation by compressing the fracture site. The advan-

FIGURE 2–9. Internal fixation devices used in conjunction with open reduction to treat a displaced unstable ankle fracture.

tages of this technique, if properly applied, include early active pain-free mobilization of the muscles and joints adjacent to the fracture without interference with bone union.

A useful variant of the internal fixation technique is the "pins and plaster" method. In this method, pins are drilled percutaneously into the shaft of the bone at some distance above and below the fracture line and are left protruding from the skin edge. After reduction, a plaster cast is applied incorporating the pins, thus enhancing the stability of the fracture reduction. This type of external skeletal fixation is beneficial in the immobilization of certain unstable fractures of long bones and occasionally in the management of open fractures.

Treatment of the Open Fracture

Open fractures are considered surgical emergencies and demand immediate treatment because of the very serious complications of infection. The skin wound may vary from a small puncture hole to a large lacerated skin defect through which bone protrudes. The wounds are frequently contaminated by road dirt, pieces of clothing and other pieces of foreign material. The soft tissue damage may be quite extensive and the blood loss significant.

Initially the wound should be covered with a sterile dressing and the part should be immobilized with the patient's immediate transport to the hospital. After hospital arrival the patient's condition, both general and local, is assessed and stabilized. Radiographs of the involved area are obtained and the patient is taken to the operating room for definitive fracture care. The total time lapse between injury and arrival in the operating room should not exceed eight hours.

At operation, a complete surgical cleansing of the wound is performed. This consists of a very thorough washing and irrigation of the wound with large amounts of sterile saline or Ringer's solution in order to remove dirt and foreign material. This is followed by surgical debridement of the wound, with excision of all devitalized skin, fat, fascia, muscle and detached pieces of bone. Emphasis should be placed on proper tissue management rather than on attempts to eradicate bacterial contaminants. Dependence can be placed on the tissue's ability to prevent the conversion of contaminants to pathogens. The surgeon's major role is to assist the injured tissue by debridement and the avoidance of premature wound closure. It is far better to accept delayed healing than to prematurely close the wound, which could create conditions for later local breakdown, thus initiating regional complications and prolonging the patient's convalescence.

A culture of the wound should be taken at the time of the debridement. If infection should complicate healing later, the potential pathogen is most likely to be isolated in the culture obtained prior to any therapy. Only broad-spectrum antibiotics that can be expected to be effective against coagulase-positive *Staphylococcus aureus* should be selected for prophylactic therapy of open fractures caused by direct trauma. Their use should be guided by sensitivity tests to detect resistant organisms. At the present time cephalothin appears to be an effective antibiotic for prophylactic therapy of open fractures due to direct trauma.

If treatment has not been unduly delayed or the wound was not too dirty, an effort may be made to close the skin wound with sutures in order to convert the open fracture to a closed one. If there was a treatment delay or the wound is extremely dirty, it is better to pack the wound open and perform delayed wound closure a few days later if there is no sign of infection.

Following surgery, the fracture is reduced and immobilized in a plaster cast, "pins and plaster," or traction, depending on its type and location. Under ordinary circumstances, internal fixation is not widely employed in the presence of an open fracture.

Fracture healing is adversely affected by extensive trauma. Open fractures heal more slowly than closed ones. The patient with an open fracture is often at risk in regard to osteomyelitis, tetanus and gas gangrene. Complete and thorough surgical wound debridement is the best prevention for osteomyelitis. Large doses of penicillin should be administered if there is concern about gas gangrene.

Tetanus is prevented by immunization. If the patient has been previously immunized by tetanus toxoid, a booster dose of toxoid should be given. If the patient has had no previous immunization or if there is inadequate available information, immediate passive immunity can be achieved by the use of 250 to 500 units of human tetanus immune globulin. Active immunity with tetanus toxoid is initiated at the same time.

Treatment of Pathologic Fracture

Pathologic fractures, even when accompanying disease states that are ultimately fatal, require treatment in order to spare the patient unnecessary pain and disability. Most pathologic fractures will unite unless the bone resorption rate caused by the underlying disease state is overwhelming. The same principles of management applying to fractures through normal bone apply to the treatment of pathologic fractures.

The single most frequent cause of the pathologic fracture seen in clinical practice is metastatic carcinoma to the skeleton. Internal fixation augmented by the use of methyl methacrylate, or "bone cement," is usually the treatment of choice when the pathologic fracture is through metastatic lesions in the long bones of the extremity. Mechanical treatment of the bone fracture should be followed by medical treatment of the tumor area, utilizing radiation therapy, hormone therapy, or chemotherapeutic agents or any combination of adjunctive treatments as indicated.

If the diagnosis of the metastatic lesion to an extremity long bone is made before fracture occurs, "prophylactic" nailing may be performed (Fig. 2–10). In this instance, the internal fixation device is inserted by means of a more simplified elective operation saving the patient the pain and misery associated with the operation performed after the bone has broken.

FIGURE 2–10. *A*, multiple lytic areas in femoral shaft due to metastatic adenocarcinoma of the breast. *B*, same femur after "prophylactic" nailing.

THE RESULT

UNION OF THE FRACTURE

Successful repair of the fracture will occur in the majority of patients in whom management of the problem has followed established principles. The number of weeks of immobilization necessary for fracture healing will vary according to the type and location of the fracture. However, the mean number of weeks required for each bone to heal in the average patient is fairly constant and has been well documented. If the healing period stretches beyond the time normally required, delayed union may be suspected.

It is a well established fact that most bones appear and feel solidly united before complete obliteration of the fracture line is noted on the x-ray film. This state is known as *clinical union*. Immobilization may be safely discontinued in most cases after clinical union has occurred.

The goals of rehabilitation in the fracture patient after successful fracture healing has occurred are: (1) to maintain or restore the range of motion of joints, (2) to preserve muscle strength and endurance, and (3) to return the patient to full function as rapidly as possible.

Internal fixation devices serve no further purpose after the fracture has united successfully. Since modern metallic appliances are completely inert in the body, they may be safely left in place. They may also be removed after the fracture has healed at the election of the physician or if they are causing symptoms to the patient by mechanical irritation due to loosening or migration.

MALUNION OF THE FRACTURE

Malunion is a term applied to a fracture that heals in a poor or abnormal position (Fig. 2–11). Two examples of poor position are (1) marked overriding of the fragments with shortening and (2) abnormal angulation of the bone. Malunion of a long bone may put the joints above and below the bone at a mechanical disadvantage and, as a consequence, frequently interferes with function of the part. The most common causes of malunion are poor reduction and inefficient immobilization.

FIGURE 2–11. *A,* fracture of tibia and fibula healed in position of malunion. *B,* osteotomy of tibia to correct malunion. Fragments held with Lottes nail.

A

B

47

If malposition of the fragments is detected before complete healing occurs, improvement in the alignment may be obtained by manipulation. If it is not detected until after complete healing occurs, improved alignment can be obtained only by a surgical osteotomy.

DELAYED UNION OF THE FRACTURE

A fracture is said to be showing delayed union when it has not successfully united after a lapse of the usual amount of time required for healing of the fracture in any given bone.

The most frequent causes of delayed union are large gaps between the fracture fragments, inefficient immobilization, poor blood supply to the fracture fragments, and extensive soft tissue damage such as might accompany an open fracture.

Delayed union is traditionally treated by prolonging complete and continuous immobilization until healing occurs. If healing does not follow this treatment, the fracture is demonstrating nonunion. In certain fractures of the lower extremity, the technique of fracture or functional bracing may be effective in treating delayed union by combining immobilization with protected weight bearing, which stresses the bone fragments and frequently stimulates bone healing.

NONUNION OF THE FRACTURE

Nonunion of a fracture means unsuccessful repair of the break. With nonunion, the callus will be found to be composed of dense fibrous tissue and fibrocartilage instead of bone. Nonunion of a fracture can be recognized on a radiograph by the presence of a fracture gap separating rounded sclerotic dense bone fragments. The marrow cavity of each fragment will be sealed closed by the dense sclerotic bone (Fig. 2–12).

The factors tending to cause nonunion include (1) large gaps between the fragments, (2) poor immobilization, (3) interposition of soft parts, usually muscle tissue between the fracture fragments, (4) metabolic disorders, such as hypoproteinemia, (5) extensive damage to the soft tissues in adjacent areas as might occur with open fractures, (6) infection in the bone, and (7) poor blood supply to the bone fragments. Poor blood supply may be an important factor in some fractures of the femoral neck, carpal navicular bone, lower third of the humerus, and lower third of the tibia. These are all areas where nonunion is a relatively common occurrence.

Treatment of fracture nonunion usually involves operative excision of the dense fibrous callus and of the sclerotic bone ends. The

FIGURE 2-12. Nonunion mid-shaft of femur with intramedullary rod in place.

marrow cavities are then reopened by reaming. Open reduction is carried out and is usually maintained by some form of internal fixation. Osteogenesis is stimulated by bridging the bone ends with an autogenous bone graft, usually taken from the patient's ilium or tibia (Fig. 2–13).

The work of a number of orthopaedic investigators has culminated in the startling demonstration that electricity can be used in the human patient to successfully treat fracture nonunion. Electric potential differences are thought to exist in all living tissue and are subject to alteration in polarity and magnitude as a result of metabolic processes, disease, injury, mechanical stress, state of consciousness, and depth of anesthesia. Mechanisms for stress-oriented bone growth may be mediated in part by bioelectric phenomena present in bone tissue.

The potentials that arise when bone is mechanically stressed are not dependent on cellular viability, arise mainly from the organic component of bone, and are electronegative in areas of compression and electropositive in areas of tension. Non-stress potentials,

FIGURE 2–13. Repair of nonunion midshaft of femur with bone graft and compression plate fixation.

known as bioelectric or standing potentials, are not stress dependent, but are dependent on cellular viability. These potentials are electronegative in areas of active growth and repair and electropositive in less active areas.

It appears that electricity, whether it be constant direct current, pulsed direct current, or magnetically induced current, can stimulate osteogenesis, but it is not yet clear which form of electrical energy is the most efficient stimulator of osteogenesis. The application of small amounts of electric current to bone stimulates osteogenesis at the site of the cathode or negative pole, but at the present time the mechanism for this favorable action is not clearly understood.

In the studies reported to date, one to three cathodes have been inserted into the fracture nonunion site. Each cathode was then connected to a separate battery pack and anode, which was kept in place for several weeks. In a surprising number of patients, this type of treatment resulted in healing of a very definite fracture nonunion.

DISLOCATIONS

A dislocation is a complete disruption of the joint so that the articular surfaces are no longer in contact. Most often the cause is trauma, and the result is a loss of structural stability of the joint. Varying degrees of tearing of the extra-articular soft tissues accompany traumatic dislocation of a joint. Like fractures, joint dislocations may be open or closed (Fig. 2–14).

The patient presenting with a traumatic joint dislocation usually exhibits pain, swelling, deformity of the part, and marked limitation of motion. A careful examination must be performed to detect accompanying damage to a major blood vessel or peripheral nerves. Adequate radiographic studies will define the problem as a joint dislocation.

Joint dislocation should be reduced as promptly as possible, preferably under general anesthesia. Most joint dislocations will reduce by means of closed reduction, but some may require open reduction. Time of immobilization will vary from three to six weeks, depending on the location of the joint and the time required for soft tissue healing to restore joint stability.

The diagnosis of joint capsule rupture can usually be documented by arthrogram.

Joint ligaments may become stretched and strained at the time

FIGURE 2-14.   Traumatic posterior dislocation of right hip.

FIGURE 2–15. *A,* fracture-dislocation of left hip. *B,* appearance of left hip after closed reduction of dislocation and open reduction and internal fixation of fracture of rim of posterior acetabulum.

of dislocation. These heal uneventfully with immobilization of the joint after reduction.

A joint ligament may also tear or rupture completely at the time of dislocation. If a torn ligament is not perceived and treated, the joint may exhibit permanent instability after reduction. After tearing, the shredded ends of the ligament retract, leaving a gap between them. If they are allowed to remain in the retracted position, healing by fibrous scar permanently elongates the ligament and contributes to continuing joint instability.

The presence of a significant joint ligament tear can usually be ascertained by stress radiographs. This involves taking an antero-posterior radiograph of the injured joint while it is being stressed with the patient under general anesthesia. The stress simulates the original injury and the radiograph will document joint instability if significant rupture is present (see Fig. 1–5).

It is believed that torn ligaments are best treated by early surgical repair in order to restore joint stability.

FRACTURE-DISLOCATION

The most severe form of injury inflicted on a joint is dislocation accompanied by fracture, usually intra-articular in type. This combination is not infrequently seen in the ankle and hip joints (Fig. 2–15). Because of the violence required to produce the injury and the accompanying articular cartilage damage, the long-term functional result achieved in the patient by treatment may be complicated by avascular necrosis or degenerative arthritis.

Fracture-dislocation of the joint is treated by prompt reduction of the dislocation, followed by selective treatment of the fracture utilizing the most appropriate of the methods discussed under fracture management.

References

Anderson, L. D., Sisk, T. D., Tooms, R. E., and Park, W. I., III: Compression-plate fixation in acute diaphyseal fractures of the radius and ulna. J. Bone and Joint Surg., 57-A:287, 1975.

Brighton, C. P., Friedenberg, Z. B., Zemsky, L. M., and Pollis, P. R.: Direct-current stimulation of non-union and congenital pseudarthrosis. Exploration of its clinical application. J. Bone and Joint Surg., 57-A:368, 1975.

Brown, P. W.: A rational approach to the avoidance of infection in open wounds. Am. Academy of Orthopaedic Surgeons Instructional Course Lectures, Vol. XXVI. St. Louis: C. V. Mosby Co., 1977.

Campbell, C. J.: The healing of cartilage defects. Clin. Orth. and Rel. Res., 64:45, 1969.

Cave, E. F.: Trauma and the orthopaedic surgeon. J. Bone and Joint Surg., *43-A*:582, 1961.

Davis, D. R., and Green, D. P.: Forearm fractures in children. Pitfalls and complications. Clin. Orth. and Rel. Res., *No. 120*. Pages 172–184, 1976.

Evans, E. B.: Orthopaedic measures in the treatment of severe burns. J. Bone and Joint Surg., *48-A*:643, 1966.

Frankel, V. H., and Burstein, A. H.: The biomechanics of refracture of bone. Clin. Orth. and Rel. Res., *60*:221, 1968.

Green, D. P.: Pins and plaster treatment of comminuted fractures of the distal end of the radius. J. Bone and Joint Surg., *57-A*:304, 1975.

Mays, J., and Neufeld, A. J.: Skeletal traction methods. Clin. Orth. and Rel. Res., *102*:144, 1974.

Mooney, V.: Cast bracing. Clin. Orth. and Rel. Res., *102*:159, 1974.

Patzakis, M. J., Harvey, J. P., Jr., and Ivler, D.: The role of antibiotics in the management of open fractures. J. Bone and Joint Surg., *56-A*:532, 1974.

Pelltier, L. F.: Fat embolism — A current concept. Clin. Orth. and Rel. Res., *66*:241, 1969.

Rang, M.: Children's Fractures, Philadelphia: J. B. Lippincott Co., 1974.

Rockwood, C. A., Jr., and Green, D. P. (Ed.): Fractures, Vol. I and II. Philadephia: J. B. Lippincott Co., 1975.

Sarmiento, A.: Fracture bracing. Clin. Orth. and Rel. Res., *102*:144, 1974.

Schmeisser, G., Jr.: A Clinical Manual of Orthopedic Traction Techniques. Philadelphia: W. B. Saunders Co., 1964.

Sim, F. H., Daugherty, T. W., and Ivins, J. C.: The adjunctive use of methyl methacrylate in fixation of pathologic fractures. J. Bone and Joint Surg., *56-A*:40, 1974.

Wade, E. A. (Ed.): Preoperative and postoperative management of musculoskeletal injuries. Clin. Orth. and Rel. Res., No. *38*, 1965.

Wray, J. B.: Factors in the pathogenesis of non-union. J. Bone and Joint Surg., *47-A*:168, 1965.

CHAPTER 3

CONGENITAL DEFORMITIES

INTRODUCTION

Congenital deformities are defined as those abnormalities of development that are present at the time of birth. It has been estimated that congenital abnormalities of various types and degrees are responsible for the death of about one-quarter of all human fetuses before or shortly after birth and handicap a certain proportion of the survivors throughout their life. Defective development of a unit of the musculoskeletal system, while rarely posing a threat to life, might seriously impair the function of the patient as a useful member of society. Although the true incidence is unknown, significant congenital deformities of the musculoskeletal system are common, being exceeded in frequency only by those of the central nervous system and cardiovascular system. Malformations seem to be more frequent now than in the past, probably because better techniques exist to detect them, the infants live longer, and the abnormalities are no longer being hidden by the family.

Some congenital deformities, such as clubfoot and torticollis, are obvious and are readily noticed by the mother, while others, such as congenital dislocation of the hip, may go undetected for a period of time. The remainder may give no clinical evidence of their presence initially until detected by radiographic examination or by the secondary effects their presence may cause. Examples of this group would be deformities of the spine, such as hemivertebra and spondylolisthesis (Fig. 3–1).

FIGURE 3–1. Congenital anomaly of fourth lumbar vertebra in 12 year old female child. There is complete absence of the posterior elements and the body of L4 is "free-floating."

It is generally recognized that congenital deformities seem to be more prevalent among the white population than among the other racial groups. Males and females appear to be affected equally, even though certain specific deformities show a definite sex predilection. Multiple births and an older mother seem to be factors in the rate of occurrence. The presence of multiple congenital deformities in the same child is not uncommon and should be constantly borne in mind.

Embryologic development is an orderly step-by-step procedure and it is thought that most congenital deformities begin early in the life of the embryo when cell division is most active. Although some congenital deformities may be due to uterine malposition, most are believed to be engendered by genetic defects, environmental influences, or a combination of both.

GENETIC FACTORS

The theoretical possibility of having to treat a patient with a congenital musculoskeletal deformity arises as soon as the male germ cell fertilizes the ovum to form the zygote. This act immediately restores the diploid chromosome number for the human (44 somatic plus 2 sex) and establishes the sex of the child. If a male germ cell carrying the X sex chromosome fertilizes the ovum, a female zygote results. If a male germ cell carries the Y sex chromosome, a male zygote is formed. The several thousand genes of each cell nucleus are located on the various pairs of chromosomes. The genes are also paired, one being inherited from the father and the other from the mother. If the genes of a pair are alike, the individual is said to be homozygous; if they are different, the individual is heterozygous.

Chromosomal abnormalities may cause congenital malformations and may be inherited or may result from mutations. Chromosomal disorders are present when there are abnormalities in the number or structure of one or more chromosomes. Down's syndrome or mongolism (Trisomy 21) is the only known common generalized malformation caused by a chromosomal anomaly and accounts for about one-third of all severely retarded children. Ninety-five per cent of children with Down's syndrome have 47 chromosomes, the extra one occurring with the twenty-first pair.

An abnormal gene may occur as a result of a mutation or may be inherited. The member of a heterozygous gene pair that expresses itself through a physical characteristic is said to be dominant; the member that does not express itself is termed recessive. Most defective sex-linked genes are recessive and so will not be expressed in a female who is heterozygous for the gene, but will be expressed in a homozygous female.

Genetic defects may be inherited from either parent or from an ancestor, or they may appear initially in a family as the result of a mutation in a chromosome or in one of the genes. The inheritance pattern of abnormalities depends upon whether the abnormal gene is dominant or recessive and also upon whether the gene locus concerned is autosomal or sex-linked. If the abnormal gene is dominant, the resultant deformity is transmitted by direct descent from affected members of a family to some of their children, who transmit it in turn (e.g., osteogenesis imperfecta). If the abnormal gene is recessive, the resultant deformity may occur in one or more siblings but less often in their children (e.g., Sprengel's deformity). If the abnormal gene is sex-linked, the resultant deformity is transmitted by clinically normal carrier females, but affects only males (e.g., hemophilia). Gene mutation is also a cause of congenital deformity. If a gene undergoes mutation in the germ plasm, the resultant abnormality will be transmitted.

ENVIRONMENTAL FACTORS

Harmful environmental factors, or *teratogens*, may alter the germ cells of either parent before fertilization or may alter the normal development of the fetus during intrauterine life, particularly during the first trimester. These factors appear to act by preventing differentiation of tissues or formation of structures within the embryo, or occasionally by causing destruction of formed organs. Extrinsic environmental factors causing fetal insult must pass the placental barrier in order to damage the developmental embryo. Fetal insult may be caused by maternal and fetal infections, maternal rubella infection, maternal ingestion of certain drugs such as thalidomide and aminopterin, and radiation.

When a congenital deformity has a genetic basis, there is a greatly increased chance that subsequent offspring will be malformed. When a congenital deformity is due to a factor that is not genetic in origin, subsequent offspring should show no greater tendency to malformation than the general population.

CONGENITAL ORTHOPAEDIC DEFORMITIES

Congenital malformations may involve any part of the musculoskeletal system and vary greatly in rate of occurrence and degree of significance. Only the most commonly seen congenital deformities are discussed here. The most important and significant congenital deformities involving the musculoskeletal system are clubfoot and congenital dislocation of the hip.

CLUBFOOT

Clubfoot is the most frequently encountered musculoskeletal congenital deformity involving the lower extremity and is estimated to occur once in every 1000 births. Family studies of large numbers of children with clubfeet implicate a genetic factor in only about 10 per cent of the children, the rest of the deformities due presumably to spontaneous mutation. Clubfoot is also known by the general term *talipes equinovarus*, which is derived from Latin and makes vague reference to the deformed position of the foot. The deformity affects males twice as often as females and occurs bilaterally in about one-half of the affected children. While there is clearly a genetic factor operating, its exact nature is undetermined. There ap-

FIGURE 3-2. Bilateral clubfoot deformity.

pears to be about a 10 per cent chance that the offspring of an affected parent will have the deformity.

Clinical Picture. A foot with this deformity is twisted inward and downward, giving the entire extremity a superficial resemblance to a club (Fig. 3-2). The foot is tight in its deformed position and resists manual efforts to readily push it back into a normal position. Closer inspection will reveal that there are actually three separate elements to the deformity:

1. *Adduction deformity of the forefoot.* In this instance, the forefoot is drawn inward in relation to the rear part of the foot. This motion takes place chiefly in the talonavicular and calcaneocuboid joints.

2. *Inversion deformity (varus)*, which is a turning in of the entire foot and heel. This motion takes place chiefly in the talocalcaneal or subtalar joint. No inversion can normally occur at the ankle joint, as the talus is securely locked in the ankle mortise. This element of the deformity elevates the medial border of the foot and depresses the lateral border.

3. *Equinus or fixed plantar flexion of the foot at the ankle joint.* This is related to tightness of the posterior capsule of the ankle joint and the heel cord. In addition, the shaft of the tibia usually exhibits an inward torsion deformity, thus increasing the inward turning appearance of the foot and leg.

The muscles on the posterior and medial aspect of the leg, particularly the calf and posterior tibial muscles, are underdeveloped and shorter than normal. The capsules of all the deformed joints are thick and contracted on the concave side of the deformity. These soft tissue contractures become progressively resistant to correction as time passes, emphasizing the importance of early corrective treatment.

It is generally believed that the bones of the feet are normally formed at first, although deformity of the shape of the talus is almost always noted at birth. The talus, os calcis, navicular and cuboid are shifted from their normal relationship in the foot by the deformed position assumed by clubfoot. The malposition of these bones can be noted on the radiograph and their replacement into normal alignment is the radiographic criterion for good correction (Fig. 3–3). Eventually, all the involved bones may become irregular in shape because of abnormal forces exerted on them by the soft tissue contractures or if the positional deformity of the foot is not corrected by the time walking begins.

Treatment. Successful treatment of clubfoot deformity is based on the principle of first obtaining complete correction of the three elements of the deformity and then maintaining the correction

FIGURE 3–3. *A*, AP view of clubfoot, showing superimposition of talus and calcaneus. *B*, same foot after four months of plaster cast treatment. Talus and calcaneus are approaching a normal relationship.

until all danger of recurrence has passed. All orthopaedists are agreed on this principle, but, understandably, there are differences in detail about the methods used to achieve this end.

The most popular methods of obtaining initial correction are the use of stretching plaster casts and the use of the Denis Browne foot plates and bar. Regardless of which treatment method is ultimately chosen, foot exercising is begun immediately after birth. The mother is taught to exercise the infant's foot at every feeding period in order to gain some flexibility over the soft tissue contractures. Treatment with a plaster cast or foot plate is done as soon after birth as possible and certainly within the first four weeks of life. Either method of obtaining initial correction can give good results if the techniques are mastered. With either method, correction must proceed in a certain sequence. In order to restore proper skeletal alignment between talus, os calcis, navicular, and cuboid, the forefoot adduction must be completely corrected before the heel varus problem is attacked. This, in turn, must be completely corrected before the equinus component of the deformity is rectified.

Once initial correction has been obtained, attention must be given to maintaining it. When all components of the deformity have been corrected and radiographic examination shows proper realignment of the affected bones, a retention cast may be applied for six to eight weeks to hold the foot in the overcorrected position for maximum stretching of the soft tissues. Initial treatment may take from three to six months to obtain full correction, depending on the rigidity of the foot. Daily stretching exercises must be given to the foot after discontinuance of the plaster cast or bar treatment. Walking is allowed in clubfoot shoes, which are high-top shoes containing outer heel and sole wedges. The child should be placed in a foot splint at nap time and during the night to aid in maintaining the corrected position. In an uncomplicated case in which correction has proceeded well, the night splint may be left on as long as it is tolerated by the child. With a docile child, this could be until at least two years of age. If the foot has been fully and permanently corrected, it should be normal in appearance and flexible and nonpainful to examination. The child should be able to wear conventional shoes without difficulty.

It must be emphasized again that clubfoot deformity may prove quite difficult to treat. Follow-up studies of large numbers of children with clubfeet treated quite adequately by the methods previously outlined show that only about 60 per cent respond satisfactorily. The remaining 40 per cent prove resistant to this type of treatment for one reason or another and require a change in treatment program to obtain correction of the deformity.

Treatment of Resistant Clubfoot. In approximately 40 per cent of children with clubfoot deformity, the soft tissue tightness and contracture about the foot is strong enough to prevent complete correction by the cast or foot plate method alone. In these patients, surgical release of the contracted soft tissue is required for correction. The most frequently used soft tissue operation is lengthening of the Achilles tendon and section of the posterior capsule of the ankle joint to lessen the equinus deformity. Surgical correction of the varus and forefoot adduction is less often required. In all instances, the plaster treatment is resumed after surgery to maintain correction.

After about six years of age, soft tissue release operations are ineffective because of the abnormal shape of the bone, and surgical procedures on the tarsal bones are required. These procedures are, of necessity, more major than soft tissue release operations and usually result in some stiffening of the foot.

In an occasional patient, the clubfoot deformity may recur some months after appearing to have been corrected by the cast or foot plate method. Although no universal agreement exists on this point, many orthopaedists believe that this type of recurrence is caused by muscle imbalance principally involving either the anterior or posterior tibial muscles. In these patients, surgical transfer of the involved tendon to the midportion of the foot helps restore a balanced foot.

Enthusiasm seems to be growing in many centers for performing complete soft tissue release operations on all involved joints of a resistant clubfoot by one year of age. Proponents of this early complete soft tissue surgery are reporting results markedly improved over those obtainable with slower and more conservative forms of treatment. Before one year of age, the foot is considered too small for adequate surgical correction unless magnification is used.

METATARSUS VARUS

This common deformity of the foot is frequently mistaken for clubfoot at first glance. Closer examination, however, shows that only the front part of the foot is involved, with the heel and heel cord maintaining normal flexibility. The actual deformity is an adduction of the forefoot in which the forefoot is drawn inward in relation to the rear part of the foot, varying greatly in severity from a flexible to a fixed deformity. An accompanying internal tibial torsion may accentuate the deformity. This condition is believed to occur more frequently than congenital clubfoot, but little evidence of an increased familial incidence exists. It is believed to be caused by an abnormal intrauterine position (Fig. 3–4).

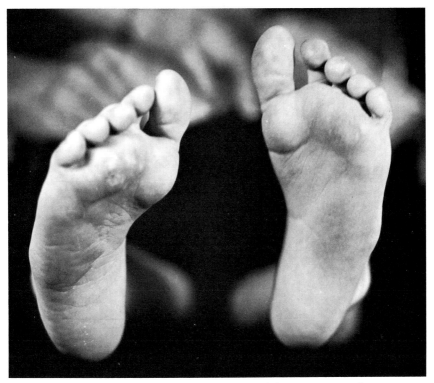

FIGURE 3–4. Untreated metatarsus varus deformity in young boy.

The five metatarsal bones appear normally formed on the radiograph, but show a positional shift to accommodate to the deformity. If the metatarsus varus deformity is not corrected by the time weight bearing begins, adaptive bone deformity of the metatarsals will develop.

Treatment. If the forefoot deformity is flexible and can be manually straightened, correction can easily be obtained by a stretching exercise performed by the mother during the child's feeding periods. If the forefoot deformity is fixed and cannot be manually straightened, correction is obtained by using stretching plaster casts.

Once correction is obtained, it must be actively maintained until the child begins to walk, because recurrence of the deformity is common. Correction is maintained by continuing forefoot stretching exercises and having the child wear "out-flare" shoes. Occasionally it is necessary for the child to wear a foot splint to bed to prevent the feet from curling under when the child lies on the abdomen.

In a child below six years of age, inability to correct the deformity completely by plaster casting is an indication for surgical soft tissue release at the five tarsometatarsal joints to obtain correction. In a child over six years of age, inability to correct the deformity completely is an indication for osteotomy through the bases of all five metatarsals to obtain correction.

CONGENITAL DISLOCATION OF THE HIP

The hip is the only joint in the body in which congenital dislocation occurs with any degree of frequency. It has been stated that one infant in 60 is born with instability of one or both hips, but 88 per cent of these recover spontaneously in the first two months of life. The remaining 12 per cent, or 1.55 per thousand, demonstrate true congenital dislocation that will persist unless it is treated.

Normally, the femoral head and acetabulum are formed from the same block of mesenchyme, insuring that the components of the hip joint are symmetrically round when formed. In congenital dislocation of the hip, the hip joint is abnormal and underdeveloped. The developmental abnormality gives rise to a characteristic pathologic, clinical, and radiographic picture (Fig. 3–5). The dislocation is thought to be present in some children at the time of birth and to occur in others shortly after birth. Although the exact cause is unknown, heredity plays a role in a significant number of patients. It is believed that ligamentous laxity, possibly genetically determined, causes hip instability and that certain environmental agents, such as abnormal intrauterine position or a breech delivery, may force the unstable hip to become displaced. Certain groups appear to carry a higher risk for congenital dislocation of the hips than the general population. These groups include: (1) persons with a positive family history for congenital dislocation of the hip, (2) children with torticollis, foot deformities or other congenital abnormalities, and (3) certain ethnic groups, such as Navajo Indians, Northern Italians, Czechoslovakians, and Japanese.

Congenital dislocation of the hip is about six times more common in girls and may be bilateral in almost half of the affected children. Since it may cause severe hip disability in adult life, it is absolutely imperative to make an early diagnosis and institute proper treatment. A direct correlation exists between the success of treatment and the age at which it is carried out. Treatment results are good in approximately 90 per cent of children in whom gentle and accurate reduction is instituted during the first three months of life. For this reason, examination of both hips should be a routine part of every newborn's first physical examination.

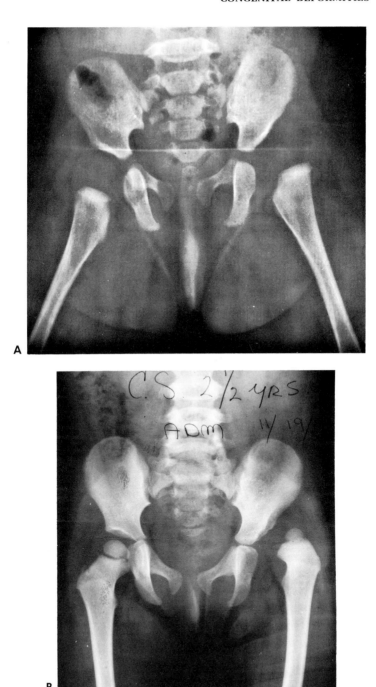

FIGURE 3–5. *A*, congenital dislocation of hip in three month old infant. *B*, congenital dislocation of left hip in 30 month old child.

Pathologic Findings. The femoral head must lie in correct relationship with the acetabulum for each to develop and grow in a normal manner. If the joint is dislocated, each component of the joint is adversely affected and growth and development proceed in an abnormal manner. In congenital dislocation of the hip, the femoral head is dislocated and lies completely out of the acetabulum. Most often it is found to lie posterior and superior to the acetabulum. The dislocated femoral head ossifies later than in a normal hip and when it does appear, it always looks smaller than normal on the roentgenogram. The roof of the acetabulum is underdeveloped, allowing the acetabulum to assume a shallow shape with its roof sloping steeply upward instead of forming a nearly horizontal shelf over the femoral head.

With the femoral head displaced superiorly and posteriorly, the hip joint capsule becomes stretched and elongated. This capsular tube may become constricted at its midpoint (hourglass contracture), trapping the femoral head in the proximal segment. The ligamentum teres may be quite thick and hypertrophied.

The empty acetabulum is frequently filled with fibrofatty tissue. The cartilaginous limbus forming the rim of the acetabulum may be enlarged and may tend to cover the acetabular opening. In some children, the tendon of the iliopsoas may be displaced laterally, passing across the mouth of the acetabulum.

The unstable hip joint resulting from a congenital dislocation predisposes to weakness of the abductor muscles, particularly the gluteus medius. Their antagonists, the adductors, become tight and contracted from the positional abnormality.

Another factor to be considered is anteversion of the femoral neck (Fig. 3–6). Normally the femoral neck and upper shaft exhibit an anterior torque angulation of 12 to 25 degrees in relation to the lower end of the femur. In congenital dislocation of the hip, the angle of anteversion is almost always increased. This means that the leg on the affected side must be twisted into marked internal rotation in order to seat the head of the femur into a normal relationship with the acetabulum.

Clinical Findings. Abnormal clinical findings in the infant are related directly to the fact that the hip is dislocated and rides upward above the acetabulum. Thus the affected leg may be shorter than the opposite leg. This can be determined by examining the child in the supine position with the pelvis level and both legs extended or by flexing both knees and hips to a right angle. In the latter position, the presence of shortening will cause the knee on the dislocated side to appear lower than on the normal side (Allis sign, Galeazzi sign) (Fig. 3–7). Shortening may also be associated

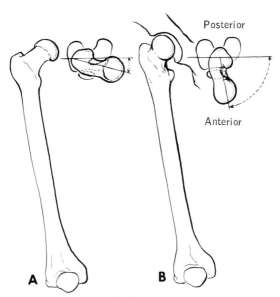

FIGURE 3-6. Angle of anteversion of femoral neck.

FIGURE 3-7. Positive Allis sign, right side.

with asymmetry of the skin folds in the buttock and upper thigh area.

Palpation reveals a prominence of the greater trochanter on the affected side and the absence of the femoral head from its normal anterior position beneath the femoral artery. When both hips are flexed to a right angle, the motion of abduction is limited on the affected side (Hart's sign) and the adductor muscle can be felt to be tight and contracted. This is frequently noted by the mother when she diapers the child. It is usually possible to internally rotate the affected hip with a greater arc than the normal side because of the increased anteversion.

If the extended thigh on the affected side is pushed towards the patient's head and then pulled back, the greater trochanter and femoral head can be felt to move up and down in the buttock. This is spoken of as "telescoping" or "piston mobility" of the femoral head. In some patients a click may be felt or heard when the thigh is abducted in flexion. The click is caused by the femoral head sliding over the acetabular rim. The click may be repeated when the head slips out of the acetabulum on the opposite maneuver. This is known as Ortolani's click or jerk.

Radiographic Findings. The roentgen findings in congenital dislocation of the hip give the impression of underdevelopment or dysplasia involving the entire hip area. The acetabulum appears shallow in depth. This appearance is accentuated by the slanting, poorly formed roof of the acetabulum, which is a reflection of the excessive slope of the ossified portion of the acetabulum. Delayed ossification of the femoral head is associated with the dislocation. As soft tissue contractures develop, the femoral head and neck are displaced upward and laterally in relation to the acetabulum.

The pelvis may appear tilted and there may be a curvature of the spine in the lumbar region. The ilium on the affected side may appear smaller or underdeveloped.

Most of the abnormalities seen on the radiograph are illustrated in Figure 3–8.

Treatment. Treatment must begin as soon as the diagnosis is made and depends, for its success, upon replacement of the femoral head into the acetabulum and maintenance of this relationship until the hip joint becomes stable. It is well established that the younger the patient at the time of treatment, the better will be the chance for the development of a normal hip. Thus it is absolutely imperative that the presence of a congenitally dislocated hip be discovered as soon after birth as possible.

Treatment will vary somewhat with the age of the child and may be conveniently considered in four age categories: (1) birth to

FIGURE 3–8. Certain lines may be traced on the radiograph to assist in establishing diagnosis of congenital dislocation of hip. *A*, Shenton's line lies along the upper margin of the obturator foramen and continues outward and downward along the undersurface of the femoral neck. *B*, line running along lateral margin of ilium and outer edge of acetabulum and extending along upper margin of femoral neck. Normally these two lines form even curves, but they are interrupted in a hip dislocation. *C*, line running horizontally through the triradiate acetabular cartilage. Normally the femoral epiphysis and metaphysis should lie below the level of this line. *D*, line drawn along roof of acetabulum to meet line *C*. These lines form acetabular angle, which is relatively obtuse in presence of congenital dislocation. Note absence of capital femoral epiphysis on dislocated side.

three months, (2) three months to two years, (3) two years to five years, and (4) over five years.

BIRTH TO THREE MONTHS. This is the golden period as far as treatment is concerned. Every effort should be made to have all affected children started in treatment before this time period has passed. The prognosis for a normal hip is good in approximately 90 per cent of children in whom gentle and accurate reduction is carried out during the first three months of life.

During this early period of life, the dislocated hip can usually be reduced by a very gentle manipulative reduction followed by maintenance of the reduced hip in a position of flexion and abduction. This position is maintained by a type of splint-brace, such as Pavlik's harness or a von Rosen splint, for a period sufficient to allow the joint capsule to tighten and the joint to become stable. Usually between four and six months are required. Successful reduction is followed by stimulation of the femoral head and acetabulum to grow and develop in a normal manner.

Some authorities favor reduction by gentle prolonged traction instead of by manipulation. Several weeks of skin traction with the leg in increasing abduction and flexion frequently result in reduction of the dislocation. The reduced position of the hip is then maintained as previously described. Open reduction is rarely required or indicated in this age group.

THREE MONTHS TO TWO YEARS. If the diagnosis is not made until the child is in this age range, it will be noted that the hip dislocation is associated with an adduction contracture. This usually requires a preliminary period of traction (skin in infants; skeletal traction in older children) in order to lengthen the contracted adductor muscles before an attempt at closed reduction is carried out. The hip should be maintained in about 45 degrees of flexion during the time in traction. Subcutaneous adductor tenotomy, followed by gentle manipulative reduction, frequently results in successful reduction of the dislocation.

If closed reduction is unsuccessful, open reduction should be performed and the hip immobilized in a plaster spica cast for an average period of six months (Fig. 3–9).

TWO YEARS TO FIVE YEARS. If the diagnosis is not made until the child is in this age range, adequate treatment becomes exceedingly difficult. By this time, the child is walking and will exhibit a typical gluteal lurch limp. If the dislocation is unilateral, the child's trunk will lurch to the side of the dislocation with each step. The gait will resemble a waddle if the dislocation is bilateral, and the child will stand with widened buttocks and an increased lordotic

FIGURE 3–9. A, congenital dislocation of left hip in 18 month old child. B, same patient nine months following open reduction of left hip.

curve of the lumbar spine. Weight bearing will tend to accentuate the soft tissue shortening and tightness about the hip and may cause secondary bone changes about the hip joint.

Several weeks of preliminary skeletal traction and a subcutaneous adductor tenotomy are required before an attempt at closed reduction can be made. On occasion, more extensive soft tissue releases combined with skeletal traction are required to bring the femoral head down to the level of the acetabulum. Open reduction of the dislocation is often necessary in this age group. The problem most frequently encountered is the difficulty of maintaining the reduction because joint malformation has rendered the joint unstable. It is frequently necessary to perform an operation on either the pelvic or femoral side of the hip joint in order to increase the stability of the reduction. Various pelvic osteotomies have been described for the purpose of redirecting the entire acetabulum so that it sits more squarely over the femoral head like a hat. An osteotomy of the femur at the subtrochanteric level may be performed to redirect the femoral head more squarely into the acetabulum. Once accurate reduction of the joint has been obtained and maintained, immobilization must be continued for a period long enough to insure joint stability.

OVER FIVE YEARS OF AGE. Satisfactory hip function is almost impossible to achieve if treatment is not started until the child is in this age range. By this time, severe secondary bone changes have occurred in association with shortening and extensive soft tissue contracture. In many of these children reduction is either inadvisable or impossible to achieve utilizing the more standard techniques. Femoral shortening, either alone or in combination with a pelvic osteotomy, would be required to effect a stable reduction. Occasionally, an operation such as a Colonna arthroplasty is indicated in an older child in order to obtain a serviceable hip joint. Most children in whom the diagnosis is not made until this age range will develop painful hips in early adult life and will require secondary reconstructive hip operations for pain relief and restoration of some hip function.

Complications. Avascular necrosis of the capital femoral epiphysis may occur as a complication after reduction, possibly because of damage to or compromise of the blood supply to the femoral head. The immobilization of the hip in an extreme or forced position of abduction or internal rotation is probably the most important cause of avascular necrosis of the femoral head. Its x-ray appearance and subsequent course will closely resemble the appearance and course of Legg-Calvé-Perthes disease (p. 97) and its treatment follows the same principles as outlined for the treatment of Legg-Calvé-Perthes disease (see p. 100).

If the child is left with incongruity of the joint surfaces after treatment is completed, the stresses of weight bearing and everyday activity on these incongruous joint surfaces may precipitate articular cartilage degeneration of the hip joint. This degeneration may progress to fully developed secondary degenerative arthritis of the hip joint in adult life, requiring secondary reconstructive hip operations for relief of pain and disability.

SUBLUXATION OF THE HIP

A newborn infant may be seen in whom the motion of abduction at the hip is limited and the adductor muscles are felt to be tight and contracted. Radiographic examination may disclose a shallow acetabulum and a small capital femoral epiphysis, but no actual dislocation. In this instance, the hip is considered unstable with the femoral head lying at the lateral edge of the acetabulum, but not actually out of the joint. Because there is no dislocation, there is no shortening of the leg. This situation is called subluxation, partial dislocation of the hip, or acetabular dysplasia.

Because there is no dislocation, no reduction is required. It is necessary, however, to seat the femoral head more squarely into the acetabulum so that pressure will influence each to develop normally. This is accomplished by the use of a device to keep the baby's legs abducted, gradually loosening the tight adductor muscles. A Pavlik harness or a von Rosen splint is a satisfactory appliance to be used for this purpose. Radiographic examination is repeated at intervals until a normal appearance of the joint is seen. As a rule, this condition is corrected quite readily.

SPRENGEL'S DEFORMITY (CONGENITAL HIGH SCAPULA)

During embryonic life, the scapula develops in the neck region and normally descends to its thoracic position during early development. If this descent fails to occur, the child is born with the scapula lying in the lower cervical and upper thoracic regions and is said to have a Sprengel's deformity. The condition is sometimes bilateral and may be associated with congenital anomalies of the cervical vertebrae and upper ribs.

As a consequence of this malformation, the scapula appears short and squat as compared with its counterpart, and the inferior angle is usually rotated medially. The supraspinous portion of the scapula tends to hook forward beneath the trapezius muscle (Fig. 3–10). In about 25 per cent of children with this deformity, the

FIGURE 3-10. Sprengel's deformity, left. (Courtesy Dr. Roshen Irani, Thomas Jefferson University Hospital, Philadelphia, Pa.)

scapula is connected to the cervical spine by a band of fibrous, cartilaginous or bony tissue called the omovertebral bone.

Clinical Picture. Because of the abnormal location of the scapula, the entire shoulder area may appear high and forward when compared with the normal side. Frequently the hooked supraspinous portion can be palpated beneath the fibers of the trapezius muscle. In most patients, the malrotation of the scapula greatly restricts abduction of the shoulder.

Treatment. Treatment is always surgical and is justified only in an attempt to obtain more shoulder motion or improve a severe cosmetic deformity. Two procedures for correction are in popular use. The first procedure calls for the removal of the "omovertebral bone" if present plus a large part of the upper portion of the scapula, including the spine and supraspinous portion. However, no attempt is made to pull the scapula down to a lower position on the chest wall.

In the second procedure, the scapula is entirely freed of its muscular attachments by subperiosteal dissection and pulled down to approximate the level of the opposite scapula. The muscles are then repositioned to provide anchorage for the scapula in its new location. Because the brachial plexus may tent over the clavicle when the scapula is pulled down from its elevated position, this procedure may be complicated by a temporary partial brachial plexus palsy. This complication can be avoided by morcellizing the middle third of the clavicle at the time of the operation.

SPINA BIFIDA

Spina bifida is a relatively common (1 to 3 per 1000 births) congenital anomaly of the spine characterized by a developmental gap or cleft in one or more of the posterior vertebral arches. Failure of the two primordia of the lamina to unite would leave the vertebral canal open dorsally. The laminar defect may range from the presence of small deformed laminae separated by a midline gap to complete absence of laminae over a wide segment such as the entire sacrum and lumbar spine. Although this developmental defect may occur at any level of the spine, it is most frequently found in the lumbosacral region. When this condition only involves the bone, it is known as *spina bifida occulta*.

Unfortunately, in many patients, the skeletal defect is also associated with neural tube defects, in which case the condition is called *spina bifida cystica*. If the skeletal gap is large enough, the contents of the spinal canal may protrude posteriorly in the midline beneath the skin of the back, with grave neurologic, urologic and orthopaedic consequences for the affected child.

The word "myelodysplasia" is a generic term that lumps together all the neural tube defects. When this posterior sacular herniation contains meninges and cerebrospinal fluid, but no nerve tissue, the condition is called *meningocele*. When the sac contains spinal fluid, spinal cord and nerve roots, the condition is called *myelomeningocele*.* The extent of the neurologic deficit depends on the level and the severity of the spinal defect and is generally more severe in myelomeningocele than in meningocele.

MYELOMENINGOCELE

This condition is the most complex treatable congenital anomaly of the central nervous system that is consistent with life. The extent of the neurologic deficit depends on the level and the severity of the neural defect and may vary from mild muscle imbalance in the legs to complete paraplegia. Paralysis in the lower ex-

---

*See also Chapter 7, p. 187.

tremities may be flaccid, spastic, or mixed, depending on the level of involvement. Extensive sensory disturbance may result in distressing trophic ulcers. Many of these children will have an associated hydrocephalus, bowel and bladder incontinence, and mental retardation. Exstrophy of the bladder and imperforate anus may also be associated complications of myelomeningocele.

Orthopaedic deformities associated with myelomeningocele depend to a great extent on the level of the lesion in the spinal cord and whether or not the resulting paralysis is flaccid or spastic in type. The most common orthopaedic deformities associated with myelomeningocele are clubfoot, dislocation of one or both hips, and severe malformations of the spine with varying degrees of scoliosis, kyphosis, and lordosis.

Treatment. Traditionally, children with myelomeningocele died in early infancy from sepsis or complications of hydrocephalus. In recent years, the use of an aggressive team approach among neurosurgeons, urologists, and orthopaedists has resulted in a dramatic decline in mortality associated with a significant rise in the functional level obtained by many of these severely handicapped children.

Closure of the sac by the neurosurgeon within the first hours of life has been shown to prevent progression of the neurologic defect. Appropriate shunting operations will decompress hydrocephalus and prevent irreversible brain damage. Urinary diversion operations protect the kidneys and, along with appropriate antibiotics, prevent ascending urinary tract infections.

The goal of orthopaedic treatment is to allow the patient to become ambulatory if possible in order to gain a measure of functional independence. In the severely involved patient, aids to ambulation such as crutches, leg or spine braces, or both may have to be utilized along with gait training to facilitate independent ambulation.

Specific orthopaedic deformities associated with myelomeningocele, such as clubfoot and dislocation of the hip, will require correction in order to make ambulation with brace support a reality. Such treatment may require the use of casts, braces, surgery, or some combination of these. Any associated sensory disturbance must be constantly borne in mind during treatment so that serious pressure sores can be avoided.

The spinal deformities associated with myelomeningocele tend to progress in severity with growth of the spine. Spinal deformity in the patient with myelomeningocele is among the most difficult to treat of all the spinal deformities of children. Occasionally, the Milwaukee spinal brace is useful in preventing rapid progress of the deformity, but most often spinal fusion is the definitive approach to spinal stabilization.

CLUBHAND

If there is a defective development of the radial elements of the limb bud, a child may be born with a partial or complete absence of the radius (Fig. 3–11). If the radial defect is substantial, the associated ulna is short and curved, causing the hand to be carried in a position of marked radial deviation. A similar primary defect in the ulna is possible, but less common. If a primary ulnar defect is present, the hand is carried in a position of ulnar deviation.

A radial clubhand (radial dysplasia, radial hemimelia) may be accompanied by deformity or absence of the thumb, the first metacarpal, and some of the metacarpal bones on the radial side of the extremity. The elbow joint may be abnormal and the humerus and scapula may be smaller than normal. Various muscle defects may be present, including absence of some arm and forearm muscles and abnormal insertion in others. The finger joints usually exhibit varying restrictions in range of motion.

Radial clubhand is believed to occur approximately once in every 55,000 births. It appears most commonly as a unilateral defect and is more frequent in males than females. Clubhand is usually a very difficult deformity to overcome. Correction requires replacement of the hand over the remaining forearm bones by stretching

FIGURE 3–11. Radial clubhand deformity. (Courtesy Dr. James Hunter and Dr. Lawrence Schneider, Thomas Jefferson University Hospital, Philadelphia, Pa.)

with plaster casts combined usually with both soft tissue and bone surgery. This position must then be maintained by protective splints for a long period of time. Some patients with absence of the thumb can be helped by pollicization — surgical construction of a thumb from a portion of the index finger.

SYNDACTYLY (WEBBED FINGERS)

Congenital webbing of the fingers is said to be the most common congenital anomaly of the hand. It is thought to be an inherited trait and is often bilateral. It may occur in association with webbing of the toes and other foot deformities. The abnormality may range from simple skin webbing between two fingers to severe webbing of all the fingers with incomplete segmentation of the bony parts and multiple joint deformities. The thumb is seldom involved.

Treatment is surgical and is undertaken only after careful study of the degree of involvement. The optimum time for treatment is thought to be between the second and fifth years of life.

POLYDACTYLY (EXTRA DIGITS)

Polydactyly is an inherited deformity often accompanied by other congenital malformations. The degree of deformity may vary from a small extra soft tissue mass not attached to bone to a complete extra digit containing all elements and attached to an extra metacarpal or metatarsal.

Extra fingers usually cause no functional difficulty in the early years of life. Extra toes may cause a shoe fitting problem.

Treatment is based upon the degree of difficulty caused by the deformity and could include surgical excision of the extra digit. Frequently, small extra skin tabs noted at birth may be ligated by the obstetrician or pediatrician and allowed to slough.

CONGENITAL PSEUDARTHROSIS OF THE TIBIA

This very disabling but fortunately rare abnormality is characterized by fracture of one or usually both bones of the leg shortly before or shortly after birth. The significant difference between this abnormality and an ordinary birth fracture is that in this condition the bone at the fracture site is abnormal and will not heal. The usual area of fracture is the lower third of the tibia and fibula, but the abnormality may also occur in the clavicle, humerus, ulna, first rib, and femur.

The cause of the condition is unknown, but may be related to a

FIGURE 3-12. Congenital pseudarthrosis of left tibia. Opposite leg is normal.

congenital deficiency of bone production or to neurofibromatosis. The bone in the area of the fracture is defective in quality and surrounded by a sleeve of dense connective tissue. On an x-ray film, the bone ends characteristically appear atrophic and tapered, bearing a resemblance to a sucked candy stick (Fig. 3-12). The false joint between the bone ends may vary from a fibrous tissue cuff to a joint-like arrangement with sclerotic bone ends, cartilage, and a joint cavity.

When the tibia is involved, anterior angulation of the leg may occur through the false joint. Shortening of the extremity may be extreme.

Treatment is aimed at securing bony union across the fracture site by the use of bone grafts and frequently internal fixation devices. Unfortunately, this happy state is quite difficult to achieve and multiple attempts at bone grafting are the rule. Not infrequently, repeated failures of bone grafting procedures leave the patient with a shortened deformed leg that is best treated by a below knee amputation.

The use of small amounts of electricity applied to bone to heal nonunion of fractures has already been described (see p. 49). Recent reports have claimed success in treating a small number of patients with congenital pseudarthrosis of the tibia using the same electrical technique. If this technique proves to be consistently successful, treatment outlook for the patient with this functionally disabling condition will become much brighter.

ARTHROGRYPOSIS MULTIPLEX CONGENITA

Arthrogryposis multiplex congenita is a syndrome of persistent joint contractures present at birth. The syndrome is relatively rare, being present in 0.03 per cent of neonates. The muscles are hypoplastic and a number of minor abnormalities, such as soft tissue webbing, may occur. The patient usually exhibits multiple congenital contractures in many limb joints, particularly in the hips, knees, elbow and wrists (Fig. 3–13). The trunk is usually unaffected, as is intelligence, but scoliosis may be present. Clubfeet, clubhands, and dislocated hips may be associated with this disorder. Some of the

FIGURE 3–13. A young man with arthrogryposis. He has joint rigidity and muscle hypotonia. (From Davidson, J., and Beighton, P.: Whence the Arthrogrypotics? J. Bone and Joint Surg., 58-B: 492, 1976. By permission.)

joint contractures are in the direction of flexion, but some, like the elbows and knees, may be in extension. Characteristically, the joints are fixed with extremely limited motion. However, apart from the limitations imposed by joint stiffness, general health is good and the disorder is neither progressive nor potentially fatal.

The term "arthrogryposis" derives from the Greek and means "curved joint." The condition has also been called *amyoplasia congenita* and *myodystrophia fetalis.*

The cause of the condition is unknown, but it is not believed to be genetically determined. Little evidence exists to suppose the basic defect is in the muscles or in the nervous system. It has been proposed that arthrogryposis multiplex congenita is the consequence of the influence of an unknown environmental agent that acts at an early stage of fetal development.

Although joint stiffness is the main characteristic of arthrogryposis, the joints themselves appear normal except for their limited motion. The major pathologic changes appear mostly in the extraarticular soft tissues. The joint capsules are thickened and contracted. The muscles may be decreased in bulk or entirely absent, being replaced by fat. Excessive fibrous tissue infiltration is found in the periarticular soft tissues as well as in the subcutaneous fat. The skin is tight and inelastic.

The goal of treatment is to make these severely handicapped children as self-sufficient as possible. For that reason, each joint is treated on an individual basis with the idea of correcting the deformity and gaining motion if possible. The incidence of scoliosis in this condition is approximately 20 per cent, with many of the curves becoming progressive, rigid, and fixed at an early age. The aim of treatment in the lower extremity is to obtain stable, well-aligned joints suitable for weight bearing. Because of the inelastic nature of the pathologic changes and the lack of muscle power, the results of treatment are often disappointing. In the presence of severe functional disability, institutional care may be required for many of these children.

References

American Academy of Orthopaedic Surgeons Symposium on Myelomeningocele, October 1971. St. Louis: C. V. Mosby Co., 1972.

Barlow, T. G.: Early diagnosis and treatment of congenital dislocation of the hip. J. Bone and Joint Surg., *44-B*:292, 1962.

Coleman, S.: Treatment of congenital dislocation of the hip in the infant. J Bone and Joint Surg., *47-A*:590, 1965.

Davidson, J., and Beighton, P: Whence the arthrogrypotics?. J. Bone and Joint Surg., *58-B*:492, 1976.

Duthie, R. B., and Townes, P. L.: The genetics of orthopaedic conditions. J. Bone and Joint Surg., *49-B*:229, 1967.

Frantz, C. H., and O'Rahilly, R.: Congenital skeletal limb deficiencies. J. Bone and Joint Surg., *43-A*:1202, 1961.

Freeman, J. M. (Ed.): Practical Management of Meningomyelocele. Baltimore: University Park Press, 1974.

Kite, J. H.: The classic: Principles involved in the treatment of congenital clubfoot. Clin. Orth. and Rel. Res., *84*:4, 1972.

Kite, J. H.: The Clubfoot. New York: Grune and Stratton, 1974.

Mayer, D. M., and Swanker, W. A.: Anomalies of Infants and Children. New York: McGraw-Hill Book Co. 1958.

Nance, W. E., and Engel, E.: Human cytogenics. J. Bone and Joint Surg., *49-A*:1436, 1967.

Ponseti, I. V., and Becker, J. R.: Congenital metatarsus adductus: The results of treatment. J. Bone and Joint Surg., *48-A*:702, 1966.

Rosen, S. von: Diagnosis and treatment of congenital dislocation of the hip joint in the new-born. J. Bone and Joint Surg., *44-B*:284, 1962.

Salter, R. B.: Innominate osteotomy in the treatment of congenital dislocation and subluxation of the hip. J. Bone and Joint Surg., *43-B*:518, 1961.

Siffert, R. S., Ehrlich, M. G., and Katz, J. F.: Management of congenital dislocations of the hip. Clin. Orth. and Rel. Res., *86*:28, 1972.

Smith, E. D.: Spina Bifida and the Total Care of Spinal Myelomeningocele. Springfield, Illinois: Charles C Thomas, 1965.

Tachdjian, M. O.: Pediatric Orthopedics, Vols. I and II. Philadelphia: W. B. Saunders Co., 1972.

Vesely, D. G. (Ed.): Clubfoot. Clin. Orth. and Rel. Res., *No. 84*, 1972.

CHAPTER 4

EPIPHYSES

INTRODUCTION

At birth, cartilage masses called epiphyses are found at each end of a long bone. The name is derived from the Greek words *epi* (upon) and *pausis* (growth). The epiphysis, a secondary center of ossification, consists of a central bony nucleus surrounded by a mass of hyaline cartilage and, with growth, enlarges by endochondral ossification of this adjacent cartilage. The part of the cartilage that lies between the bony nucleus and the metaphysis constitutes the *growth plate*, which is the source of longitudinal growth in a long bone (Fig. 4–1). Endochondral ossification occurs in the growth plates in the same manner as that which occurred originally when the primary center of ossification was formed. Longitudinal growth occurs by the continued addition of cartilage at the top of the plate and the continued replacement of calcified cartilage by bone at the bottom of the plate. In late adolescence the growth plate progressively narrows until all growth ceases. At the completion of bone growth at the time of skeletal maturity, the growth plate and epiphysis are completely ossified except for the layer of cartilage that surrounds the epiphysis and persists as adult articular or joint cartilage.

Two types of epiphyses are found in the extremities: *pressure epiphyses* and *traction epiphyses*, also called *apophyses* (Fig. 4–2). Pressure epiphyses are found at the end of long bones and are considered articular elements. They are subjected to pressures transmitted through the joint of which they are a part. The growth plate of pressure epiphyses provides for longitudinal growth of the long

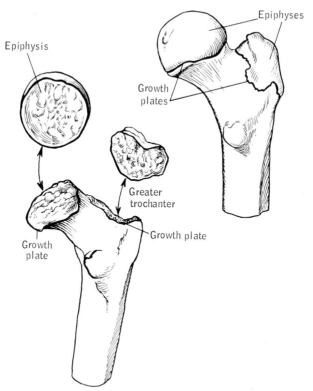

FIGURE 4–1. Upper end of femur, showing capital femoral and greater trochanteric epiphyses.

FIGURE 4–2. Types of epiphyses.

bone. After skeletal maturity is obtained, pressure epiphyses persist as joint components covered with articular cartilage. Examples are the femoral and humeral head epiphyses.

Traction epiphyses or apophyses are the site of origin or insertion of major muscles or muscle groups and are, therefore, subjected to traction rather than pressure. They do not enter into the formation of joints and hence are not covered with articular cartilage. Traction epiphyses contribute to bone shape, but not to longitudinal growth of the bone. Examples are the tibial tubercle, lesser trochanter of the femur, and humeral condyles. The growth plate has the same anatomical appearance and responds to the same physiologic influences in both types of epiphyses.

Bone Growth

Longitudinal growth of bone is primarily a function of the growth plate of pressure epiphyses. Affections of bone growth, therefore, are essentially those of the growth plate. The physiologic mechanisms governing or controlling the activities of the growth plate are not well known, but it would appear that the basic controlling and monitoring mechanism of growth is hormonal. Although there are underlying genetic limitations to skeletal stature, many aspects of growth — such as maintenance of rate, growth spurts, and time of cessation — are regulated primarily by anterior pituitary function. The gonads and thyroid, either by their direct influence on the plate or, more likely by their effects on the pituitary, have been implicated in explaining the growth spurt at puberty and the plate closure that occurs at skeletal maturity.

As an organ system specifically concerned with the single function of longitudinal bone growth, the plate is sensitive to the biochemical, physiologic, and pathologic changes that occur in the body as a whole. In addition to its response to growth hormone, it would appear that the growth plate is sensitive to many stimuli, and several clinical conditions are encountered that are accompanied by acceleration of the longitudinal growth of a long bone. These conditions would include those states associated with local hyperemia, trauma, infection, or tumor. Recent experiments have shown that the growth plate can also be stimulated with a high degree of consistency by an electrical field of appropriate voltage. On the other hand, other alterations of physiologic conditions or the influence of other stimuli result in degenerative changes in the plate instead of growth acceleration. Malnutrition, starvation, and severe chronic illness deprive the plate of adequate protein and other substances necessary for rapid growth. Longitudinal growth is retarded as a result of diminished cellular activity and matrix production in the growth zone. Normal growth processes resume promptly when an adequate diet or normal health is restored.

Abnormal pressure applied to the plate may often result in retardation of growth. Angulation of the shaft of a bone, asymmetrical pressures as a result of abnormal muscle pull or laxity, or the application of corrective braces or casts that produce angular forces may cause deformity by slowing growth on the side of compression.

The normal growth plate as seen in standard histologic sections can be divided into various zones. The most proximal zone in the growth plate is called the *zone of small size cartilage cells.* This is followed in succession by the *zone of cell columns,* the *zone of hypertrophic cells,* and the *metaphysis* (Fig. 4–3). The zone of cell columns is the proliferative region of the growth plate, and the zone of hypertrophic cells is believed to relate to calcification of the cartilage matrix. The space between the cells is filled with cartilage matrix or intercellular substance. The intercellular substance, not

FIGURE 4–3. Normal human growth plate showing the various layers. *A*, resting cells. *B*, proliferating cells. *C*, hypertrophying cells. *D*, endochondral cells (metaphysis). (From Salter, R. B.: Injuries involving the epiphyseal plate. J. Bone and Joint Surg., 45-A:587, 1963. By permission.)

the cells, provides the strength of the growth plate, particularly its resistance to shear. In the first two layers of the plate the matrix is abundant and the plate is strong. In the third layer the matrix is scanty and the plate is weak. Thus, it is through this third layer that the plane of cleavage occurs in traumatic epiphyseal separations.

Growth is accomplished by proliferation of cartilage cells from the zone of small size cartilage cells, also called the *germinal layer* (Fig. 4–4). Subsequent changes in the area are concerned with preparation of the newly formed cartilage for replacement by bone. Complex, incompletely understood physiologic mechanisms are involved in this preparation and are all geared towards rendering the matrix calcifiable. Conditions interfering with these basic physiologic mechanisms, or inborn errors of metabolism, may result in failure of the matrix to prepare for calcification or in lack of normal os-

FIGURE 4–4. Diagram of the growth plate of a long bone. The vascular supply to the germinal cells, which are concerned with chondrogenesis, enters through the epiphysis and penetrates the osseous end-plate. The vascular supply to the metaphysis plays no role in the nutrition of the plate but participates in the removal of the cellular and matrix end-products of chondrogenesis, in osteogenesis, and in remodeling. Actual longitudinal growth occurs only in the growth zone (interstitial growth) as a result of cell reproduction and elaboration of intercellular matrix. In the zone of cartilage transformation, complex physiological and biochemical processes are concerned with preparation of the cartilage matrix formed in the growth zone for later replacement by bone in the zone of ossification. Widening of the plate (appositional growth) and later external remodeling are the functions of the perichondrial ring. (From Siffert, R. S.: The growth plate and its affections. Am. Academy of Orthopaedic Surgeons Instructional Course Lectures, Vol. XVIII, J1, 1962–1969, p. 27. By permission.)

teogenesis with consequent skeletal deformity. Similarly, nonavailability of the necessary bone salts, as in rickets, will interfere with orderly osteogenesis by making calcification impossible.

Blood is supplied to the epiphysis and growth plate by two sets of vessels. The epiphyseal vessels enter the bony secondary center of ossification and arborize to ultimately reach the growth plate. Metaphyseal vessels are the terminal branches of the nutrient arteries and penetrate into the bony portion of the growth plate. The cartilaginous component of the growth plate apparatus, however, remains relatively avascular. The growth and survival of the epiphyseal cartilage and growth plate are dependent upon the blood supply from the epiphyseal side. Interference with the vascular supply to the germinal cells results in failure of chondrogenesis and complete failure of growth.

The possibility of restoring or providing increased length of a bone or an extremity through the transplantation of a growing epiphysis has intrigued clinicians and challenged researchers for years. The generally unfavorable experimental results reflect the difficulties researchers have encountered in developing techniques to maintain an intact epiphyseal circulation. It is this loss of blood supply that probably causes failure of epiphyseal transplants. Interference with the epiphyseal circulation is also thought to be the pathophysiologic basis of avascular necrosis of an epiphysis, a situation encountered clinically in Legg-Calvé-Perthes disease (p. 97) and sometimes as a complication after a slipped capital, femoral epiphysis (p. 90).

The metaphyseal vessels arise from the nutrient and periosteal vessels of the diaphysis. The rich and relatively abundant circulation on the metaphyseal side of the growth plate plays a much less vital role in the growth process. It can even be interrupted for short periods by such clinical problems as fracture or epiphyseal separation with only, at most, a temporary growth alteration. The metaphyseal blood supply is apparently involved in osteogenesis through the appositional laying down of new bone in the metaphysis.

CLINICAL CONSIDERATIONS

From the foregoing discussion it can easily be recognized that skeletal growth is a complex mechanism subject to the perfect operation of many variables. Disruption of one or more of the variables may have disastrous effects on human form and function. Developmental abnormalities of growth are assumed to be hereditary disorders of metabolism involving essential physiologic and biochemical complexes. Varying degrees of involvement, mixed disorders of chondrogenesis and matrix formation, and enzymatic errors can produce marked alteration in normal growth and unlimited variations of clinical patterns of these diseases. Two developmental disorders in which specific defects have been identified are achondroplasia (p. 106) and osteogenesis imperfecta (p. 108).

Local conditions that exert some deleterious effect on the growth plate are seen fairly frequently in clinical practice. A force applied to growing bone may cause the intact epiphysis to shear off at the growth plate with a clinical result similar to a fracture of the bone. Of all injuries to the long bones during childhood, approximately 15 per cent involve the growth plate.

Disuse of an extremity can cause shortening by removal of the normal weight bearing stresses needed for orderly growth. Theoretically this could be brought about by prolonged immobilization in a plaster cast or traction apparatus. Diseased states in children associated with severe muscular paralysis could be accompanied by retardation of bone growth with possible extreme shortening.

Growth disturbance secondary to abnormal pressure effects on the epiphysis may be seen with cerebral palsy or congenital dislocation of the hip. Pronation of the feet may exert abnormal pressure effects on the epiphyses of the knees, resulting in the development of a secondary knock-knee deformity.

Infection can directly involve the epiphysis and cause its destruction with resultant shortening of the bone. The growth plate which forms an effective barrier to the spread of infection in older children forms no such barrier in infants. In infants the cartilaginous growth plate itself is resistant to infection, but, since the metaphyseal vessels penetrate it, the exudate can easily spread to the epiphysis from the metaphyseal focus. The epiphyseal center of ossification can, therefore, be destroyed by the actual infection, or the development of the epiphysis may be impaired by thrombosis or interruption of its blood supply. One condition characterized by this epiphyseal impairment is pyogenic arthritis of infancy (p. 181).

Since hyperemia in the region of the growth plate may act as a stimulus to growth, a pocket of infection localized in a bone shaft adjacent to an epiphysis could stimulate the epiphysis to overgrow and lengthen the bone.

TRAUMA

The cartilage of the growth plate has the primary function of providing for longitudinal growth of bone, but it must also distribute the forces and loads placed on the osseous units. However, because the strength of cartilage is less than that of bone, the growth plate is a weak link in the immature skeleton. A shearing or avulsing force applied to a growing bone may cause the intact epiphysis to separate from the bone through the growth plate with a clinical result similar to a fracture of the bone. The cartilaginous growth plate is weaker than the joint capsule or normal ligaments and tendons; thus, injuries that produce joint dislocation or major tendon rupture in the adult produce epiphyseal separation in the child. Epiphyses most commonly involved are distal radius, proximal radius, proximal humeral, and distal tibial. The child notes immediate pain, and disability and clinical deformity may be present. Radiographic examination defines the problem as one involving the epiphysis.

Trauma to traction epiphyses may give rise only to locally painful conditions of limited significance because these epiphyses do not contribute to longitudinal bone growth. The real orthopaedic problems involve disturbances to pressure epiphyses.

The three main types of injuries sustained by a pressure epiphysis are separation of the epiphysis through its growth plate, fracture that crosses the growth plate, and crushing injury of the growth plate itself. Separation of the epiphysis is more common than the other two types of epiphyseal trauma (Fig. 4–5). The separation al-

FIGURE 4–5. *A*, traumatic displacement of distal radial epiphysis at wrist. *B*, normal position of distal radial epiphysis on lateral radiographic view.

most invariably occurs on the diaphyseal side of the growth plate through the area of hypertrophied cartilage cells, the area of greatest structural weakness. In the majority of instances, it is possible to replace the epiphysis into proper alignment by a gentle manipulative maneuver. In this type of injury, the growth cells remain intact with the separated epiphysis, and the prognosis for renewed growth after replacement is good unless the injury simultaneously damages the nutrient vessels to the epiphysis. If that occurs, avascular necrosis may complicate the problem.

The other two types of epiphyseal injury carry with them a generally more serious prognosis with regard to growth disturbance. Fractures crossing the growth plate often result in gaps in the plate that fill with bone if the integrity of the plate is not anatomically restored by either closed or open reduction. Crushing injuries carry

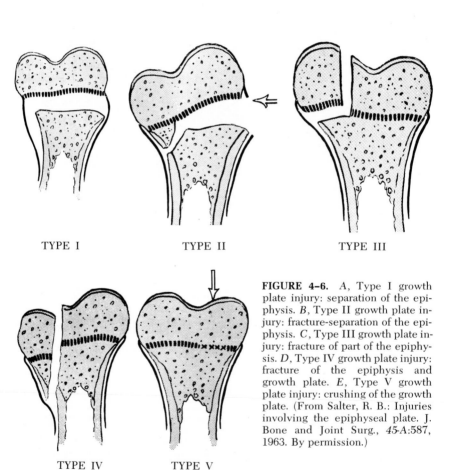

TYPE I   TYPE II   TYPE III

TYPE IV   TYPE V

FIGURE 4–6. *A,* Type I growth plate injury: separation of the epiphysis. *B,* Type II growth plate injury: fracture-separation of the epiphysis. *C,* Type III growth plate injury: fracture of part of the epiphysis. *D,* Type IV growth plate injury: fracture of the epiphysis and growth plate. *E,* Type V growth plate injury: crushing of the growth plate. (From Salter, R. B.: Injuries involving the epiphyseal plate. J. Bone and Joint Surg., 45-A:587, 1963. By permission.)

FIGURE 4–7. Premature closure of distal radial epiphysis following crushing injury to growth plate (Salter Type V).

the worse prognosis since they invariably allow bony bars to grow across the growth plate, leading to premature closure.

Epiphyseal injuries have been classified by Salter and Harris into five types (Fig. 4–6). Injuries of Type I, II, and III carry a good prognosis for growth, provided the blood supply to the epiphysis is intact. Type IV injuries have a bad prognosis unless the growth plate is completely and accurately realigned. Type V injuries are associated with actual crushing of the growth plate and carry the worst prognosis (Fig. 4–7).

If the entire growth plate ceases to grow, the result is progressive shortening without angulation. If growth ceases in one part of the plate but continues in the rest, progressive angular deformity occurs (Fig. 4–8). If the involved bone is one of a parallel pair such as tibia and fibula or radius and ulna, progressive shortening of the one bone will produce progressive deformity in the neighboring joint.

FIGURE 4–8. Carrying angle deformity of right elbow secondary to growth plate damage.

The clinical problems produced by complications associated with this type of injury are generally more serious in the lower extremity. The distal femoral epiphyseal growth plate, for example, contributes 70 per cent of the longitudinal growth of the femur and 40 per cent of the length of the lower extremity. Any injury that completely or partially arrests this growth potential may lead to significant shortening or angular deformity of the extremity. The younger the child at the time of such an injury, the greater will be the potential for these undesirable sequelae. Interference with longitudinal growth, persistent angular deformity, and loss of joint motion are recognized as possible complications of these injuries.

CORRECTION OF EPIPHYSEAL DISTURBANCES

Developmental abnormalities affecting the growth plate are puzzling conditions. In most instances, the specific defect remains obscure and definitive treatment is lacking. Occasionally local surgical treatment, such as osteotomy, may be required to improve the form or function of an extremity.

Except for the use of human growth hormone in children with hypopituitarism, no medical therapy is available that will reliably and safely add to the ultimate stature of short children or reduce the ultimate height of excessively tall ones. The orthopaedist is most frequently called upon for advice when local disturbances affect the growth plate.

After injury to a growth plate, local growth may either cease immediately or continue at a retarded rate for a time before stopping. In addition, a growth disturbance may involve either the entire growth plate or only part of it. The main types of clinical deformities that may develop are shortening of the bone, angulation of the bone, or a combination of the two. In any case, the resultant deformity is progressive until the end of the child's growth period. Because of the secondary tilting effect on the pelvis and spine, shortening of more than one inch becomes a problem when it involves the legs. Shortening of less than one inch can be accepted and adequately compensated for by the use of a heel lift in the shoe. Shortening of the upper extremity may be cosmetically objectionable, but it usually causes no functional problem.

Unequal length of the extremities can also develop from causes other than epiphyseal damage. Fractures through the shaft of a long bone that are allowed to heal with the fragments in an overlapped position can result in shortening. Injury or disease causing loss of bone substance can have the same effect. However, in many instances it is possible to surgically correct significant leg length inequality or angulation if certain criteria are met.

Recently success has been reported in the treatment of partial epiphyseal plate closure (Salter Type IV injuries) by surgically excising the bone tissue occupying the damaged portion of the growth plate and replacing it with a silicone rubber implant or a free fat graft. A fairly normal growth pattern appears to resume in the majority of patients reported. If the above technique is not applicable, progressive angulation of a bone at a joint is best treated by osteotomy of the bone so that the growing potential of the undamaged portion of the growth plate may be preserved and some lengthening of the extremity may be gained. When progressive angulation exists in a very young child, it may be necessary to perform osteotomy more than once during the growth period.

The orthopaedist's most frequent challenge in this regard is to correct for progressive shortening of the lower extremity, which can give rise to significant leg length discrepancy if allowed to continue. There are, theoretically, five methods of obtaining length equalization:

1. *Stimulation of growth of the short leg.* Such stimulation may

follow the hyperemia induced by a fracture, a surgical osteotomy, or surgical stripping of the periosteum. The effect operates for only a short period of time and the results are unpredictable. Attempts to stimulate growth artificially have usually either failed or proved impractical. Recent experiments have shown that the growth plate can be stimulated with a high degree of consistency by an electrical field of appropriate voltage, but no convincing clinical evidence has been reported as yet.

2. *Elongation of a short bone.* Bone lengthening operations should be restricted to older children and adolescents. A one-stage procedure is fraught with the danger of vascular and nerve complications. Gradual lengthening of the femur or tibia and fibula over a period of weeks using a special frame and skeletal traction devices is feasible and has been carried out successfully.

3. *Shortening of a long bone.* Bone shortening operations may be performed in the femur and tibia, but should be reserved for patients who have completed or nearly completed their growth.

4. *Amputation and prosthetic replacement.* This is usually reserved for patients with the extreme shortening most frequently associated with congenital limb defects.

5. *Retardation of growth of the long bone.* This is the method most commonly employed.

To retard the growth of the long bone, the epiphyses of the normal leg must be operated upon so that its growth may be delayed and the short leg may have time to catch up in length. At the time of the epiphyseal surgery on the longer leg, it is possible to permanently or temporarily inhibit its growth, depending upon which type of operative procedure is carried out.

To be a candidate for this type of surgery, the child must have enough growth potential left to make the procedure worthwhile. The surgery must be performed at just the right age in order to allow time for this growth "catching up" to occur. The proper time to perform epiphyseal surgery is decided after determining the patient's bone age and after consulting growth prediction charts. These charts indicate the amount of correction expected by arrest of each epiphysis at various ages. A long-term plan must include careful study of growth prediction charts, determination of bone age, and, if possible, a longitudinal study for several years prior to any growth retardation operation. The rate of growth should be graphed and projected into the future so that accurate determination of the desired shortening will be obtained. Since 70 per cent of the longitudinal growth of the leg comes from the epiphysis around the knee, the lower femoral and upper tibial and fibular epiphyses are the ones usually chosen for surgery.

Two types of growth retardation operations are in general use. The growth plate can be permanently arrested by a procedure called epiphysiodesis. The selected growth plates of the long leg are prematurely arrested by destroying the germinal cells with surgical curettage. The epiphysis is then prematurely fused to the shaft by the insertion of multiple small bone grafts across the destroyed growth plate. The epiphyses of the short leg continue to grow and gradually the leg length inequality lessens. Growth of the shorter leg is the factor that corrects the discrepancy. This procedure is useful when maximum retardation must be obtained.

Temporary arrest of growth can occasionally be obtained by straddling each side of the growth plate with three metal staples (Fig. 4–9). If the staples are properly placed and if they do not loosen or break, this procedure can effectively inhibit the activity of a growth plate. Stapling causes a quantitative retardation of growth averaging between 70 and 90 per cent of normal. It was originally believed that growth would resume after removal of the staples, thus

FIGURE 4–9. Temporary growth arrest obtained by stapling growth plates of lower femur and upper tibia at knee joint.

apparently giving this procedure the advantage of reversibility over the operation of epiphysiodesis. However, careful long-term studies have shown that epiphyseal stapling has not been reliable in reversibly arresting growth.

THE OSTEOCHONDROSES

The term osteochondrosis refers to a curious self-limiting disorder affecting pressure epiphyses during the growth period. This disorder has been described in nearly every pressure epiphysis in the body, and unfortunately, the describers' names have clung as identifying tags. The unwary might suppose that the terms Legg-Calvé-Perthes disease, Freiberg's disease, and Scheuermann's disease, for example, have little in common. The truth of the matter is that these terms all describe the same underlying pathologic process, the only difference being the functional importance of the involved pressure epiphysis. Legg-Calvé-Perthes disease, for example, is an osteochondrosis of the capital femoral epiphysis; Kohler's disease involves the tarsal navicular bone; Freiberg's disease involves the head of the second metatarsal bone, while Scheuermann's disease is an osteochondrosis of the vertebral body epiphysis.

The pathologic process in an osteochondrosis is an avascular necrosis of the developing epiphysis produced by causes that are still unknown. Whatever the underlying cause, interference with the epiphyseal circulation occurs, resulting in avascular necrosis involving the epiphysis. The bone of an epiphysis so affected softens, dies, and is gradually absorbed. However, the cap of articular cartilage surrounding the epiphysis remains intact and unaffected because its nutrition is derived from the synovial fluid. Because the bony tissue contained within the cartilage cap is soft and degenerating, the epiphysis may collapse and flatten under the pressure of the body weight. The body attempts to repair the damage almost immediately, and gradually the dead bone is replaced by new bone growing in from the adjacent viable bone. This process of repair is known as "creeping substitution."

Any pressure epiphysis so affected then undergoes avascular necrosis, but always heals spontaneously with some permanent residual flattening or deformity. Factors producing the derangement of the epiphyseal circulation that cause the avascular necrosis are presently unclear; but trauma, infectious diseases, endocrine imbalance, faulty metabolism, and nutritional and hereditary predisposition have been mentioned as possible etiologic agents. To many, trauma seems to be the most plausible factor initiating the ischemic process. This can occur either by direct injury to the vessels or vascular occlusion secondary to a traumatic synovitis, but the evidence in support of this theory is more indirect than proved.

LEGG-CALVÉ-PERTHES DISEASE

Osteochondrosis of the capital femoral epiphysis bears the name of three physicians who described it independently about 1910. Also known as *coxa plana* (flat hip), it is one of the important causes of painful limp in childhood. The incongruity of the hip joint secondary to the residual flattening of the femoral head caused by this disorder may lead to a painful osteoarthritis of the hip during adult life (Fig. 4–10). For this reason it is the most important of the osteochondroses.

The underlying pathologic process in Legg-Calvé-Perthes disease, as in all of the osteochondroses, is an avascular necrosis resulting in massive necrosis of the bone of the capital femoral epiphysis with the articular cartilage covering the femoral head

FIGURE 4–10. Osteoarthritis of the left hip, which has developed in a mechanically imperfect joint. Patient had Legg-Calvé-Perthes disease in both hips as a child.

remaining intact. Almost immediately bone repair begins with new bone from the adjacent viable bone invading the *necrotic* epiphysis and gradually replacing the dead bone. This process of "creeping substitution," the method employed by bone tissue to heal an area of avascular necrosis, gives the self-limiting character to an osteochondrosis and accounts for the distinguishing radiographic changes. Complete healing will occur, but the contour of the epiphysis flattens and the shape and appearance of a completely normal epiphysis are never regained. It usually takes from 12 to 36 months for healing to be completed.

Clinical Features. Legg-Calvé-Perthes disease affects children between the ages of four and ten years and is more common in boys. It is usually unilateral, but may be bilateral. It frequently affects children of low birth weight who are not quite "up to par" physically as compared with their peers. It rarely occurs in the black race. The attack rate is approximately one in 800 male children and one in 4500 female children. The disease has two striking characteristics: a clinical onset within a relatively narrow age range, usually between four and eight years, and the marked predilection for boys.

The initial complaint is usually vague discomfort in and about the affected extremity with pain possibly referred to the thigh or knee. The child limps in an effort to avoid or lessen the pain (antalgic gait). Examination reveals restriction of hip motion on the involved side as compared with the unaffected side. Usually the first hip motion lost is that of rotation. Spasm of the adductor muscles may be present.

Serial radiographs disclose the changes in the epiphysis brought about by necrosis and repair in the manner characteristic of this disorder (Fig. 4–11). Early, the epiphysis appears to thin out or flatten. It then appears to break up or fragment. Dense areas representing dead bone appear in the head, but these later disappear as healing progresses. Neighboring bone is hypervascularized and therefore osteoporotic, particularly in the metaphysis. The diminished density of the osteoporotic bone causes, by contrast, an apparent increase in the density of the necrotic bone. The fragmented epiphysis tends to coalesce into a single mass of healing bone as repair proceeds. The femoral neck tends to shorten and broaden. The acetabulum tends to alter its shape to fit the contour of the femoral head. When healing is completed, there is almost always some residual deformity of the femoral head varying from slight flattening to complete collapse with mushrooming of the head about the neck. The younger the patient at the onset, the better will be the ultimate clinical and radiographic result. The amount of final

FIGURE 4–11. *A*, Perthes disease of left hip. Capital femoral epiphysis is undergoing necrosis and fragmentation. *B*, same hip, five years later, showing residual flattening of femoral head.

shortening depends to a great extent on the amount of residual deformity.

Treatment. Catterall, an English orthopaedist, made a significant contribution to the understanding of this disease when he published a study of a large number of treated and untreated patients reviewed to determine if there was any correlation between the radiographic appearance of the affected hip and the final outcome. He was able to classify Legg-Calvé-Perthes disease into four groups based upon the radiographic appearance, and he showed that the patient's prognosis varied indirectly with the amount of necrosis present in the femoral head. The outcome was worse with a flattened, deformed femoral head with a segment of the head subluxed beyond the confines of the acetabulum.

Studies such as these have led to a change in the philosophy of treatment over the past decade. It was formerly thought that efforts directed towards reducing weight bearing pressures on the affected femoral head would usually be sufficient to minimize permanent femoral head deformity since the disease process is self-limiting and healing always occurs. Modern treatment is more aggressive and has as its purpose not to minimize femoral head deformity, but to prevent it. The key to prevention of femoral head deformity is to maintain the femoral head totally contained within the acetabulum during the treatment period. Total containment assures a congruous and spherical femoral head and prevents subluxation of the head in relation to the acetabulum. Uncorrected subluxation will lead to further collapse of the femoral head and premature closure of the growth plate with resultant deformity. If the femoral head is kept properly contained within the acetabulum during the revascularization and reossification phase of healing, it will tend to mold into a more normal shape (biologic plasticity). It has also been shown that if containment can be maintained at all times, weight bearing will not be detrimental to the hip joint. In general, there are two methods in use to obtain and maintain containment: (1) the use of abduction-containment plasters or braces or (2) operative treatment.

When the child with Legg-Calvé-Perthes disease is seen initially, there is frequently a great deal of pain and muscle spasm about the hip secondary to an associated synovitis. It is considered best to hospitalize the child for a short time for complete bed rest with the extremity placed in Buck's traction with the hip in slight flexion until the spasm subsides. An arthrogram is helpful in determining the proper position of the leg in the brace in order to completely contain the femoral head within the acetabulum. An arthrogram will occasionally reveal enlargement of the femoral head not adequately demonstrated by plain radiographs. Once the proper brace has been selected, constructed, and placed on the child and total containment in the brace can be demonstrated, the child can begin ambulation in the device. If the brace can satisfactorily "contain the hip," it must be kept on 23 hours out of each 24 until complete healing occurs.

If for some reason, adequate containment cannot be obtained or maintained by the brace, then surgical methods to obtain proper containment must be considered. The operations in use are based on the same principle defined for the use of the brace: that is, to provide containment of the femoral head during the necrotic and revascularization phases by correcting subluxation so that femoral head remodeling will occur. One could obtain this result by operating upon either the femoral or pelvic side of the hip joint. A varus osteotomy could be performed through the subtrochanteric area of the femur. This would permit deeper placement of the femoral head in the acetabulum. An innominate osteotomy (see p. 71) could be performed through the pelvic side of the joint. This would allow the roof of the acetabulum to be placed more squarely over the femoral head. Both procedures give the better relationship between femoral head and acetabulum so necessary for normal contouring.

Most patients with Legg-Calvé-Perthes disease, given adequate treatment, can be expected to heal with relatively minimal femoral head deformity. Long-term follow-up studies show that only the occasional patient with severe residual femoral head deformity develops secondary painful hip symptoms during adult life.

SCHEUERMANN'S DISEASE

Osteochondrosis of vertebral body epiphyses is known as Scheuermann's disease. It has also been called *vertebral epiphysitis* and *adolescent kyphosis* or *round back*. The area of the spine most frequently involved is the thoracic segment. The pressure of weight bearing on an affected spinal segment will cause anterior wedging and some flattening of the softened vertebrae. If this is sufficiently severe, a kyphotic deformity or "hump" will appear in the thoracic segment of the spine. This disorder is the most common cause of "round back" deformity in children (see p. 334).

Symptoms usually appear between the ages of 10 and 16, with involvement being about twice as common in girls. The initial symptom is usually back pain or fatigue. This may be followed by the gradual appearance of the "round back" deformity. Radiographic examination shows involvement of the vertebral epiphysis with or without flattening of the body, depending on the stage of the avascular necrotic process. The affected vertebrae appear wedge-shaped with undulating end plates.

Mild cases of Scheuermann's disease may be treated by hyperextension spinal exercises to counteract the tendency for anterior vertebral body wedging and kyphosis. If any degree of deformation of the spine is present, the back should be first immobilized in a plaster body jacket and then supported by a long spinal brace with shoulder straps to hold the spine erect until healing occurs. An occasional patient will develop a severe kyphotic deformity. This is unacceptable, not only cosmetically, but also because of the possibility of developing spinal cord compression or kinking. These patients should have the deformity corrected surgically, combining spine fusion with Harrington rod fixation.

A section of the spine affected by Scheuermann's disease during the growth period may in adulthood develop degenerative changes secondary to the vertebral deformation. Pain in the thoracic segment of the spine during adult life not infrequently has its origin in adolescent Scheuermann's disease.

BLOUNT'S DISEASE (TIBIA VARA, OSTEOCHONDROSIS DEFORMANS TIBIAE)

Blount's disease, a curious localized condition affecting the proximal tibial epiphysis, is a fairly common cause of bowleg deformity in the child. In spite of its relative frequency, the cause remains conjectural at the moment. The medial portion of the upper tibial growth plate displays abnormal growth, which results in delayed ossification, allowing the lateral portion to overgrow. Characteristically, a beaklike projection of bone is seen on the radiograph in the superior medial metaphyseal area. The clinical deformity at the knee does not increase after closure of the growth plate.

The disorder may be seen as an infantile type occurring during the second year of life. These children are frequently overweight and the disorder occurs bilaterally in one half of the patients. The adolescent type occurs between six and twelve years of age and is most often unilateral.

Although spontaneous correction may occasionally occur, most children with this disorder require active treatment. Depending on the age of the child, the stage of the disease, and the severity of the clinical deformity, treatment may utilize bowleg braces or surgical osteotomy through the proximal tibia.

Questionable Osteochondroses

Two other painful conditions occurring in children, one involving the tibial tubercle and the other the os calcis, were in the past frequently classified with the osteochondroses. Authorities now question their right to belong in this category since neither involves a pressure epiphysis and bone biopsy material has failed to disclose evidence of avascular necrosis. It is now considered that both conditions represent simply a tendinous attachment strain on a traction epiphysis.

OSGOOD-SCHLATTER DISEASE

This condition, characterized by a painfully tender and enlarged tibial tubercle, is seen most commonly in boys between 10 and 15 years of age. It is caused by pull of the patellar tendon on the tibial tubercle epiphysis. Pain is accentuated by local pressure, such as in kneeling, and by any activity that causes forceful contracture of the patellar tendon on the tubercle, such as running, stair climbing, or bicycle riding. The disease may occur bilaterally.

Radiographic examination may reveal some fragmentation and what appears to be separation of the tibial tubercle, but serial films will not show the gamut of changes characteristic of avascular necrosis and "creeping substitution."

The condition is self-limited and the ultimate prognosis is excellent. However, the knee pain suffered by the patient during the acute phase is often severe enough to require treatment. Mild cases may respond favorably to simple restriction of activities, such as prohibiting kneeling, running, and bicycling. In more severe cases, it may be necessary to immobilize the extremity in a plaster walking cylinder for six weeks. Extreme local tenderness about the tubercle may respond to local injections of hydrocortisone. The local pain and tenderness disappear with time, but residual enlargement of the tibial tubercle may be permanent.

SEVER'S DISEASE

This condition causes painful heels, usually in boys between the ages of seven and ten. Also known as apophysitis of the os calcis, it is caused by pull of the Achilles tendon on this traction epiphysis. Pain is brought on by walking, especially on the toes, and causes a limp. The back of the heel is locally tender to palpation.

Radiographic examination may be interpreted as showing a "dense fragmentation" of the epiphysis, but not too much significance has been ascribed to this interpretation. True avascular necrosis does not occur.

If the heel of the shoe is raised one-half inch on the affected side, painful pressure on the heel is usually relieved. Removal of the back counter of the heel portion of the shoe is also useful in relieving pressure. It is frequently beneficial to gouge out the heel of the shoe to form a foam rubber-filled saddle for the os calcis. The condition is entirely self-limited and can be treated quite satisfactorily by combination of symptomatic treatment and restriction of activity.

References

Anderson, M., Green, W. T., and Messner, M. B.: Growth and prediction of growth in the lower extremities. J. Bone and Joint Surg., *45–A*:1, 1963.

Bright, R. W.: Operative correction of partial epiphyseal closure by osseous-bridge resection and silicone-rubber implant. An experimental study in dogs. J. Bone and Joint Surg., *56–A*:635, 1974.

Bright, R. S., and Burstein, A. H.: Epiphyseal plate cartilage. A biomechanical and histological analysis of failure modes. J. Bone and Joint Surg., *56–A*:688, 1974.

Brighton, C. P.: Clinical problems in epiphyseal plate growth and development. Am. Academy of Orthopaedic Surgeons Instructional Course Lectures, Vol. XXIII. St. Louis: C. V. Mosby Co., 1974.

Catterall, A.: The natural history of Perthes disease. J. Bone and Joint Surg., *43–B*:37, 1971.

Kember, N. F., and Sissons, H. A.: Quantitative histology of human growth plate. J. Bone and Joint Surg., *58–B*:426, 1976.

Kopits, S. E.: Orthopaedic complications of dwarfism. Clin. Orth. and Rel. Res., *114*:153, 1976.

Langenskiöld, A.: An operation for partial closure of an epiphyseal plate in children and its experimental basis. J. Bone and Joint Surg., *57–B*:325, 1975.

Salter, R. B., and Harris, W. R.: Injuries involving the epiphyseal plate. J. Bone and Joint Surg., *45–A*:587, 1963.

Siffert, R. S.: The growth plate and its affections. J. Bone and Joint Surg., *48–A*:546, 1966.

Stephens, D. C., and Louis, D. S.: Traumatic separation of distal femoral epiphyseal plate. J. Bone and Joint Surg., *56–A*:1383, 1974.

Tachdjian, M. O.: Pediatric Orthopaedics, Vols. I and II. Philadelphia: W. B. Saunders Co., 1972.

CHAPTER 5

DISTURBANCES IN SKELETAL DEVELOPMENT

INTRODUCTION

In this chapter are described the relatively rare but frequently bizarre orthopaedic conditions brought about by abnormal influences on bone tissue. These abnormal influences are of generalized character and include errors in calcium metabolism, errors in tissue metabolism, dietary or nutritional errors, endocrine dysfunction, and congenital errors in bone tissue development either transmitted by established patterns of inheritance or arising as a result of a fresh mutation.

Constitutional diseases of bone with a known pathogenesis include chromosomal aberrations, metabolic abnormalities, and the mucopolysaccharidoses. Constitutional diseases of bone with an unknown pathogenesis include abnormalities of cartilage or bone growth and development, disorganized development of cartilage and fibrous components of the skeleton, malformation of individual bones, singly or in combination, and abnormalities of density of cortical diaphyseal structure, of metaphyseal modeling, or of both. Bone abnormalities may also arise secondary to a disturbance in an extraskeletal system, as in the endocrine, hematologic, neurologic, renal, gastrointestinal, or cardiopulmonary systems.

105

FIGURE 5–1. Achondroplastic dwarf. (Courtesy Dr. Beckett Howorth, Greenwich, Conn.)

CONDITIONS ASSOCIATED WITH GENETIC ABNORMALITIES

ACHONDROPLASIA

Achondroplasia is a congenital dwarfism resulting from a developmental error of enchondral ossification in which there is failure of normal ossification of the long bones, but not of the flat bones. Skeletal changes are usually noticeable at birth, which is frequently premature. Subsequent growth results in the formation of a dwarf with short limbs and a relatively large head (Fig. 5–1). Epiphyseal closure usually occurs at the normal time. The adult height of an achondroplastic dwarf is seldom more than 4 feet. As a rule, mental and sexual development are normal. Achondroplasia is probably the most commonly seen cause of dwarfism.

The deformity is transmitted by an autosomal dominant gene. However, 90 per cent of all cases are sporadic and are believed to arise as the result of a fresh mutation. The underlying defect is a failure of longitudinal growth in the cartilage of the growth plate. The exact nature of this error of localized cartilage growth is unknown. Parents of an achondroplastic child are unlikely to have a second such child. However, because the pattern of inheritance is autosomal dominant, the child of an achondroplastic parent has a 50 per cent chance of being affected.

Orthopaedic treatment is sometimes required for associated skeletal deformities. The achondroplastic dwarf may have marked lumbar lordosis with low back pain. The incidence of spinal stenosis is high in achondroplasia. Bowleg deformity, deformities about the hips, and deformities about the elbow may require corrective treatment.

MULTIPLE EXOSTOSES (DIAPHYSEAL ACLASIS)

Multiple exostoses is the result of a developmental error that restricts metaphyseal remodeling during longitudinal growth. Multiple outgrowths of bony exostoses or spurs capped with cartilage gradually develop from the abnormally broad metaphyseal region of long bones. These exostoses always point away from the adjacent epiphysis (Fig. 5–2).

The deformity is transmitted by an autosomal dominant gene.

FIGURE 5–2. Multiple broad-based exostoses projecting from both the proximal and distal ends of the tibia and fibula.

The underlying defect is believed to be an absence of the normal osteoclastic activity in the process of remodeling the metaphysis during longitudinal growth. This not only results in the formation of the exostoses but also may cause shortening and bowing of some long bones.

The patient may exhibit many exostoses of varying size usually found at the ends of long bones, at the knee, wrist or shoulder, or at both ends of the fibula. These changes are infrequent in the bones of the hands and feet. As a rule, the exostoses stop growing and their cartilage caps ossify after skeletal bone growth ceases.

Radiographic examination reveals the presence of multiple broad-based exostoses projecting from the shafts of the affected bone. The parent long bones are frequently thickened and distorted in shape.

Most exostoses produce no symptoms and do not require surgical removal. Some are associated with pain caused by local pressure against tendons, nerves, or other such tissues. Those exostoses causing pain should be excised. The development of chondrosarcoma in an exostosis has been reported in adults, but it is quite rare.

This condition must not be confused with the presence of a single solitary osteochondroma, which is considered a benign tumor of bone (see p. 219).

Osteogenesis Imperfecta (Fragilitas Ossium)

Osteogenesis imperfecta is a crippling condition associated with weakness and fragility of all bones of the body and, at times, blue sclera and deafness. As a result, the bones are soft and fragile and multiple fractures are the rule.

The pattern of inheritance is usually autosomal dominant but, occasionally, may be autosomal recessive. The recessive form usually leads to early death. The underlying defect is believed to involve bone matrix and to be associated with an impaired maturation of collagen fibers or possibly with the synthesis of an abnormal collagen. It results in inability to form bone matrix and causes, among other things, ligamentous laxity and thinning of the sclerae. Some evidence suggests a qualitative defect in the osteoblasts resulting in excessive osteoclasia.

Osteogenesis imperfecta may be apparent at birth or may appear shortly thereafter. Many infants survive only a few weeks. In many patients with this condition, a very definite China blue coloration of the sclerae may be noted.

FIGURE 5-3. Characteristic long bone deformity seen with osteogenesis imperfecta.

Radiographic examination reveals slender, frequently deformed osteoporotic bones with very thin cortices and sparse trabeculae (Fig. 5-3).

Surviving patients may sustain multiple fractures that usually heal surprisingly well following immobilization. Prolonged immobilization must be avoided, however, since it adds the problem of disuse atrophy to the already weak bones.

The skeletal deformity that results from bone softening and multiple fractures may cause dwarfism and structural abnormalities of the extremities, spine, and pelvis. Severe bowing of long bones can be corrected by performing multiple segmental osteotomies through the bone and using intramedullary metal rod fixation as internal support until bone healing occurs.

OSTEOPETROSIS (ALBERS-SCHÖNBERG DISEASE, MARBLE BONES)

Osteopetrosis is a rare condition characterized by the formation of extremely hard, dense bones throughout the skeleton. The formation of abnormally dense bone continues until skeletal growth ceases. The markedly increased bone density gives rise to the synonym *marble bone disease.*

The pattern of inheritance is autosomal recessive. The essential pathologic defect is believed to be failure of osteoclastic resorption of bone, resulting in an abnormal increase in bone mass.

Radiographic examination reveals the excessive density of all the affected bone.

The dense sclerotic bone may compromise the marrow cavity, causing an aplastic anemia that may be fatal. Optic atrophy may be noted. Pathologic fracture through these bones may occur. Healing of this type of bone tissue may be slow and delayed union of the fracture is relatively common.

NEUROFIBROMATOSIS (VON RECKLINGHAUSEN'S DISEASE)

Neurofibromatosis is a bizarre developmental anomaly characterized by multiple light brown pigmented spots on the skin (café au lait spots), multiple fibrous pedunculated tumors in the skin and soft tissues, and multiple neurofibromata of peripheral, cranial, or spinal nerves.

The pattern of inheritance is usually autosomal dominant. The disease may appear at any age and affects males more frequently than females. It is also known as *Von Recklinghausen's disease,* and the reader should be aware that occasionally hyperparathyroidism is also known as Von Recklinghausen's disease.

Orthopaedic interest is focused upon the skeletal complications of neurofibromatosis, which develop in about one-half of the afflicted patients. Fibromatous lesions within bone usually appear on the radiograph as circumscribed radiolucent defects and, occasionally, actual cysts may be found within the bone substance. Severe scoliosis is frequently an associated deformity. Neurofibromatosis has been suspected as a cause of congenital pseudarthrosis of the tibia. Occasionally growth enlargement or gigantism of all or part of an extremity is seen. Symptoms and signs resulting from peripheral nerve involvement vary according to the particular nerve affected. The tumors possess a definite tendency to undergo secondary sarcomatous change with an ultimately fatal outcome.

THE MUCOPOLYSACCHARIDOSES

In 1919 Gertrude Hurler, a German pediatrician, described two children suffering from a disease characterized by mental retardation, skeletal dysplasia, and a gibbus. Hurler's syndrome, which is autosomal recessive, and the X-linked form described by Hunter became the prototypes of mucopolysaccharidoses, a group of related heritable disorders of connective tissue with skeletal manifestations of varying severity. A genetic defect in connective tissue metabolism that impairs or alters the metabolism of mucopolysaccharides results in widespread deposition of specific mucopolysaccharides in the tissues and their excessive excretion in the urine.

These patients are usually normal at birth with the stigmata of their disease frequently not appearing until after the first year of life. A striking feature in the history is the progressive nature of these diseases. As a result of the biochemical abnormality, these patients develop varying and progressive degrees of mental retardation and severe skeletal disorders. Hurler's syndrome usually terminates fatally at a young age.

To date, six distinct syndromes have been described and the specific mucopolysaccharide identified.

Type	Mucopolysaccharide
Hurler's syndrome	Heparan sulphate and dermatan sulphate
Hunter's syndrome	Heparan sulphate and dermatan sulphate
Sanfilippo's syndrome	Heparan sulphate and chondroitin sulphate
Morquio's syndrome	Chondroitin sulphate and keratan sulphate
Scheie's syndrome	Heparan sulphate and dermatan sulphate
Maroteaux-Lamy syndrome	Dermatan sulphate

The diagnosis of mucopolysaccharidosis is made by the characteristic historical, clinical, and biochemical findings. Biochemical analysis to determine the specific mucopolysaccharide excreted in excess in the urine aids in early diagnosis. Fibroblast cultures are also helpful for diagnosis and genetic counseling. These studies take advantage of the tendency of the intracellular mucopolysaccharides to stain pink with toluidine blue dye. Clinically normal-appearing carriers also show a high incidence of pink-staining fibroblasts. This information is useful in genetic counseling.

Various skeletal abnormalities may be encountered. Skeletal dysplasia is present in all mucopolysaccharidoses but varies markedly in severity, being mild in Sanfilippo's syndrome and severe in patients with Hurler's and Morquio's syndromes. Spine deformities may be a problem in patients with Morquio's and Maroteaux-Lamy syndromes. Odontoid dysplasia and cord compression has been seen in these patients. Occasionally, a patient with Morquio's syndrome may develop progressive quadriparesis or die suddenly while sleeping or during the induction of anesthesia.

Bowing of the lower extremities is seen mostly in patients with Morquio's syndrome. This deformity can be corrected by osteotomy. Flexion-contractures are found in all the mucopolysaccharidoses except Morquio's syndrome, in which patients tend to be loose-jointed. Carpal tunnel syndrome and cavus feet have been reported in patients with Scheie's syndrome.

GAUCHER'S DISEASE

Gaucher's disease is a rare reticuloendothelial disease due to an inborn error of lipid metabolism. In this disease, proliferating macrophages in the spleen, liver, lymphoid tissue, and bone marrow are filled with kerasin, a lipid. These large lipid-filled macrophages are called *Gaucher's cells*. The disease is characterized by a relatively slow course, enormous enlargement of the spleen, anemia with leukopenia, hemorrhagic tendencies, and bone lesions. The more severe forms of Gaucher's disease seen in early childhood have a worse prognosis than the forms encountered later in life.

Gaucher's cells infiltrate the bone marrow and cause localized osteolytic lesions of bone. Avascular necrosis of the femoral head is a frequent finding in patients with Gaucher's disease. Gaucher's cells are found in the marrow spaces of the viable cancellous bone about the bone infarct, but are not seen within the infarcted segment itself. Gaucher's disease is usually associated with a mottled appearing enlargement or expansion at the lower end of the femur. It is said that when viewed on a radiograph, the lower end of the femur in Gaucher's disease resembles an Erlenmeyer flask.

Diagnosis is made by demonstrating Gaucher's cells in bone marrow obtained by marrow aspiration.

No specific curative treatment exists, although radiation therapy is usually effective in decreasing the size of the bone lesions. Patients with symptomatic avascular necrosis of the femoral head may require orthopaedic treatment for this complication (see p. 399).

CONDITIONS ASSOCIATED WITH DIETARY OR METABOLIC ABNORMALITIES

CALCIUM DEFICIENCY DISEASES

The bony skeleton of vertebrates serves two principal functions. It gives a rigid structural protection for the soft tissues of the body, and it provides a calcium reservoir for maintaining calcium homeostasis in the living organism. Normally, the body's major source of calcium is the diet. Calcium, however, is poorly absorbed from the gut, and vitamin D is required to increase the rate of calcium absorption from this area. The actual rate of calcium absorption from the intestine is regulated by calcium ion concentration of the extracellular fluid. A type of feedback control system operates constantly to maintain a normal calcium ion concentration. The agent maintaining this feedback system is thought to be parathyroid hormone.

In the normal individual with adequate calcium intake, the physiologic balance between bone remodeling and calcium homeostasis is maintained. Any imbalance, either slight or severe, in the mechanisms regulating plasma calcium levels, if uncorrected, may be expected to lead to metabolic bone disease. The basis for metabolic bone disease is a disturbance in the metabolism of bone tissue that may follow either renal or endocrine malfunction, genetic abnormality, or nutritional deficiency. Three basic types of metabolic bone disease are recognized: (1) osteopenic diseases — characterized by a generalized decrease in bone mass, (2) osteosclerotic diseases — characterized by an increase in bone mass, and (3) osteomalacic diseases — characterized by normal bone mass but an increase in the ratio of the organic fraction to the mineralized component.

The metabolism of vitamin D and its mechanism of action are quite complicated and not yet completely understood. Vitamin D in the human is derived from the diet and from the skin. It appears that 7-dehydrocholesterol is synthesized from steroids in the body and converted at an unknown anatomic site in the skin to cholecalciferol (vitamin D_3). Cholecalciferol is then metabolized in the liver to the 25-hydroxycholecalciferol form. This is the circulating biologically active form of vitamin D carried in the blood stream on an alpha globulin. The amount of this form circulating, however, is self-regulating. When the amount in the blood reaches a set concentration, further hydroxylation by the liver is reduced.

The next step occurs in the kidney where the 25-hydroxy form is further hydroxylated and a metabolite known as 1,25-dihydroxycholecalciferol is produced. The amount present in the kidney is dependent upon the hormonal and ion content of the blood passing through the kidney. This is the more potent form for stimulation of intestinal absorption of calcium and for action on bone. Small amounts of the vitamin metabolites along with sufficient calcium are necessary to calcify bone matrix properly.

Bone tissue, because of its calcified collagenous intracellular substance, serves an important bodily function by acting as a storage depot for calcium. As a result of physiologic demands, bone tissue may release some of its stored calcium to meet the immediate needs of the patient for this ion and to maintain a normal calcium ion concentration in the extracellular fluids.

The body will readily sacrifice structural integrity of the skeleton to maintain serum calcium levels. When the physiologic demands become abnormal, serum calcium homeostasis is maintained at the expense of intact skeletal development and calcium deficiency diseases may appear.

The calcium deficiency disease of infants and children is called rickets. The same disease appearing in the adult is called osteomalacia. Both rickets and osteomalacia can be found in association with renal disease in addition to appearing independently.

Rickets. Rickets, the calcium deficiency disease of infants and children, is caused by vitamin D deficiency or dietary lack of calcium and phosphorus. Improved infant nutrition has now made nutritional rickets a medical curiosity except in the underdeveloped areas of the world. Most cases of rickets presently seen result from metabolic abnormalities. Malabsorption may cause a nutritional rickets in spite of adequate dietary intake of vitamin D by preventing the intestinal mucosa from absorbing the available vitamin D. Gluten sensitive enteropathy or celiac disease, liver disease, such as congenital biliary atresia, and fibrocystic disease with pancreatitis are among the disorders predisposing to malabsorption. The calcium deficiency allows the infant's bones to soften and become deformed.

This physiologic abnormality causes a relative increase throughout the body of osteoid tissue, which is the protein base in which calcium and phosphorous have failed to deposit. This results in craniotabes or frontal and parietal bossing of the skull; epiphyseal thickening noted particularly about the wrist, ankle, and knee; enlargement of the cartilage of the costochondral junctions, giving a beading effect known as the rachitic rosary; generalized weakness and lethargy; and delayed milestones of sitting, standing and walking.

The pull of the diaphragm produces a horizontal depression on the thorax called "Harrison's groove." The thorax may become flattened laterally, producing a pigeon breast deformity, and in severe cases the thoracic deformities may seriously compromise pulmonary ventilation. Once sitting commences, a kyphoscoliosis may develop. Once walking commences, deformities in the long bones may occur with the stress of weight bearing. Knock-knee, bowleg, and coxa vara deformity are not uncommon (Fig. 5–4). Greenstick fracture of long bones may occur. Because of the involvement of epiphyseal cartilage, rickets may affect longitudinal bone growth.

The distinctive histological features of rickets are the persis-

FIGURE 5–4. *A*, Severe bowleg deformity in patient with hypophosphatemic rickets. *B*, same patient after correction of deformity by femoral and tibial osteotomies.

tence of excessive uncalcified bone seen as wide osteoid seams. Calcification of cartilage at the epiphyseal plate is defective with excessive proliferation of cartilage cells.

The radiographic findings in rickets are distinctive. There is a generalized osteoporosis and a thinning of the cortices and bone trabeculae. Affected epiphyses may appear irregular and fuzzy, with widening of the growth plate. The metaphyses may appear frayed, widened, and occasionally cup-shaped (Fig. 5–5). The areas of most rapid bone growth show the greatest involvement. These areas include distal radius and ulna, distal femur, proximal tibia, proximal humerus, and the costochondral junctions.

Laboratory examination usually reveals a low serum phosphorus and a high serum alkaline phosphatase. Although rickets is a calcium deficiency disease, the serum calcium is usually maintained at a normal level through withdrawals of calcium from the skeletal storage depot by parathyroid hormone.

Treatment of active rickets includes the use of a high calcium diet, large doses of vitamin D, and exposure to sunlight or ultraviolet rays. Many of the skeletal deformities spontaneously regress with correction of the physiologic defect. Some orthopaedic deform-

FIGURE 5–5. Radiograph of lower extremities of patient with hypophosphatemic rickets. Note the irregular, fuzzy, and broadened growth plates at the knee and ankle joints and the typical bowing of the tibiae.

ities may be corrected by the use of braces. Persisting deformities of the long bones frequently require surgical correction by osteotomy.

Osteomalacia. Osteomalacia (the term means "softening of the bone") is the adult form of rickets. The main difference is that in osteomalacia epiphyseal cartilage and longitudinal bone growth are unaffected because onset of the disease occurs after closure of the growth plates. Since it occurs after growth is complete, it usually follows a more chronic course and results in fewer skeletal manifestations. Osteomalacia is now primarily a secondary disease. It may be caused by dietary calcium deficiency, chronic diarrhea, excessive calcium demands of pregnancy and lactation, long-standing lack of sunshine, renal acidosis, or following gastrectomy or intestinal disease.

An early symptom of this disease is often muscular weakness, but bone pain and fractures occur as the disease develops. Osteomalacia is usually accompanied by some degree of hyperparathyroidism. The characteristic histologic finding is excessive osteoid tissue.

Renal Disease (Renal Rickets, Renal Osteodystrophy). A definite physiologic relationship exists between chronic renal insufficiency and the appearance of abnormal skeletal changes. Although several different clinical states exist the general relationship was, in the past, described by the loose term renal rickets. Severe renal insufficiency is associated with a renal acidosis. All available calcium is used by the body to neutralize the renal acidosis. When this supply proves insufficient, a compensatory parathyroid hyperplasia occurs to increase the amount of circulating parathyroid hormone. This hormone releases calcium from the skeletal storage depot. The skeleton, thus deprived of calcium, undergoes abnormal changes. If this process occurs in children, rickets results. If it occurs in adults, osteomalacia is produced. In addition to the changes of rickets or osteomalacia, the secondary parathyroid hyperplasia may promote osteoclastic resorption and fibrosis of bone with the production of cystic changes and bone destruction resembling the changes seen with osteitis fibrosa cystica (see p. 123).

Skeletal changes are now known to occur with two broad categories of disease. Therefore, the term renal rickets should be abandoned in favor of more specific nomenclature.

The first category consists of renal diseases associated with *impaired glomerular filtration.* The primary cause may be chronic glomerulonephritis, chronic pyelonephritis, congenital anomaly of the kidney, obstructive uropathy, or heavy metal poisoning. These patients present with chronic renal failure and uremia. The skeletal disturbance accompanying this state has been referred to as renal osteodystrophy.

The second category consists of renal diseases associated with *defective function of the renal tubules.* At least seven different clinical states have been determined to fit this second category. The commonest is familial hypophosphatemia or hypophosphatemic rickets inherited as a sex-linked dominant trait. This disease was formerly known as vitamin D resistant rickets because it requires large doses of vitamin D for treatment. The onset is usually in early childhood. It is characterized by very low plasma phosphate values and is accompanied by bone pathology similar to rickets. Because of the low phosphate there is a generalized lack of growth, in addition to the picture of rickets in bone.

Fanconi's syndrome is a less common clinical state associated with renal tubular defects and skeletal changes. In this condition there is failure to resorb phosphates, glucose and amino acids normally, and acidosis is frequently present. Serum calcium is normal or low; phosphorus is low; and alkaline phosphatase is increased. Dwarfism and skeletal deformity may be severe.

VITAMIN INFLUENCES ON BONE TISSUE

Vitamin A. Vitamin overdosage may result in chronic vitamin A intoxication that, in children, may cause disturbances of bone growth because of this vitamin's specific effect on osteoblasts, osteoclasts, and epiphyseal chondroblasts of growing bone. Short, thick bones result from cortical thickening and premature epiphyseal closure. The prognosis for normal development is excellent after correction of the vitamin overdosage.

Vitamin C (Scurvy). Scurvy is a nutritional disease caused by a lack of vitamin C in the diet. Vitamin C is an important factor in regulating the formation of intracellular substances such as osteoid, collagen, and ground substance. Deficiency of this essential vitamin causes an abnormality of the intracellular matrix, particularly of cells and tissues of mesodermal origin. The specific defect appears to be the inability of the tissue to hydroxylate proline. As a consequence, less collagen is formed and it is of poorer quality. The disease is characterized by hemorrhagic tendencies, particularly beneath mucous membranes and the periosteum. Wound healing is poor in patients with scurvy.

Subperiosteal hemorrhages are the characteristic orthopaedic phenomena of scurvy and involve the knee and shoulder areas most frequently. The growth plate may weaken, sometimes allowing affected epiphyses to displace from their normal position. The effects of scurvy may cause a delay in osteogenesis with a resulting decrease in the density of the bone tissue. Pathologic fractures may occur.

Treatment consists of the addition of citrus fruits, fruit juices, and ascorbic acid to the diet. Specific orthopaedic treatment is rarely required for skeletal complaints.

Vitamin D. The human organism requires vitamin D to influence the rate of absorption of ingested calcium from the gastrointestinal tract. This is absolutely essential to maintain normal calcium and phosphorus levels in the blood without making abnormal physiologic demands on the skeletal system. Abnormally low concentrations of this ion lead to tetany. Abnormally elevated concentrations lead to coma. As previously discussed, deficiency of vitamin D causes rickets and osteomalacia.

OSTEOPOROSIS

Osteoporosis is a type of metabolic bone atrophy with an unknown mechanism of causation that results in loss of bone mass.

The bone tissue is qualitatively normal, but there is too little of it as a result of a deficiency in protein matrix formation caused by decreased osteoblastic activity combined with increased osteoclastic resorption of bone — in other words, the rate of bone formation is less than that of bone resorption. This results in a marked decrease in the total amount of bone in the skeleton. The principal cell causing the bone loss in osteoporosis is the osteoclast.

Osteoporosis is the commonest metabolic affection of bone tissue and involves mostly the vertebral bodies, the pelvis, and areas containing large amounts of cancellous bone. It has been estimated to be radiologically detectable in 50 per cent of all persons over 65 years of age. It is believed that approximately 20 per cent of elderly persons develop symptoms attributable to osteoporosis because bone tissue that is lost by normal catabolism is not replaced in equal measure by new bone.

Calcium and phosphorus metabolism are unaffected in osteoporosis. The bone trabeculae become thin and sparse, with the result that compact bone is transformed into spongy bone with more open texture. Bone mineral content is normal, but the matrix is insufficient. The most important clinical implication of osteoporosis, of course, is that affected bones are prone to fracture.

There are many causes of osteoporosis: disuse of a part, prolonged immobilization, protein deficiency states, hormone deficiency (including post-menopausal) states, conditions associated with negative calcium balance, and prolonged corticosteroid therapy. General immobilization results in more widespread osteoporosis, and balance studies have shown losses of up to 9 per cent of the total body calcium, sometimes accompanied by hypercalcemia. The condition of weightlessness associated with prolonged space flight has also been shown to be accompanied by a similar loss of calcium. The most frequently encountered cause of osteoporosis, however, is senility. The condition is seen more than twice as often in women as in men and is frequently manifested as an impairment of the bony strength of the spine.

Spinal osteoporosis, the result of the decreased osteoblastic activity that may accompany senility and post-menopausal states, may lead to pain and deformity. Compression fractures in the thoracolumbar segment are common. Progressive loss of height of the vertebral bodies due to compression of the softened bone may produce kyphosis or round back deformity or actual shortening of the patient's stature.

On radiographic examination the vertebral bodies appear translucent and there is loss of the normal trabecular pattern (Fig. 5–6). The thoracic vertebrae become wedge-shaped and the bodies of

FIGURE 5-6. Lateral radiograph of lumbar spine, illustrating the biconcave appearance and compression of vertebral bodies in senile osteoporosis.

lumbar vertebrae appear biconcave as a result of pressure of the intervertebral discs on the softened bone. Often spontaneous compression fractures are seen in the thoracic and lumbar spine.

In senile or post-menopausal osteoporosis, serum levels of calcium, phosphorus, alkaline phosphatase, and CO_2 and the level of urinary hydroxyproline are usually normal.

The treatment is empiric and generally unsatisfactory because the mechanism of causation is not understood. The principle objectives in the treatment of osteoporosis are the alleviation of pain and the prevention of fractures. Brace support for the spine may be necessary in the presence of painful compression fractures. A diet high in protein, calcium, and phosphorus with vitamin D supplement helps obtain a positive calcium balance. The administration of estrogens and androgens alone or in combination is thought to be indicated because of the anabolic effect of these hormones on bone tissue. Their use is helpful in relieving bone pain, but does not demonstrably result in increased bone production. Currently there is clinical interest in using fluoride to treat osteoporosis because of its supposed ability to strengthen the apatite crystal of bone. No convincing long-term therapeutic results have yet appeared. The hormone calcitonin produced by the thyroid has been shown to be able to produce increased density of bone in many mammals if given over long periods of time. Its use in the treatment of osteoporosis has been recommended by some authorities and denied by others. It is not clear at the present time whether or not calcitonin is effective in the treatment of human osteoporosis.

CONDITIONS ASSOCIATED WITH ENDOCRINE DYSFUNCTION

Dysfunction of certain endocrine glands may have far-reaching orthopaedic implications because of the effect of the imbalance on skeletal tissue. The specific effect exerted on the skeleton will depend largely on the age of the patient at the time the particular endocrine dysfunction arises. As a rule, the younger the patient at the time of onset, the more profound will be the effect on skeletal tissue.

Pituitary, thyroid, and parathyroid gland problems are generally associated with the greatest changes in skeletal tissue. Hypersecretion of growth hormone by the anterior lobe of the pituitary may cause acceleration of bone growth resulting in overgrowth and increased stature. On the other hand, decreased secretion of either growth hormone or thyroid hormone may have the opposite effect on bone growth, resulting in undergrowth and dwarfism. Oversecretion of parathyroid hormone may give rise to a curious medical disease called generalized osteitis fibrosis cystica, which is characterized by diffuse skeletal osteoporosis, cystic changes in bone, and certain abnormalities in blood chemistry. Thyroid hormone has an effect on the maturation of bone tissue in children.

HYPERPITUITARISM

Hypersecretion of growth hormone is caused by an eosinophilic adenoma of the anterior lobe of the pituitary gland. If this tumor appears during childhood, the excessive growth hormone stimulates the growth plate to a remarkable degree to cause bone overgrowth and gigantism. Growth hormone exerts no particular delaying effect on the growth plate, so epiphyseal closure usually occurs at the normal time. Children so affected often show subnormal sexual development. The condition may be accompanied by slipping of the capital femoral epiphysis (see p. 385).

Excessive growth hormone in the adult cannot affect longitudinal bone growth but does affect circumferential bone growth, resulting in thicker bones. If hypersecretion of growth hormone occurs in the adult, a condition known as *acromegaly* results. The bones of the skull, face, and jaw, and those of the hands and feet become thick and enlarged. Enlargement and thickening of the soft tissues of the face, hands, feet, and viscera contribute to the physical deformity that characterizes an acromegalic patient.

HYPOPITUITARISM

Hyposecretion of growth hormone may be caused by a tumor or a suprasellar cyst compressing the anterior lobe of the pituitary gland. Deficiency of growth hormone causes marked undergrowth of skeletal tissue and dwarfism. The dwarfism may be present at birth or may appear during the first year of life.

Some patients with hypopituitarism may exhibit dwarfism associated with normal body proportions and normal mental development (Lorain type of dwarfism). Other patients may exhibit relatively normal growth associated with obesity, subnormal sexual development, and a predilection to develop slipping of the capital femoral epiphysis (*dystrophia-adiposa-genitalis*, *Fröhlich's syndrome*).

HYPOTHYROIDISM

Congenital hypothyroidism in children results in a condition known as *cretinism*. The cretin typically has a dull, sleepy facial expression, thick lips, a thick, protruding tongue, and mental and sexual retardation.

Deficiency of thyroid hormone delays ossification of skeletal tissue and retards longitudinal growth of bones. The epiphyses appear later than normal and may remain open for many years past regular closure time, but they do not make a significant contribution to longitudinal bone growth. For this reason, a cretin may be a dwarf. If this condition is diagnosed early and treated by thyroid extract for life, significant improvement can be anticipated.

Hypothyroidism in the adult produces a condition called *myxedema*. There are usually no specific associated skeletal abnormalities in the adult.

HYPERPARATHYROIDISM

Tumors of the parathyroid glands, usually occurring in adults, may produce excessive secretion of parathyroid hormone that can result in hypercalcemia, renal stones, and morphological changes in bone as a result of excessive bone resorption. However, if dietary calcium is plentiful, bone disease may be very slow in developing.

If the metabolic effects of increased parathyroid hormone on the skeletal system are profound, a rare clinical condition known as *generalized osteitis fibrosa cystica* may be produced.

Excessive parathyroid hormone sometimes causes excessive osteoclastic resorption of bone with marrow fibrosis, usually upsets calcium and phosphorus metabolism, and commonly results in generalized osteoporosis and decrease in bone density. Hyperparathyroidism is characterized by a loss in bone mass, as well as an increase in the ratio of the organic fraction to the mineral fraction. This, then, represents a mixture of osteopenia and osteomalacia. Fibrous lined cysts of a regular size and distribution may appear in any bone, but are most frequently seen in the bones of the extremities and pelvis. Growths resembling giant cell tumors may be found at the ends of long bones. The bones are softened by the osteoporosis, decreased density, and cystic changes. Actual bone absorption may be noted on the radiographs (Fig. 5–7).

FIGURE 5–7. Hyperparathyroidism. Note subperiosteal absorption of bone. This is seen only with hyperparathyroidism.

The patient with primary hyperparathyroidism may complain of severe skeletal pain. The bone softening may result in skeletal deformities and pathologic fractures. Between 50 and 75 per cent of patients may have associated renal complications including hematuria, kidney stones, and renal failure with uremia.

Laboratory examination reveals elevation of serum calcium and alkaline phosphatase, a decrease in serum phosphorus level, and increased urinary phosphate excretion.

Primary hyperparathyroidism with skeletal changes must be differentiated from osteoporosis, osteomalacia, polyostotic fibrous dysplasia, Paget's disease, multiple myeloma, and metastatic carcinoma. Treatment is surgical removal of the adenoma or excessive glandular tissue.

Secondary hyperparathyroidism may be seen in patients with chronic renal insufficiency. Severe renal insufficiency is associated with a renal acidosis. All available calcium is used by the body to neutralize the renal acidosis. When this supply proves insufficient, a compensatory parathyroid hyperplasia occurs to increase the amount of circulating parathyroid hormone so the extra calcium can be released from the skeletal storage depot. The skeleton thus deprived of calcium may undergo abnormal changes. Long-standing low-grade hyperparathyroidism may lead to excessive bone resorption (see p. 117).

CONDITIONS CAUSED BY UNKNOWN FACTORS

RETICULOENDOTHELIOSIS (HISTIOCYTOSIS X)

Under the heading of reticuloendotheliosis are listed a group of unusual granulomatous conditions, implicating the skeletal system, believed to be abnormalities of the reticuloendothelial system. Although clinically these conditions differ considerably, they are believed to be related because of fundamental pathologic and microscopic similarities. Proliferation of reticuloendothelial cells within bone may produce disseminated granulomatous lesions throughout the skeleton characterized histologically by the presence of histiocytes.

1. Eosinophilic Granuloma

Eosinophilic granuloma is a localized benign form of reticuloendotheliosis developing as a granulomatous lesion in bone resulting in focal areas of bone destruction. The lesion is composed of masses of histiocytes filled with cholesterol and interspersed with multiple eosinophiles. These lesions cause pain and most frequently affect children and young adults. Although it has been described in almost every bone in the skeleton, it is most commonly found in the ribs, flat bones, vertebrae, and shafts of long bones.

Although it is most common to see a single lesion, multiple lesions and involvement of several bones have been described. The growth of this granulomatous tissue within the bone substance may cause pain and local tenderness. Pathologic fracture may occur through the lesion, but healing of the fracture always follows.

On radiographic examination, eosinophilic granuloma resembles an oval or circular cyst within the medullary area of the bone showing clear-cut margins and no surrounding reactive bone formation (Fig. 5–8). These lesions may be mistaken for osteomyelitis, osteoid osteoma, Ewing's sarcoma, osteogenic sarcoma, multiple myeloma, bone cyst, and giant cell tumor.

The natural history of these lesions seems to indicate gradual spontaneous healing. Frequently biopsy is carried out to rule out the other conditions often confused with eosinophilic granuloma. Excision or curettage of the lesion induces healing. Radiotherapy may also be curative when surgical treatment cannot be carried out.

2. Hand-Schüller-Christian Disease

This is a relatively rare chronic granulomatous type of reticuloendotheliosis with an onset during early childhood. It is characterized by multiple destructive lesions in the skull, spine, pelvis,

FIGURE 5–8. Large esosinophilic granuloma of humeral shaft. (Courtesy Dr. Albert Berg, Staten Island, N.Y.).

and long bones. In addition, the patient may have exophthalmos and diabetes insipidus.

Histologically, granulomatous tissue from a Hand-Schüller-Christian disease lesion contains histiocytes laden with cholesterol.

Radiation therapy may induce healing of the skeletal lesions, but the disease is often fatal in a patient with extensive involvement.

3. Letterer-Siwe Disease

This is a very rare, generalized form of reticuloendotheliosis of infancy that some authors regard as an acute form of Hand-Schüller-Christian disease. The disease is characterized by an acute onset, typically short course, and invariably fatal outcome. The patient usually succumbs to the disease before significant bone lesions develop.

ENCHONDROMATOSIS (DYSCHONDROPLASIA, OLLIER'S DISEASE)

Enchondromatosis is a rare condition resulting from an unknown developmental error affecting cartilage cells at many growth plates. Masses or nests of cartilage cells in varying stages of development become displaced into the metaphyses of affected bones instead of being calcified and ossified in the normal manner.

Curiously, the lesions caused by this developmental error tend to involve one side of the body more than the opposite side. These cartilage-filled spaces in abnormal skeletal locations may cause shortening, deformity, or pathologic fracture of the affected bone. If enchondromatosis is associated with multiple skin hemangiomas, the condition is called *Maffucci's syndrome.* Chondrosarcomatous degeneration is considered more common in enchondromatosis than in solitary enchondroma.

The lesions of enchondromatosis are most often found in the hands and feet and at the growing ends of the long bones. Disturbances of development at the growth plate may result in a knock-knee or bowleg deformity, clubhand deformity, or cubitus varus deformity at the elbow (see pp. 421, 76 and 274).

Radiographic examination reveals mottled cystic spaces of irregular size and shape in the metaphyses of affected bones (Fig. 5-9). Enchondromatosis should not be confused with benign enchondroma, which is a single enchondroma in bone and is classified as a benign bone tumor.

There is no specific treatment for enchondromatosis. Leg length equalization operations or osteotomy to correct angular deformities may be indicated occasionally.

FIGURE 5–9. Multiple irregular cyst formation and bone deformity typical of enchondromatosis.

FIBROUS DYSPLASIA

Fibrous dysplasia is a peculiar skeletal anomaly believed to represent some type of maturation defect in bone tissue. Normally, bone tissue is constantly dying and being replaced by new bone. Fibrous dysplasia arises when some bone tissue is replaced instead by an irregular mass of tissue containing bone spicules and masses of cartilage embedded in a fibrous tissue matrix. The etiology of the disorder is unknown. A basic question regarding the developmental or neoplastic nature of fibrous dysplasia remains unanswered.

Clinically, fibrous dysplasia may be encountered in several forms. It may be confined entirely to one bone, in which case it is termed *monostotic fibrous dysplasia*. Monostotic lesions occur most commonly in the femur, tibia, and rib. If more than one bone is involved, it is referred to as *polyostotic fibrous dysplasia*. Polyostotic lesions occur most commonly in the femur, tibia, fibula, ilium, metacarpals, metatarsals, ribs, and humerus. A particularly severe form of polyostotic fibrous dysplasia, accompanied by irregular patches of café au lait skin pigmentation and precocious puberty, may be encountered in young girls. This triad of abnormal findings is known as *Albright's syndrome.*

The characteristic radiographic appearance of a monostotic lesion is a diaphyseal defect with cortical expansion, but no sign of bone destruction (Fig. 5–10). Although the central portion of the defect is usually radiolucent, a trabeculated or multicystic change may occur. In some instances, these features are accompanied by a pathologic fracture.

Differential diagnosis should include enchondroma, unicameral bone cyst, nonossifying fibroma, aneurysmal bone cyst, and giant cell tumor. Diagnosis is frequently not established until late childhood or young adulthood, but should be confirmed by biopsy. There appears to be a female predilection for fibrous dysplasia.

The lesions of fibrous dysplasia grow slowly, frequently deforming bone, and causing premature closure of epiphyses. The dis-

FIGURE 5–10. Fibrous dysplasia involving bones of right forearm. Left forearm normal.

order may affect any bone, but involvement of long bones is most common. The clinical effects may be pain, enlargement or deformity of bone, or pathologic fracture. The fractures usually heal well except those of the upper third of the femur. Severe femoral deformation is the rule after multiple fractures in this area, causing some of the most crippling features of the disease. Sarcomatous transformation of fibrous dysplasia has been reported, but it is regarded as rare. It has been noted to occur most often in long bones, particularly the femur and tibia. Osteosarcoma is the most common type of malignant transformation, but chondrosarcoma, fibrosarcoma, and anaplastic tumors have been described.

There is no specific treatment for fibrous dysplasia. It might be feasible to perform resection or wide excision of the area. In other instances, it might be preferable to scrape out the abnormal tissue surgically and fill the resulting bone defect with fresh bone chips from the ilium.

These surgical techniques are not feasible in the presence of polyostotic fibrous dysplasia, however. Treatment in this instance is directed toward correcting deformities brought about by pathologic fracture such as bowing of long bones or nonunion of the fracture. Corrective osteotomy and bone grafting may be indicated.

PAGET'S DISEASE (OSTEITIS DEFORMANS)

Paget's disease is a fairly common skeletal abnormality of obscure etiology frequently characterized by progressive structural deformities in the pelvis, femur, tibia, lower spine, and skull. It is commonest in males between the ages of 50 and 70. It is estimated to affect 3.5 per cent of the population over 45 years of age, with most patients asymptomatic and the disease discovered only as an incidental finding on a routine radiographic examination. In some patients only a single bone may be affected, while in others many bones may be involved. Whether single or multiple, the lesions are focal, being clearly demarcated from the adjacent uninvolved bone tissue. In occasional patients, the disease may appear in an active phase associated with bone pain and skeletal deformity.

Pathologic Findings. The structural changes in Paget's disease are brought about by a disorderly and disorganized combination of accelerated osteolysis and excessively abnormal bone regeneration resulting in disordered, but active, bone remodeling. Grossly, these changes cause irregular thickening of the affected bones, which present rough irregular cortical surfaces. Histologically, the irregular, wavy cement lines that separate areas of bone formed at different periods give rise to the jigsaw or mosaic bone pattern that is typical of this disease. The serum calcium and phosphorus are usually within normal limits, but active disease is accompanied by increased excretion of hydroxyproline in the urine and elevation of the alkaline phosphatase concentration in the blood. The first is usually considered an index of bone resorption and the second measures osteoblastic activity.

Clinical Picture. Paget's disease may cause skeletal pain usually referred to the lower back area or the legs. Involvement of the weight bearing long bones leads to thickening and deformity. The tibia usually bows anteriorly, while the femur tends to bow anteriorly and laterally. Despite the progressive deformity, however, the bones usually remain strong enough for weight bearing, even in the advanced stages of the disease. Involvement of the spine with Paget's disease may be associated with deformity and compression of the vertebral bodies in a kyphosis or scoliosis deformity. Involvement of the spine may be complicated by the development of spinal stenosis with nerve root or spinal cord compression. Progressive thickening of the external cortex of the skull may lead to enlargement of the head. The lesions of Paget's disease are sometimes extremely vascular and there can be a great increase in blood flow through affected bones creating, in effect, arterial venous shunts. In extreme cases, the consequent increase in cardiac output can result in cardiac failure.

If none of the potentially serious complications develop in a patient with Paget's disease, prognosis for length of life is good.

Radiographic Findings. On radiographic examination bones affected by Paget's disease appear thickened and frequently curved. The bone substance appears sclerotic and contains porous, thick trabeculae that frequently give the involved bone a dense honeycombed or cystic appearance (Fig. 5–11). Paget's disease generally begins at one end of a long bone and may spread towards the other end.

Differential Diagnosis. The osteoblastic skeletal metastases from a primary prostatic carcinoma may closely resemble the sclerotic bone lesions of Paget's disease. The findings of an abnormally high serum acid phosphatase value rules out Paget's disease and makes almost certain the diagnosis of prostatic carcinoma with metastases. In all bone diseases except those due to prostate carcinoma, it is only the serum alkaline phosphatase value that is increased.

Treatment. At the present time there is no known cure for Paget's disease and treatment is mostly symptomatic and supportive. Salicylates, aluminum acetate, parathormone, and radiation therapy have been used in the past for the relief of pain.

FIGURE 5–11. Extensive Paget's disease involving pelvis and both hips.

Recently reports have appeared in the literature assessing the beneficial effects of both mithramycin and calcitonin, the calcium-lowering hormone of the thyroid, in the treatment of Paget's disease and some of its complications. It would appear that both drugs are effective, especially when given together, in relieving bone pain and causing a decrease in the serum alkaline phosphatase level and the urinary hydroxyproline level.

Evidence is also accumulating that indicates that some diphosphonate salts are also effective agents in treating this disease. Diphosphonate salts apparently slow the rapid bone turnover characteristic of Paget's disease and aid in relieving pain. Histologically, the bone pattern tends to revert to normal and the elevated biochemical indices are lowered.

Complications. Two serious complications of Paget's disease are pathologic fracture and malignant degeneration. Pathologic fracture is the commonest complication and may be the earliest clinical sign of Paget's disease. The convex side of the deformed long bone is the usual site of fracture. As a rule, the fractures heal but are notoriously slow in uniting.

Paget's disease is a precancerous condition and malignant degeneration may develop in 20 to 30 per cent of patients with Paget's disease. Osteosarcoma is the malignancy most commonly observed, but chondrosarcoma and fibrosarcoma may also be found. The bone tumors in Paget's disease are highly malignant, and the usual life expectancy after its development is about one year.

References

Amstutz, H. C., and Carey, E. J.: Skeletal manifestations and treatment of Gaucher's disease. J. Bone and Joint Surg., 48-A:670, 1966.

Barry, H. C.: Paget's Disease of Bone. Edinburgh: E. & S. Livingstone Ltd., 1969.

Bauze, R. J., Smith, R. and Francis, M. J. O.: A new look at osteogenesis imperfecta. A clinical, radiological and biochemical study of 42 patients. J. Bone and Joint Surg., 57-B:2, 1975.

Fairbank, H. A. T.: Atlas of General Affections of the Skeleton. Baltimore: Williams & Wilkins Co., 1951.

Falvo, K. A., Root, L., and Bullough, P. G.: Osteogenesis imperfecta: Clinical evaluation and management. J. Bone and Joint Surg., 56-A:783, 1974.

Hadjitavlou, A. G., Tsoukas, G. M., Siller, T. N., Danai, S. S., and Greenwood, F.: Combination drug therapy in treatment of Paget's disease of bone. Clinical and metabolic response. J. Bone and Joint Surg., 59-A:1045, 1977.

Harris, W. H., Dudley, H. R., Jr., and Barry, R. J.: The natural history of fibrous dysplasia. An orthopaedic, pathological and roentgenographic study. J. Bone and Joint Surg., 44-A:207, 1962.

Harris, W. H., and Heaney, R. P.: Skeletal Renewal and Metabolic Bone Disease. Boston: Little, Brown and Co., 1969.

Henry, A.: Monostotic fibrous dysplasia. J. Bone and Joint Surg., 51-B:300, 1969.

Lichtenstein, L.: Histiocytosis X (Eosinophilic granuloma of bone, Letterer-Siwe disease, and Schüller-Christian disease). J. Bone and Joint Surg., 46-A:76, 1964.

McKusick, V. A.: Heritable Disorders of Connective Tissue. St. Louis: C. V. Mosby Co., 3rd edition, 1966.

Mankin, H. J.: Rickets, osteomalacia, and renal osteodystrophy. Review article. Part I. J. Bone and Joint Surg., 56-A:101, 1974.

Mankin, H. J.: Rickets, osteomalacia and renal osteodystrophy. Review article. Part II. J. Bone and Joint Surg., 56-A:352, 1974.

Reiss, E.: Primary hyperparathyroidism: A simplified approach to diagnosis. Med. Clin. North Am., 54:131, Jan., 1970.

Rodrigues, R. J., and Lewis, H. L.: Eosinophilic granuloma of bone. Review of literature and case presentation. Clin. Ortho. and Rel. Res., 77:183, 1971.

Stein, I., Shapiro, B., Ostrum, B., and Beller, M. L.: Evaluation of sodium etidronate in the treatment of Paget's disease of bone. Clin. Ortho. and Rel. Res., 122:347, 1977.

CHAPTER 6

DISORDERS OF JOINTS

INTRODUCTION

Hyaline articular cartilage caps the bones that form a synovial joint and provides a smooth gliding surface for movement. The cartilage is nourished by diffusion through the matrix of materials derived from capillaries in the perichondrium. Joint cartilage, not believed to be innervated, is bathed with synovial fluid, a dialysate of plasma derived from a moderately vascular synovium, which functions as the perfect lubricant and as an additional source of nutrition for articular cartilage. Under normal conditions, synovial fluid is viscous and serous in appearance, containing few polymorphonuclear leukocytes and no crystalline elements. The glucose levels of normal joint fluid and plasma are similar. Fluid aspirated from normal joints does not clot spontaneously. The precipitate formed by adding normal synovial fluid to dilute acetic acid is characteristically discrete and firm in appearance ("mucin" clot test). These characteristics of normal synovial fluid may be altered in various disease states of joints.

The classic pathologic response to a noxious stimulus affecting a joint is inflammation characterized by local heat, redness, swelling and pain. The degree of the inflammatory response will depend greatly upon the type and extent of the offending stimulus, its location, and the state of the host tissue. By its nature, the inflammatory response cannot involve the musculoskeletal system exclusively. The reticuloendothelial system, the cardiovascular system and connective tissue are intimately concerned in this response. Consequently, the inflammatory response frequently makes itself known as a systemic illness characterized by malaise, prostration, fever, and finally, localized pain.

Joint inflammation starts in the synovial membrane, which, as a consequence of the irritation, may secrete large amounts of fluid into the joint cavity together with numerous inflammatory cells. This resulting synovial effusion is usually painful and interferes with normal joint function. The inflammatory joint fluid is characterized by an increased content of serum proteins, decreased viscosity, and a decreased content of hyaluronic acid. Cloudiness of the fluid results from increased numbers of white blood cells. Fluid obtained from inflamed joints clots because of the presence of fibrinogen, which enters an inflamed joint by means of increased vascular permeability. In most types of inflammatory joint disease, the "mucin" test shows a flocculation instead of a discrete, firm mucin clot.

The inflammatory joint response runs the gamut from a mild effusion to a severely destructive process causing permanent joint damage. Trauma to a joint frequently irritates the synovium to evoke an outpouring of synovial fluid and a joint effusion. Rheumatoid arthritis is characterized by chronic joint inflammation. Bacterial joint infection may be accompanied by joint cartilage destruction if the chondroid matrix is digested by proteolytic enzymes. The final result may be irreversible, permanent joint damage.

Emphasis must be placed upon identification of the cause of the inflammatory joint response at the earliest possible moment. Adequate and timely treatment can greatly modify the joint response and mitigate its harmful effect. The laboratory reflection of joint inflammation includes an elevated serum uric acid in gout, leukocytosis in bacterial infection, and a persistent elevation of the erythrocyte sedimentation rate in the serum of the patient with rheumatoid arthritis. Additional diagnostic information may be obtained from an examination of the aspirated synovial fluid with reference to color and appearance, culture, cell count, sugar content, acid-phosphatase activity, and the presence or absence of crystals. Joint and synovial tissue biopsy may be required to establish a diagnosis.

ARTHRITIS

Arthritis is a nonspecific term denoting acute or chronic inflammation of the joint. Theoretically, any lesion or disorder associated with or causing inflammation of a joint may be said to produce a form of arthritis. The diagnosis in most patients seen clinically because of "arthritis" will fall within the following groups:

1. Rheumatoid arthritis (including juvenile rheumatoid arthritis and ankylosing spondylitis)
2. Arthritis due to rheumatic fever
3. Osteoarthritis (degenerative joint disease)
    (a) primary
    (b) secondary
4. Arthritis due to infection (pyogenic arthritis, tuberculous arthritis)
5. Metabolic disease affecting joints (gout)
6. Neuropathic joint disease (Charcot joint)
7. Monarthritis
8. Special forms
    (a) hemophilic arthritis
    (b) psychogenic rheumatism

In terms of total number of victims, arthritis leads all other diseases as a cause of crippling and resulting economic loss to the community. It actually results in more lost work days than accidental injury. The total number of people affected can be expected to increase as the life span lengthens, because osteoarthritis — the most frequently seen form of arthritis — is predominantly a disease of middle and old age.

RHEUMATOID ARTHRITIS

Rheumatoid arthritis, a chronic inflammatory disease of undetermined etiology and pathogenesis, is systemic in nature and characterized by the manner in which it involves the synovial membrane of joints, tendons or bursae.

The disease is seen most commonly in those between the ages of 25 and 50, but it may also be seen in children and in the aged. It shows a sex ratio of three women affected for each male. There is a slight tendency for the disease to be familial. The incidence of rheumatoid arthritis in the United States is believed to be 1 to 3 per cent of the adult population. Psychogenic factors are thought to be of some importance in the precipitation or exacerbation of the disease in many patients. This is the most feared form of arthritis because of the profound crippling that may result.

Pathologic Features. The major target organ for rheumatoid involvement is the synovial tissue. Inflammatory disease may be present wherever synovium is found. The disease is thus not limited to synovial joints, but may also occur in tendon sheaths and bursae. Because this primary site of the disease is vascular and innervated, it can react to noxious stimuli with the full range of exudative and proliferative inflammatory changes. The ensuing damage to the articular cartilage is secondary to the synovial inflammatory response.

Despite extensive study, the etiology of rheumatoid arthritis remains obscure. It is generally accepted, however, that immune mechanisms play an important role in the initiation and perpetuation of this disease. Immunologic reactions have been shown to underlie the pathogenesis of a number of rheumatic diseases, and studies on immunologic reactivity are being intensely pursued in most of the other inflammatory connective tissue disorders. It seems quite likely that cell-mediated immune reactions may be central to the pathogenesis of many of the rheumatic diseases. The articular changes, once started, become self-perpetuating because of the mechanisms within the synovial membrane itself. Presumably, an antigen-antibody reaction takes place directly within the synovial cavity, causing injury to and marked proliferation of the synovium. This diseased synovium damages the articular cartilage and adjacent tissues, primarily by the release of proteolytic enzymes. These enzymes cause further injury to the synovium, as well as perpetuating the disease process.

Joint involvement is heralded by synovial inflammation with effusion. The inflammatory changes may also involve the capsule and periarticular soft tissues, causing the swelling, tenderness, and painful motion seen in the joints clinically. There is regional atrophy of bone and muscle. Joint effusion is present in the active stage, but this disappears during remissions and in the chronic stage. Although the synovial tissues are densely infiltrated by mononuclear cells, the synovial fluid typically contains thousands of neutrophils, giving it a cloudy appearance. Hyaluronate is reduced in the fluid and the "mucin" test shows a flocculation instead of a clot.

Since there is as yet no definitive treatment for rheumatoid arthritis, the initiating antigen persists and evokes a chronic stage of inflammation. Round cells, particularly lymphocytes, and plasma cells become the predominant cell type in the synovium. The synovium proliferates extensively and becomes a permanently thickened, hyperemic densely cellular membrane with enlarged erythematous villi. This thickened granulomatous tissue contributes to the formation of an eroding and invading membrane known as a *pannus*.

The excess joint fluid derived from the inflammatory synovium precipitates a layer of fibrin that coats the synovial and articular surfaces. This fibrin layer gradually becomes organized into a high-

FIGURE 6–1. Rheumatoid knee joint exposed at surgery. Note marked destruction of articular cartilage.

ly vascular, spreading, granulation tissue membrane or pannus by the growth into it of cells and vessels from the synovium. The pannus gradually spreads over the joint surfaces, eroding and pitting the underlying cartilage and bone (Fig. 6–1). A reasonable hypothesis about the mechanism is that lysosomal hydrolases and other enzymes released from the proliferating rheumatoid synovium in contact with cartilage gain access to the cartilage matrix and degrade it, thus preparing the way for the actual invasion of the cartilage and the underlying subchondral bone by the pannus.

Pannus formation is characteristic of rheumatoid pathology. Pannus destroys articular cartilage and may even erode subchondral bone, resulting in progressive and crippling joint deformity and permanent loss of motion. This destructive pathologic process renders the joint quite unstable and muscle pull across the joint may cause flexion or extension contractures, subluxations, or even joint dislocations.

As the acute inflammatory process subsides, the granulation tissue may become converted to dense scar, causing fibrous ankylosis of the joint. If this fibrous scar is converted to bone, a true ankylosis results. The fibers of associated skeletal muscles undergo localized or diffuse degenerative changes, with the degenerated muscle being gradually replaced by fibrous tissue. The involved bones show osteoporosis or bone rarefaction.

Clinical Features. Most often rheumatoid arthritis has an insidious onset. Joint involvement is usually symmetrically distributed, with the proximal interphalangeal joints of the fingers being especially susceptible. Frequently, one or just a few joints become swollen and painful at the onset, with other joints becoming affected later. In many patients rheumatoid arthritis is relatively mild and remission occurs before extensive joint damage has taken place. In advanced rheumatoid arthritis, chronic deformities include contractures, subluxation, and ankylosis, and gross local distortion of joints may be found.

The painful swelling in and about the joint limits motion. The thickening of the periarticular tissues, combined with the muscle atrophy above and below, gives the joint a characteristic spindle-shaped appearance. The proliferating connective tissue tends to overgrow and erode the joint cartilage and to invade the supporting cancellous bone, leading to severe disability and deformity — often with ankylosis of the joint. These changes are most likely to be seen in the hands, wrists, knees, hips, and feet, but almost every

FIGURE 6-2. Typical changes in the hand caused by rheumatoid arthritis.

joint in the body may be involved (Fig. 6–2). Involvement of a joint by the rheumatoid inflammatory process may lead to weakening of the joint capsule, and herniation of the synovium when the effect of increased intra-articular pressure is added. This may result in the characteristic para-articular synovial cyst frequently found in the popliteal space.

As the disease progresses, the patient may experience fatigue, exhaustion, lassitude, vasomotor disturbances, paresthesias, generalized morning stiffness of one or several hours' duration, and general debility. Underweight frequently accompanies rheumatoid arthritis. Muscular weakness and atrophy are prominent. The skin of the extremities may become smooth, glossy, and atrophic. Constitutional manifestions may include elevated temperature, tachycardia, generalized lymphadenopathy, and malnutrition with bodily wasting. Other extra-articular manifestations may include a systemic vasculitis or a necrotizing panarteritis. Amyloidosis occurs in 5 to 10 per cent of patients and may lead to renal insufficiency.

Subcutaneous nodules are a characteristic pathologic finding in rheumatoid arthritis and can be noted in about 25 per cent of patients. The nodules are firm and nontender and most often develop in the periarticular tissues such as joint capsule, tendon sheath, and bursae. It is believed that the rheumatoid nodule results from fibrinoid necrosis of blood vessels with ischemic breakdown of collagen. Nodules generally appear relatively late in the disease process and almost invariably in patients with rheumatoid factor in their sera. Nodules indicate active disease and a poor prognosis.

Spontaneous subluxation of the cervical spine is a well-recognized and not uncommon complication of rheumatoid arthritis. It occurs most commonly at the atlanto-axial level, but may also occur at lower levels in the cervical area. Although many of these patients are free from symptoms or complain only of increasing neck pain, cord pressure with tetraplegia can ensue.

Radiographic Features. A single film of the hand and wrist is usually more useful diagnostically in peripheral rheumatoid arthritis than a view of any other part (Fig. 6–3). However, radiographic changes other than soft tissue swelling may not appear for several months after the onset of the disease.

The degree of radiographic change will vary with the stage of the disease and can be summarized as follows:

Early Stage
1. Soft tissue swelling
2. Osteoporosis or bone rarefaction
3. Loss of joint space without alteration of contour

FIGURE 6–3. Radiograph of hands, exhibiting bone and joint changes typical of rheumatoid arthritis.

Intermediate Stage
1. Bone erosion at the margins of the articular cortices
2. Subchondral cyst formation
3. Progressive osteoporosis
4. Progressive loss of joint space
5. Joint contracture deformities
   Late Stage
1. Severe osteoporosis
2. Complete destruction of the joint resulting in subluxation, dislocation, or ankylosis

Laboratory Features. There are no laboratory tests that are specifically diagnostic for rheumatoid arthritis. Aspirated joint fluid is often cloudy and of reduced viscosity. The "mucin" test of synovial fluid shows a flocculation instead of a clot. The joint fluid contains an increased number of polymorphonuclear leukocytes, but this finding is not pathognomonic. A high titer of rheumatoid factor may be present in the synovial fluid.

Most patients exhibit an elevated erythrocyte sedimentation

rate, particularly during periods of disease activity. Positive C-reactive protein and a low serum iron may be found on examination of the blood. A secondary anemia with a normal white cell count is frequently found.

Serum from patients with rheumatoid arthritis contains a substance of unknown composition called the *rheumatoid factor*, produced by the plasma cells and the rheumatoid synovial membrane. Many authorities believe that the rheumatoid factor represents a response to immunization to an unknown antigen in the joint, with the plasma cells throwing off rheumatoid factor as a by-product of this process. Rheumatoid factor in the presence of gamma globulin is capable of agglutinating certain strains of streptococci, sensitized sheep cells, and latex particles. This reaction forms the basis for the latex flocculation test and the sheep cell agglutination test, both of which will ultimately be positive in a high percentage of patients with rheumatoid arthritis.

Management of the Patient. Most rheumatologists today will agree that the two major advances in the treatment of rheumatoid arthritic patients over the past decade have been the growing recognition of the need for a team approach in the rehabilitation of these patients and the increasing participation of the orthopaedic surgeon as a member of that team. It should be emphasized once again that rheumatoid arthritis is a systemic disease of unknown etiology and no curative drug is known at the present time. Treatment is directed both at the general care of the whole patient and locally to the affected joint. The principal therapeutic objectives are control of the inflammatory process and preservation of joint function. Mechanical damage, muscular weakness, fluctuation of disease activity, and the psychological behavior of the patient all play relative roles in the assessment of functional disability. Ideally, the treating team should consist of a rheumatologist, a physiatrist, and an orthopaedist — who bring together for the patient's benefit the principles of medical care, rehabilitation, and orthopaedics. The orthopaedist's responsibility as a member of the team is directed toward the musculoskeletal system in an effort to prevent or correct joint deformity.

Rest and the application of heat to the affected part are of great help in relieving joint and muscle pain and stiffness. A number of drugs may be helpful in controlling the inflammatory process. These include aspirin, gold salts, chloroquine, primaquine, phenylbutazone, indomethacin, immunosuppressive agents, and corticosteroids administered both systemically and by intra-articular injection. Most of these drugs have potentially serious side effects and must be given under close medical supervision.

Maintenance of joint function is of prime importance in the

treatment of rheumatoid arthritis. Preservation of range of motion in affected joints must be emphasized during the treatment program. Active exercise must be part of the program in order to maintain muscle tone. Strengthening exercises may prevent disuse atrophy and restore wasted muscles. If muscle tone is very poor, the joint may have to be protected temporarily by bracing. Fixed flexion contractures about the joints may require traction, wedging casts, or open surgical release for their correction. Forced manipulation of joints under anesthesia is not favored because of the brittle nature of the bone.

The progressively destructive nature of rheumatoid arthritis frequently leads to permanent joint crippling or even complete invalidism for the patient. Early in the disease a patient may voluntarily assume the "position of comfort" for a joint in order to relieve the pain caused by the joint inflammation. Usually this means a flexed position. If not constantly watched for and guarded against by the attending personnel, this "position of comfort" may become a permanent fixed flexion contracture. Every effort should be made to keep the joint in the "position of function," even by resorting to traction, splints, casts, or braces, if necessary.

Surgery may play an important role in the treatment and rehabilitation of the patient with rheumatoid arthritis who is not responding adequately to nonoperative measures. Operations on joints can be very effective in preventing some deformities, in relieving pain, and in improving overall function. Many types of operations have proved successful in the past, and new operations have been developed which promise success in the future. It is no longer held necessary to wait until the disease is "burned out" to operate if it is believed surgery can help the patient. In general, the best results from surgery are achieved when the medical treatment, orthopaedic management, and physical care are coordinated by careful planning on the part of the physicians involved. Surgery not only is playing an ever-increasing role in the rehabilitation of the handicapped patient but also is being used to prevent deformities.

Since the major target organ for rheumatoid involvement is the synovial tissue, the operation of *synovectomy*, the surgical removal of the inflamed synovium, has a well-established place in the rehabilitation of patients with rheumatoid arthritis. Persistent, unresponsive synovitis is the primary indication for synovectomy and relief of pain seems to be the principal benefit derived by the patient. Although synovitis may recur after synovectomy, approximately 60 per cent of the patients would appear to maintain significant long-term pain relief.

To produce the best functional result, synovectomy should be performed early in the course of the disease prior to the onset of signs of joint destruction on the radiograph. If synovectomy can indeed prevent progressive joint destruction, it is clearly of great importance in the selected patient and must be thought of as a conservative rather than radical measure. However, although the short-term results are encouraging, few long-term studies have been reported as yet. The joints that lend themselves most readily to surgical synovectomy are the knee, elbow, wrist, shoulder, ankle, and metacarpal phalangeal joints of the hands. Attempts to perform medical synovectomy using cytotoxic drugs have generally failed.

Once joint destruction has occurred, the operation of synovectomy loses much of its effectiveness. Late synovectomy may relieve pain, but does not help restore functional effectiveness to the joint. Restoration of motion and function to a destroyed joint can only be affected by operations on bone. The joints most frequently requiring surgical attention because of destructive articular changes are the hip, knee, and joints of the forefoot (Fig. 6–4).

FIGURE 6–4. Destruction of medial compartment of knee secondary to rheumatoid arthritis.

A stiff, painful destroyed hip joint is best treated by an operation designed to restore motion to the joint. Total hip replacement arthroplasty would be the procedure of choice for most patients. Cup arthroplasty is occasionally used for this purpose in younger patients.

A stiff, painful, unstable, and severely affected knee would also require some type of replacement arthroplasty for its treatment. Many types of total knee replacement devices are available and their ability to restore painless function to destroyed knee joints has been quite encouraging over a short-term observation.

Since rheumatoid arthritis is a polyarthritis with an almost unpredictable course, even in the face of adequate medical management, surgical fusion of a major joint is rarely performed. Present day surgical emphasis is on attempting to restore relatively painless motion to the joint provided joint stability can be maintained.

Rheumatoid arthritis frequently affects the forefoot, with the development of stiff, painful feet. Typically, the forefoot broadens, the metatarsal heads are depressed into the sole of the foot, and a cock-up deformity of the toes develops (Fig. 6–5). Surgical removal of all the metatarsal heads relieves the forefoot pain and allows the toes to drop down into a more functional position.

FIGURE 6–5. Typical forefoot deformity in rheumatoid arthritis.

JUVENILE RHEUMATOID ARTHRITIS

Rheumatoid arthritis having an onset before 16 years of age is considered to be the juvenile form. It is a chronic arthritis that may appear in different forms, even beginning as a fulminating systemic process known as Still's disease. Although the systemic aspects of the disease may be more severe in the adult, the joints in the juvenile form have the same appearance and there may be the typical subcutaneous nodules. The streptococcus agglutination test is usually negative. Involvement of the cervical spine is common in this form of arthritis. The inflammatory reaction within the joints frequently destroys the growth cartilage, thus arresting longitudinal growth of bone.

Juvenile rheumatoid arthritis can have a polyarticular onset similar to that observed in adult patients or can present as a single joint disease that may or may not progress to polyarticular arthritis. The most valid criterion for diagnosing juvenile rheumatoid arthritis is the persistence of joint involvement for several months in a patient who has no other demonstrable disease. The laboratory tests for rheumatoid factor, useful in diagnosing adult rheumatoid arthritis, are not often positive in the juvenile form. It has been estimated that approximately 50 per cent of patients recover from juvenile rheumatoid arthritis without disability after receiving only nonsurgical treatment.

Synovectomy in children has not received universal approval, partly because of concern about interference with bone growth as a result of surgical trauma and partly because of isolated examples of serverely restricted range of joint motion following operation. Recent studies, however, show that short-term results in children are no less favorable than those in adults. Indeed, the danger of abnormal bone growth as a result of a rheumatoid inflammation is believed to be one of the indications for synovectomy by its proponents. This is believed to be especially true in a child with unilateral involvement of the knee. It is probable that the joint stiffness sometimes encountered after synovectomy derives from the difficulty of obtaining a young child's cooperation in postoperative exercises. If synovectomy is to be considered in a patient with juvenile rheumatoid arthritis, the question of timing and patient selection is especially important in view of the fact that half or more of the patients recover from the disease with little or no residual disability.

MONARTHRITIS

Occasionally a patient, either child or adult, presents with signs of an inflammatory response confined to one joint, frequently the knee or ankle. It should be noted that in some patients monarthritis is rheumatoid in nature and progresses to a typical polyarthritis, while in other patients no such progression occurs and the diagnosis remains unclear. In these patients, arthrotomy and synovial biopsy should be performed. A lengthy period of observation is often necessary before a definitive diagnosis can be made, and in a substantial number of patients the diagnosis is never made. In a few patients, complete resolution of the monarthritis occurs.

ANKYLOSING SPONDYLITIS (MARIE-STRUMPELL DISEASE)

Ankylosing spondylitis is a chronic, progressive polyarthritis characterized by involvement of the sacroiliac joints, the spinal apophyseal or synovial joints, and the adjacent soft tissues. Some patients may develop a peripheral joint involvement clinically indistinguishable from that seen in rheumatoid arthritis, but peripheral joint involvement is much less common in this disorder than in rheumatoid arthritis. Approximately 90 per cent of the patients are males between the ages of 20 and 40. The most frequent presenting complaint is back pain.

The cause of ankylosing spondylitis is unknown. It is not clear at the moment whether it is a variant of rheumatoid arthritis or exists as a totally different entity. Rheumatoid arthritis is seen about fifteen times more frequently than ankylosing spondylitis. The essential pathologic joint changes characterized by proliferative chronic synovitis are indistinguishable in the two diseases, but the majority of patients with ankylosing spondylitis have a negative rheumatoid factor. A high association of a histocompatibility antigen HL-AW27 has been reported in patients with ankylosing spondylitis and provides an important diagnostic adjunct in the work-up of patients suspected of having this disease.

Inflammatory synovitis appears to begin at the sacroiliac joints and goes on to involve the apophyseal joints of the spine and the costovertebral joints, giving rise to the characteristic complaint of backache. As the disease progresses, cartilage and bone destruction results in fibrous and bony ankylosis of the spine. This causes the back stiffness or "poker spine" deformity that is the hallmark of this disease. One additional pathologic feature adds to the rigidity of the spine: calcification occurs beneath the anterior and posterior longitudinal spinal ligaments. As this process progresses, it may encase the entire vertebral column in a calcium shell, giving rise to the characteristic "bamboo spine" effect seen on radiographs (Fig. 6–6).

FIGURE 6-6. Ankylosing spondylitis of spine. Note bamboo effect on AP view and bony encasement of vertebral bodies on lateral view.

The course of the disease as measured by the progression of radiologic characteristics is not modified by any available form of treatment. Mild or moderately severe disease with progressive ankylosis of the lumbar, thoracic, and cervical spine is the rule.

No treatment known at present will effectively check the progression of the arthritic process and ankylosing spondylitis. Treatment is directed towards relieving pain and keeping the spine erect. The overall prognosis for pain relief and maintenance of function is generally good. About three-quarters of the patients manage to work full time in light occupations, supporting themselves and their families.

The main goal of treatment is to insure that the patient does not develop severe flexion contractures of the neck and back. Most patients tend to flex the spine voluntarily in order to relieve pain during the acute stages of the disease. If this tendency is not fought and corrected, the patient's spine may be permanently ankylosed in a flexed position. The patient must be instructed in the dangers of the flexed position and kept on a program of hyperextension spinal exercises. Brace support is occasionally indicated. Anti-inflammatory drugs orally and roentgen therapy locally seem effective in curtailing pain and making an exercise program more tolerable.

Occasionally, a severe, fixed flexion deformity of the spine can be corrected by a surgical osteotomy through the dorsolumbar junction. A few patients will develop significant peripheral joint involvement, particularly the hip joint, which frequently progresses to bony ankylosis. Because of the extreme functional disability caused by a stiff spine and stiff hips, restoration of some hip joint motion by total hip replacement arthroplasty, either unilaterally or bilaterally, would be indicated.

ARTHRITIS DUE TO RHEUMATIC FEVER

Rheumatic fever, an inflammatory disease occurring as a delayed sequel to infection with Group A streptococci, is an acute febrile illness mostly affecting children and frequently associated with a painful polyarthritis. Patients may have painful swollen joints due to synovial inflammation and effusion, but since the articular cartilage is not affected, no permanent joint damage is produced. Treatment of the underlying problem restores the joint to normal. Whatever permanent damage is associated with this disease is localized to the cardiac valves.

It is generally believed that the incidence of rheumatic fever, like that of streptococcal sore throat and scarlet fever, has been decreasing for several years, the rate of decrease presumably having been accelerated by the wide use of antimicrobial therapy. Rheumatic fever, however, remains a worldwide disease prevalent wherever poor economic conditions, overcrowding, and substandard housing prevail.

OSTEOARTHRITIS (DEGENERATIVE JOINT DISEASE)

Osteoarthritis, also known as degenerative joint disease, is a common progressive disorder characterized pathologically by degeneration of articular cartilage and proliferation of subchondral bone. It is a disease mainly of middle and old age and affects females more frequently than males. It strikes most weight-bearing joints, particularly the cervical and lumbar spine, the hip, and the knee, giving rise to the clinical complaints of joint pain and stiffness. The distal interphalangeal joints of the fingers frequently show nodular thickenings known as *Heberden's nodes* (Fig. 6–7). Factors such as trauma, poor posture or body mechanics, obesity, and occupational strain may precipitate or aggravate symptoms. Health statistics from the United States Department of Health, Education and Welfare have shown that of the people unable to work for more than six months because of arthritis, 56 per cent had osteoarthritis and only 27 per cent had rheumatoid arthritis.

FIGURE 6-7. Patient with osteoarthritis showing Heberden's nodes.

The term osteoarthritis is actually somewhat of a misnomer since it implies inflammation. At the present time, inflammation is not believed to play a significant role in the pathologic picture of osteoarthritis. The current concept of osteoarthritis implies biochemical deterioration in diarthrodial or synovial-lined joints. Normally, degenerative changes found in joints are associated with the aging process. These changes, if solely related to age, are usually nonprogressive. These joint changes are quite distinct from the more severe and progressive process of cartilage degeneration and osteophyte formation characterizing osteoarthritis. There are also appreciable biochemical differences between osteoarthritic articular cartilage and that of the unaffected elderly. Both aging and osteoarthritis are associated with a depletion of total protein polysaccharides, but with a difference. Normal cartilage in the aged contains increased keratin sulfate and decreased chondroitin-4 sulfate, while osteoarthritic cartilage contains diminished keratin sulfate and elevated chondroitin-4 sulfate.

Articular cartilage, unlike most other tissues, is avascular and its cells are entirely dependent on a copious water-rich matrix for their metabolic exchanges. The matrix is a composite material in which the fibrous component is collagen and the filler is proteoglycan ground substance. The collagen gives cartilage its tensile strength. Joints have a limited capacity to respond to trauma, inflammation, and biochemical challenge. The development of wear changes in the articular surfaces of joints is related in part to their ability to resist the compressive forces applied by activity. The capacity of a subchondral bone–articular cartilage system to withstand compressive, dynamic forces is the joint's principal defense against these day-to-day pressures.

Most authorities believe that the first evidence of osteoarthritis is found in articular cartilage where one of the earliest changes is diminution of chondroitin sulfate, an acid mucopolysaccharide, relative to the collagen of the matrix. This results in depletion of the ground substance and "unmasking" of the collagen, which in itself is probably stable. Normally, the matrix dissipates stresses hydrostatically, but when the collagen is "unmasked" its fibers may rupture because they are subjected to excessive bending and torsional stress. This produces the characteristic lesions of early osteoarthritis: flaking, fibrillation, fissuring, and erosion of articular cartilage with loss of metachromatic staining. Subchondral bony sclerosis in the weight bearing areas, osteoporosis in the non–weight bearing areas, cysts, and marginal osteophyte formation are regarded as secondary phenomena produced by the loss of articular cartilage in the transmission of mechanical forces to the more labile bony tissues.

The way in which the articular cartilage is depleted of mucopolysaccharides is uncertain, but an enzymatic pathway is suspected. A hyaluronidase-like enzyme has been identified in the synovial fluid of patients with osteoarthritis. Some investigators believe that a break in the surface layer of articular cartilage exposes the cartilage matrix to this enzyme and digestion of chondroitin sulfate results. Stresses on the weakened cartilage will produce more cracks in the surface, allowing entry of additional enzyme-laden synovial fluid and increased destruction. Other investigators favor an enzyme theory, but believe the chondrocytes release lysosomal hydrolases that degrade the protein polysaccharide. The major weakness of this theory is that no such enzyme has, as yet, been isolated from articular cartilage.

Pathologic Features.   Both cartilage and bone are altered in osteoarthritis, but changes in other articular or periarticular structures are minimal. Degenerative change in the articular cartilage seems to be the primary pathologic lesion, with proliferation of bone of the joint margins and in areas of denuded bone occurring as a secondary effect.

Available data indicate that primary arthritis of weight bearing

FIGURE 6-8. Femoral head specimen, showing cartilage denudation seen with osteoarthritis.

joints is a focal disease demonstrating marked variation in histologic, biochemical, and metabolic parameters.

As we have seen, the earliest articular cartilage lesions show decreased concentration of chondroitin sulfate relative to the collagen of the matrix. The loss of polysaccharide from the cartilage matrix results initially in loss of elasticity, contributing to further breakdown of cartilage through physical stress. The normally smooth, translucent cartilage becomes dull and opaque. Later, affected areas become roughened and soft. Fraying and fibrillation of the cartilage appear. Loss of cartilage substance progresses ultimately to denudation of underlying bone (Fig. 6-8).

Where the articular cartilage is thinned, the subchondral bone shows a proliferation of fibroblasts and new bone formation that appears on radiographs as subchondral bone sclerosis. Subcortical trabeculae also thicken. Subchondral cysts filled with fibrous tissue may appear (Fig. 6-9). Periosteal bone proliferation occurs at the joint margins at the site of ligamentous and tendinous attachments forming bony spurs or ridges called osteophytes (Fig. 6-10).

Synovial changes include villous proliferation with an increase in the number of surface cells and encroachment of synovia on the margins of the articular cartilage. The subsynovial areolar tissue is

FIGURE 6–9. Femoral head slice, showing cysts seen in osteoarthritis.

FIGURE 6–10. Femoral head slice, showing marginal osteophytes seen in osteo-arthritis.

replaced by fibrous tissue, and chronic inflammatory cells may be evident throughout the synovium. With further progression, the capsule becomes markedly thickened by fibrous proliferation and adheres to adjacent structures. The joint space, as seen radiographically, is diminished owing to loss of surface cartilage, as well as to the advance of the subchondral bone into the deeper layers of existing cartilage.

It has long been held that the appearance of degenerative joint changes is commensurate with the aging process. However, there is presently sufficient evidence of focal, histologic, chemical, and metabolic changes, as well as of genetic and environmental influences to permit the conclusion that degenerative joint changes, although correlated with age, are not necessarily an accompaniment of aging.

Clinical Features. In clinical practice, osteoarthritis can be seen in a primary form or as a secondary form. Osteoarthritis is said to be primary when it arises apparently de novo and when its onset is unexplainable by the current knowledge of predisposing factors. A high proportion of patients with primary osteoarthritis and multiple joint involvement maintain comfortable function on adequate medical treatment programs and never require surgical intervention.

Osteoarthritis is defined as secondary when degeneration occurs in a joint previously damaged by a congenital defect, a prior joint disorder or disease, or by trauma. Legg-Calvé-Perthes disease, slipped capital femoral epiphysis, congenital dislocation of the hip, and intra-articular fractures are well known precursors of secondary osteoarthritis of the affected joint later in life. Articular cartilage has almost no capacity to regenerate once it is injured. The wear and tear of normal activity leads to mechanical abrasions of the articular cartilage and damage to the joint surface, which can be progressive in time. Damage is accelerated if the joint margins have been permanently distorted by prior deformity or trauma. Frequently, a weight bearing joint afflicted with secondary osteoarthritis will require surgical intervention.

When present, the symptoms typically consist of pain, stiffness, and swelling in the affected joint. The pain tends to be of an achy nature and is definitely correlated with the stiffness. Characteristically, the pain and stiffness are brought on by immobility of the part and are relieved by mobility of the part only to return with prolonged activity. This is why these patients feel worse after prolonged sitting and can relieve their stiffness to some extent by walking around. Where there is a large volume of synovial tissue, as in the knee joint, there may be a profuse effusion causing increased pain through the mechanism of joint distention. With acute onset of disease, the part may appear swollen, warm and extremely tender.

The joints most frequently affected are the lumbar spine, knees, hips, and elbows. Around the shoulder area the glenohumeral joint is usually spared, but the acromioclavicular joint is frequently affected. In the hand the pattern of joint involvement is exactly opposite that of rheumatoid arthritis. In osteoarthritis, the distal interphalangeal joints (Heberden's nodes) and the first carpometacarpal joints are primary affected.

Radiographic Features. The radiographic changes seen in most patients with osteoarthritis are quite striking and prove an invaluable aid to diagnosis. It is well to bear in mind, however, that in general there is no particular correlation between the severity of the radiographic findings and the degree of clinical distress. Frequently joints show striking changes on radiographs, but few or no symptoms clinically.

The actual changes seen radiographically result mainly from bony proliferation; thus one sees subchondral sclerosis, which gives the bone its dense appearance on the radiograph. This is usually associated with spur formation around the joint margins. Occasionally subchondral bone cysts are seen. The joint space becomes narrow and, to a certain extent, deformed. Unlike rheumatoid arthritis, however, the general outlines of the joint are preserved and the bone texture remains normal (Fig. 6–11).

FIGURE 6–11. Severe osteoarthritis of knee joint.

Management of the Patient. Even in the face of distressing symptoms and a frightening radiographic appearance, the joints in this condition generally retain a surprising degree of motion and do not go on to bony ankylosis as might occur in rheumatoid arthritis. This is basically because osteoarthritis is not associated with the formation of a pannus to eat away articular cartilage and the underlying subchondral bone. Flexion contractures may develop, however, particularly in the hip and knee.

Effective treatment of joints afflicted with osteoarthritis revolves around physical modalities (such as moist heat, exercise, splint and occasionally brace support), medical treatment (particularly with the salicylates and anti-inflammatory drugs), and surgical procedures in carefully selected instances. The indicated surgical procedures will be discussed more fully in the regional chapters.

The changes in the hands, although typical, usually do not progress to a functional deformity and rarely require specific treatment. A notable exception is involvement of the first carpometacarpal joint. Pain and stiffness in this joint can lessen the efficiency of the entire hand and may require intermittent immobilization, intra-articular hydrocortisone, or joint surgery for relief.

Involvement of the lumbar spine is heralded by pain and stiffness in this area (see page 361). Since most of these patients are overweight, a weight reduction program is a necessary accompaniment of treatment. Exercise within toleration is helpful in maintaining muscle tone and joint mobility. Support from braces and corsets should be avoided if at all possible, because of their tendency to increase the sensation of spinal stiffness. It will be remembered that these joints tend to stiffen with immobility and generally do better if kept flexible. Various physical therapeutic measures, such as diathermy and massage, are also helpful in allaying symptoms.

There are drugs available to aid in combating the symptoms of pain and the sensation of stiffness. Systemic treatment with salicylates is usually of benefit because of its analgesic effect. Many of the anti-inflammatory drugs have proved to be very effective in controlling pain and stiffness in this condition, but patients receiving them must be closely watched and the medical contraindications observed. The systemic use of the corticosteroids has failed to help this condition consistently, and their routine use is to be avoided.

As a rule, surgery plays little part in the treatment of osteoarthritis of the lumbar spine. Spinal fusion is usually not feasible since the process invariably involves several vertebrae and their associated joints. The most notable exception is the presence of nerve root compression secondary to an arthritic spur encroaching upon the intervertebral foramen. If the compression occurs in the lower lumbar segment, the patient will develop a distressing sciatica that may have to be relieved surgically by a nerve root decompression operation.

Involvement of the knee is signified by the complaint of pain and stiffness in the joint and frequently also in the thigh, calf, and popliteal area. A yellowish-clear viscid effusion is often noted in the knee joint. Some decrease in the range of motion of the joint may be noted, but it is rarely as significant as that seen in the knee afflicted with rheumatoid arthritis. Subpatellar crepitus is frequently found. Fixed flexion contractures may be observed in joints in which the disease is longstanding. Angular deformities of the joint, either genu varum or genu valgum, develop fairly often in osteoarthritis of the knee because quite frequently in this disease only one side of the joint is affected, while the other side is spared (Fig. 6–12).

Medical treatment for a knee joint afflicted with osteoarthritis could include frequent periods of rest for the part, use of local moist heat, or the use of intra-articular corticosteroids injected after aspiration of the effusion. Local treatment to the joint could be combined, if necessary, with systemic salicylates or other anti-inflammatory drugs.

FIGURE 6–12. Angular deformity of knees with osteoarthritis.

FIGURE 6-13. Angular deformity of knee secondary to osteoarthritis corrected by proximal tibial osteotomy. Staple used for internal fixation.

Fixed flexion contractures may have to be stretched in traction or plaster casts.

Surgery may be required for the knee joint that fails to respond to adequate medical management (see p. 425). The development of angular deformity of the knee can be particularly troublesome because the mechanical malalignment of itself accelerates joint deterioration and increases pain. Angular deformity at the knee should be corrected by an osteotomy performed through the proximal tibia. This operation is designed to straighten the knee and shift the weight bearing stress back into proper balance. In most patients, the benefit is relief of pain and frequently a slowing down of the degenerative process (Fig. 6–13).

If the degenerative process is too advanced to be benefited by an osteotomy and the patient is severely disabled, the choice would have to be made between arthrodesis — surgical fusion of the joint that would totally and permanently stiffen the joint — and a total knee replacement arthroplasty. In this operation a metallic surfacing unit is cemented to overlie the femoral condyles and a high density polyethylene surfacing unit is cemented to overlie the tibial plateaus (Fig. 6–14). Short-term results of total knee arthroplasty are encouraging, but no

FIGURE 6–14. A type of total knee arthroplasty. The metallic femoral condylar rings fit into plastic tibial runners when knee is extended.

significant number of long-term results have been reported as yet. Complications of this procedure could include mechanical loosening of the components or infection that might result in dire functional consequences for the patient.

Involvement of the hip joint is probably the most serious complication from a strict orthopaedic viewpoint because of the crippling effect on the patient of a stiff, painful hip (see page 394). An osteoarthritic hip joint may assume, in time, a flexed, adducted, externally rotated attitude that adds to the deformity and accentuates the painful limp. If the hip joint is not damaged too severely, symptoms of pain and stiffness can often be controlled by intra-articular corticosteroids and systemic salicylates or other anti-inflammatory drugs. If shortening is present, it should be compensated for by a heel lift. The use of a cane in the opposite hand as a walking aid is frequently helpful in relieving pain.

Surgical treatment is necessary more frequently in the hip joint than in any other joint affected by osteoarthritis (see p. 396). Basically, the operations available for the hip joint are the same as discussed for the knee joint. Early in the course of the disease, medial displacement osteotomy performed in the intertrochanteric area may relieve pain, but it does not usually result in the regaining of lost motion.

In the advanced case, most orthopaedists would advise total hip replacement arthroplasty rather than hip fusion. It is a much kinder operation for the older patient and the follow-up results have been sufficiently encouraging to recommend it with increasing confidence. Total hip replacement arthroplasty can be performed bilaterally, whereas hip fusion should only be performed unilaterally.

GOUTY ARTHRITIS

Gout is a disorder of uric acid metabolism with familial predisposition and significant joint implications. The acute form of gouty arthritis is initiated by the deposition of sodium urate crystals within the joint space. The chronic form is characterized by the deposition of urate crystals in the subcutaneous tissue, cartilage, bone, and kidney. Uric acid precipitation within the renal collecting system leads to stones in many gouty patients.

Although there are other causes besides gout for hyperuricemia, all patients with gout have hyperuricemia resulting from overproduction of uric acid, defective excretion of uric acid, or both. Renal retention of uric acid is caused by the failure of renal tubules to secrete uric acid after it has been filtered at the glomerulus and reabsorbed. Uric acid is the metabolic end product of purine precursors, mainly adenine and guanine, which usually occur as components of the nucleic acids DNA and RNA. Hyperuricemia may be produced by excessive synthesis of purines or, in some patients, may be due to decreased ability of the kidney to excrete uric acid rather than increased synthesis. Regardless of whether hyperuricemia results from overproduction of uric acid or from renal retention, when the saturation point of the serum is exceeded, crystallization may occur and the stage is set for gouty arthritis. Ninety-five per cent of those affected are male, usually in the fourth, fifth, and sixth decades, and may be of any race, nationality, or social level. Acute gouty arthritis is typically a severe arthritis marked by an abrupt onset involving one or more joints and exhibiting natural periods of remission. The joints most often involved are peripheral. Gout should always be suspected in the presence of swollen, painful and hot fingers, toes, wrists or ankles. It is occasionally seen about the knees and elbows, infrequently in the shoulders, and rarely in the spine. In the classic description of gout, involvement of the great toe is cited. However, other areas of the foot, notably the fifth toe, tarsal, and ankle regions can be involved (Fig. 6–15). In the hand, the interphalangeal joints are most often affected and the joint swelling is fusiform with exquisite tenderness.

If the diagnosis is not made early, urate salts may actually precipitate in a collection, called a *tophus*, located in and about the joint and in

Urate deposits

Urate deposits
Metatarso-
phalangeal
joint

Urate
deposits

FIGURE 6-15. Urate deposits about the joints of the toe in gout.

other bony regions. Tophi occur commonly about the interphalangeal joints of the fingers, the wrists and the toes, and in bursae such as the radiohumeral, olecranon, subdeltoid, prepatellar, trochanteric, and ischial. Many times this amorphous material in the soft tissues is mistakenly reported as "calcification" on the radiograph. It is believed that about 20 per cent of gallstones and renal calculi have their origin in gout. Deposits of urate may form bone tophi. These are seen as cystic areas in the bone near the joint margin.

An acute gouty arthritis can be precipitated in a patient with quiescent gout by surgery, trauma, or dietary indiscretion. Acute gouty arthritis may progress to the chronic type.

Radiographic Features. If tophi are absent, the radiographic findings may be negative. If present, tophi may be seen in the soft tissues about the joint or in the bursae. Cystic areas may be noted in the bone at the articular margin.

Laboratory Features. Although hyperuricemia is not diagnostic of gout, the blood urate is usually elevated before, during, and after an acute attack. Acute gout is usually accompanied by leukocytosis and an elevated sedimentation rate and C-reactive protein. In patients with the metabolic overproduction of urate, the urine uric acid is elevated, whereas patients with renal tubular lesions have a depressed urine uric acid. If synovial fluid can be harvested from a joint, demonstration of sodium urate crystals in the fluid by the polarizing microscope confirms the diagnosis of gout.

Management of the Patient. The basic treatment for gout is medical and is well documented in standard texts. Two therapeutic approaches are used, the choice depending upon whether acute or chronic gouty arthritis is being treated. Acute attacks can be controlled by the use of anti-inflammatory agents (colchicine, indomethacine, phenylbutazone, or corticosteroids). Chronic gout is best controlled by uricosuric agents that act to lower the serum uric acid level (probenecid, sulfinpyrazone, and allopurinol).

Specific orthopaedic care is reserved for those occasional patients requiring surgical excision of tophi.

Neuropathic Joint Disease (Charcot Joint)

The term neuropathic joint disease or Charcot joint indicates a form of chronic progressive degenerative arthropathy affecting one or more peripheral or spinal joints. This represents a complication of various neurologic disorders, the common feature of which is a disturbance in sensation in the affected joints. Charcot joint occurs most commonly in men past 40 years of age.

The underlying neurologic disorders that may give rise to Charcot joint include tabes dorsalis of syphilitic origin, diabetic neuropathy, syringomyelia, myelomeningocele, spinal cord compression, peripheral nerve section, leprosy, and congenital absence of pain syndrome. The distribution of joints affected is determined by the basic neural lesion. In tabes dorsalis the knees, hips, ankles, and vertebrae are involved. In diabetic neuropathy destructive changes occur in tarsal and metatarsal joints; in syringomyelia, the shoulder or elbow is involved. The main feature that these conditions have in common is absence or depression of pain sensation in the presence of continued physical activity. The patient loses the protective reaction in the joint to the minor traumata of everyday living, usually made worse by the underlying neurologic disorder. Being thus unprotected, the joint is subjected to repeated sprains, hemarthroses, and fractures, leading to progressive joint destruction, debris formation, relaxation and stretching of supporting ligaments, and chronic instability of the joint (Fig. 6–16). If mechanical destruction outstrips the process of repair, the consequence is marked swelling, hemorrhage, debris formation, and local heat. Pain causes normal individuals to protect the area and prevent further trauma — with the result that healing takes place. In patients with neuropathy, however, the damage may go on until the joint is totally destroyed.

Clinical Features. The outstanding clinical feature of neuroarthropathy is the presence of an obviously abnormal joint that is clinically unstable. When the condition is related to tabes, the joints most often affected are the knees, hips, ankles, and spine. Involvement is frequently multiple. The typical patient is a male past 40 years of age.

FIGURE 6–16. AP radiograph of knee, showing destruction secondary to neuropathic arthropathy (Charcot joint).

The affected joints are usually swollen and are typically unstable owing to severe relaxation of the supporting structures. These joints are not always absolutely painless. Patients frequently complain of joint discomfort, particularly if swelling is present. However, the discomfort is disproportionately mild compared with the dramatic clinical and radiographic appearance of the joint. A careful neurologic examination will usually unearth evidence of the underlying neurologic disorder.

Radiographic Features. The changes seen in a Charcot joint are considered similar to those seen in exaggerated osteoarthritis: marked erosion of joint cartilage, destruction and fragmentation of subchondral bone, and large spurs of the joint margins. The spur formation may be flamboyant and bizarre in appearance. Compression fractures and free bodies in the joint cavity are frequent. The soft tissues are thickened and may contain scattered calcification. Joint effusion is common.

Management of the Patient. Careful clinical studies clearly indicate that inadequately protected fractures, sprains, and effusions of neuropathic joints are often the precursors of joint destruction. It has also been shown that these lesions, if adequately treated, generally heal without secondary joint damage. The key to proper treatment of neuroarthropathy, therefore, is the prevention of these injuries by early recognition of the problem and adequate protection of the joint even to the extent of bracing.

Unfortunately, many patients are not seen until the damage has already been done. The outstanding clinical feature in these patients is an obviously abnormal joint that is clinically unstable. Often sufficient stability can be obtained by the use of protective and supportive braces.

A Charcot joint exhibits a poor tolerance to surgery because of the difficulty of obtaining efficient postoperative immobilization. Operations on neuropathic bones are notorious for poor healing and nonunion. If a joint seems beyond salvage, fusion may be indicated, but it must be recognized that fusion is difficult to achieve and that nonunion is common. The main problem in a Charcot joint is instability, and for this reason arthroplasty operations, which tend, by their very nature, to cause instability, are never indicated. In selected instances, amputation may the treatment of choice.

SPECIAL FORMS OF ARTHRITIS

Hemophilic Arthritis. In a patient afflicted with hemophilia, repeated joint hemorrhages may lead to degenerative changes in the bone and cartilage associated with marked fibrous tissue contractures. The degree of degeneration and disability is directly proportional to the severity and frequency of the joint hemorrhage. It is not at all unusual to see severe arthritic changes at an early age in a hemophilic patient with severe bleeding tendencies.

Repeated joint bleeding leads to hemosiderosis of the synovial membrane and subsequently to shrinking and fibrosis of the joint capsule. The articular cartilage undergoes degenerative changes with thinning and, ultimately, total or partial disappearance. The bone becomes atrophic and its structure becomes coarse. The articular surfaces are deformed by abnormal growth at the growth plate. Subchondral bone cysts, probably formed by the resolution of old hemorrhage, may be present.

The joints most frequently affected are the knee, ankle, and elbow. The changes visible on radiographs resemble those of a type of secondary osteoarthritis, often with superimposed osteoporosis.

Psoriatic Arthritis. Psoriasis occurs in about 3 per cent of patients with typical rheumatoid arthritis. Conversely, in certain instances of psoriasis, arthritic changes appear in the terminal phalangeal joints of those fingers showing psoriatic nail lesions.

Psychogenic Rheumatism. This term refers to a common form of nonarticular rheumatism thought to represent the rheumatic manifestations of a psychoneurosis. Psychoneurotic patients in emotional conflict caused by psychic trauma, fear, anxiety, apprehension, or sorrow may experience arthralgia, muscle and tendon aches, stiffness, interference with joint motion, and other rheumatic symptoms that resemble some form of arthritis. The absence of true joint changes on clinical and radiographic examination and the concurrent evidence of psychoneurosis usually suffice to differentiate this condition from organic arthritis. Vague, nonspecific diagnoses such as myositis, fibrositis, and neuritis are frequently assigned to these patients.

BURSITIS

A bursa is a closed sac differentiated out of areolar tissue. Its delicate walls are normally separated from each other by a film of slippery fluid. Bursae exist as lubricating devices to diminish the friction of movement and are found beneath the skin, beneath tendons, and overlying joints. There are believed to be about 52 bursae in the human body.

Inflammation of a bursa is a common clinical occurrence, and its cause may be trauma, unusual use of the part, infection, gout, or rheumatoid arthritis. As a response to the stimulus of inflammation, the lining membrane may produce excess fluid causing distention of the sac. In the case of trauma, the fluid may be bloody and in the case of gout, urate crystals will be present. The symptoms produced by the inflammation are, in large measure, conditioned by the anatomic location of the bursa. Some of the more common are described.

PREPATELLAR BURSITIS

The prepatellar bursa lies superficial to the distal pole of the patella and the upper half of the patellar tendon. It may become acutely inflamed and swollen from local trauma or may be chronically involved by repeated or prolonged kneeling. For that reason, this condition has also been known as "housemaid's knee" or "nun's knee." Clinically, a localized, well-circumscribed fluctuant mass is seen lying over the anterior aspect of the knee. The knee joint proper is not involved. Treatment consists of aspiration of the fluid, local instillation of corticosteroids, and application of a pressure dressing. If the cause of the inflammatory response is infection, incision and drainage with proper antibiotic coverage are indicated. Occasionally, chronic recurrent enlargement justifies surgical excision of the bursal sac.

OLECRANON BURSITIS

Trauma to the point of the elbow frequently results in marked swelling of the olecranon bursa, giving rise to a large knob in this area (Fig. 6–17). Following an acute trauma, the fluid in the bursal sac is frequently bloody and the bursal walls may become permanently thickened. Tender swelling of the olecranon bursa may also be seen with gout and rheumatoid arthritis. Repetitive minor trauma to the olecranon bursa, such as long periods of leaning on the elbow, may lead to chronic, relatively nontender enlargement of the bursa. Chronic enlargement has been known as "bartender's elbow." The treatment for olecranon bursitis is the same as that outlined for prepatellar bursitis.

TROCHANTERIC BURSITIS

Inflammation of the bursa overlying the greater trochanter of the femur is a frequent occurrence. It may appear as a primary entity

FIGURE 6–17. Distended olecranon bursa.

following trauma, unusual use of the legs, or gout, or may be associated with degenerative arthritis of the lumbar spine.

Typically, involvement of this bursa gives pain along the postero-lateral hip and thigh area, particularly on direct palpation or when the hip abductors are tightened. The patient may find it painful to cross the involved leg over the opposite one or to lie on the involved area. Frequently the pain will run along the course of the tensor fascia lata to the knee and will be described as a burning sensation.

Diagnosis is made by reproducing the pain by direct manual pressure on the greater trochanter in the absence of any physical findings referable to the hip joint proper. Trochanteric bursitis does not cause any restriction of passive motion of the hip joint. Radiographic examination is usually negative, but occasionally small calcium deposits may be seen adjacent to the trochanter.

Superficially the pain caused by trochanteric bursitis could be mistaken for sciatica or for pain originating in the hip joint proper. Careful examination will clearly disclose the absence of any objective physical signs of sciatica and the presence of unrestricted hip motion.

Local injection of hydrocortisone into the bursa usually suffices to alleviate the condition. Moist heat to the painful area is beneficial. Rarely, the bursa may have to be excised.

BURSITIS OF THE HEEL

Several bursae are found in the region of the heel that may become painful when inflamed. One bursa lies subcutaneously between the skin and the Achilles tendon, and another lies between the Achilles tendon and the os calcis. Either can become inflamed, enlarged, and painful, particularly by irritation from a shoe or by excessive walking or running.

The patient usually obtains some relief by removing the counter of the shoe and using a heel pad to raise the painful area from the back of the shoe. The inflamed bursa can be treated definitively by local injection of hydrocortisone or by surgical excision.

A third bursa is located on the plantar aspect of the heel at the origin of the plantar aponeurosis and the short flexor muscles as they arise from the os calcis. Symptoms in this area are caused by direct pressure on the heel and the inflamed plantar bursa. This condition, seen most frequently in male adults, has been called "postman's heel" or "policeman's heel" and is the most common cause of heel pain in the adult patient. Occasionally, on the radiograph a small bone spur may be seen arising from the plantar surface of the os calcis, but in these cases symptoms are more likely to be caused by inflamed overlying plantar bursa than by the small bone spur itself.

Treatment consists of local injections of corticosteroids into the inflamed bursa. A sponge rubber heel cushion with a hole cut in the center glued in the heel of the shoe frequently helps to relieve local pressure on the painful area.

SUBDELTOID OR SUBACROMIAL BURSITIS

The physician will frequently hear a patient complain of "bursitis" of the shoulder. In this particular area, bursitis is too often used as an all-inclusive term to explain away all shoulder pain.

Although it is true that a primary subdeltoid or subacromial bursitis may occur, other causes of shoulder pain, often called bursitis by mistake, are far more frequent. These other causes of shoulder pain are covered in detail in Chapter 10, Disorders of the Shoulder.

References

Cathcart, E. S., and Cohen, A. S.: Synovial fluid and synovial membrane abnormalities in arthritis of the knee joint. Am. Academy of Orthopaedic Surgeons Instructional Course Lectures, Vol. XX:231. St. Louis: C. V. Mosby Co., 1971

Coventry, M. B.: Osteotomy about the knee for degenerative and rheumatoid arthritis — indications, operative techniques and results. J. Bone and Joint Surg., 55-A:23, 1973.

Gutman, A. B.: View on the pathogenesis and management of parimary gout, 1971. J. Bone and Joint Surg., 55-A:357, 1972.

Hammerman, D., Rosenberg, L. C., and Schubert, M.: Diarthrodial joints revisited. Review article, J. Bone and Joint Surg., 52-A:725, 1970.

Laurin, C. A., Desmarchais, J., Daziano, L., Gariépy, R., and Derome, A.: Long-term results of synovectomy of the knee in rheumatoid patients. J. Bone and Joint Surg., 56-A:521, 1974.

Linscheid, R. L.: Surgery for rheumatoid arthritis — timing and techniques: The upper extremity. J. Bone and Joint Surg., 50-A:587, 1968.

Mankin, H. J.: The articular cartilages—a review. Am. Academy of Orthopaedic Surgeons Instructional Course Lectures, Vol. XIX. St. Louis: C. V. Mosby Co., 1970.

Peterson, L. F. A.: Surgery for rheumatoid arthritis — timing and techniques: The lower extremity. J. Bone and Joint Surg., 50-A:587, 1968.

Rana, N. A., Hancock, D. O., Taylor, A. R., and Hill, A. G. S.: Atlanto-axial subluxation in rheumatoid arthritis. J. Bone and Joint Surg., 55-B:458, 1973.

Simon, W. H. (Ed.): The Human Joint in Health and Disease. Philadelphia: University of Pennsylvania Press, 1978.

Wilson, F. C. (Ed.): The Musculoskeletal System. Philadelphia: J. B. Lippincott Co., 1975.

CHAPTER 7

SKELETAL INFECTION

INTRODUCTION

Bone tissue infection and joint infection present special problems depending on the type of organism involved and the anatomy of the area invaded. As with infection in general, infection in bone depends on an intimate interplay between the parasite (usually bacteria) and the host. Bacterial considerations include area of entry, localization, virulence, and colonization of the area. Host consideration includes the anatomic properties of the involved bone, cellular and humoral immune mechanisms, and the reparative power of the damaged area. The complexities associated with bone infection are mainly the result of host factors, especially certain peculiarities of bone. These include limitation of a soft tissue space, a vascular supply that favors massive bone necrosis, and an inadequate resorption mechanism for necrotic bone that results in incomplete healing. The most common infection is that caused by a pyogenic organism. If the infection is localized to the structure of the bone, the condition is called *osteomyelitis*. If the infection is confined to the joint, it is termed *pyogenic arthritis*. Even when the invading organism is the same, the two conditions produced are different and are dissimilar in clinical course, prognosis, and management. Under some circumstances, the use of antimicrobial agents to combat bone or joint infection is curative, while under other circumstances such

168

use is only supportive to judicious surgery and is directed chiefly at preventing septicemia and fulminating local sepsis.

The tubercle bacillus may attack bone and joints, which are the locus of about 3 per cent of all tuberculous infections. Bone can also be infected with *Treponema pallidum,* resulting in congenital and acquired bone syphilis. Although less common, fungus infections, particularly coccidioidomycosis, blastomycosis, and actinomycosis, can occur in bone.

PYOGENIC INFECTIONS

The most common bacterial invaders of the musculoskeletal system are *Staphylococcus aureus, Proteus, Pseudomonas, Aerobacter,* colon bacillus, *Salmonella,* and *Streptococcus,* with occasional infections caused by pneumococcus, meningococcus, gonococcus, influenza bacillus, and *Serratia marcescens.* Infection of a part of the skeletal system with a pyogenic organism is more common in infants and young children than in adults. The acute form of the disease is usually blood-borne and has a predilection for the rapidly growing child.

Infection of bones and joints was expected to fade into comparative insignificance with the coming of the antibiotic era, but this surmise proved false. The mortality has decreased from about 20 per cent to 2 per cent since the introduction of antibiotics, but the morbidity remains high. This decrease is mainly due to the diminished frequency and mortality of septic hematogenous osteomyelitis. One of the results of early, but sometimes inadequate, antibiotic therapy is the masking of symptoms and altering of the natural course of the disease — reducing the mortality but not eliminating the morbidity due to tissue destruction. This appears to be a consequence of late diagnosis of the condition as a result of the administration of antibiotics to children with fevers of uncertain etiology.

Although the mortality associated with severe bone infections has been dramatically reduced by antibiotic treatment, reported studies have shown a steadily increasing rise in the incidence of bone and joint infections over the past two decades. Two factors have been identified as contributing to the increased incidence: One is the masking of the early signs of infection by the indiscriminate use of antibiotic therapy and the other is the emergence of antibiotic-resistant strains of organisms. Since *Staphylococcus aureus* can be implicated as the causative agent in 65 to 70 per cent of bone and joint infections, the incidence of strains of penicillin-resistant staphylococci is of serious concern. It has been found in clinical situations that when staphylococci are resistant to penicillin, they are invariably penicillinase producers. More recently concern has also been expressed about the relative increase in gram-negative infections.

Antibiotics are delivered to the bone or joint either through the blood stream or by local irrigation. It has been found that bone antibiotic concentrations are directly related to serum concentrations. To be effective in treatment, the proper drug with minimal side effects must be chosen, and it must be delivered to the site of the organism at a concentration of from four to ten times the minimal inhibitory concentration.

Acute Osteomyelitis

When pyogenic organisms directly invade the substance of a bone, the condition is called osteomyelitis. This inoculation may be the result of erosion from a neighboring infection or the organisms may be introduced directly into the bone by contamination accompanying open fractures or gunshot wounds. By far, the most frequent form of osteomyelitis, however, is the acute hematogenous form in which the infection is spread by the blood stream to the bone from a distant focus such as infected tonsils, boils, abscessed teeth, or upper respiratory infections. The disease, therefore, is a systemic infection or bacteremia of which the bone involvement is only a local manifestation.

Acute osteomyelitis is usually a blood-borne disease and is most frequently seen in the rapidly growing child. Boys are affected more frequently than girls. The bones most often involved are the tibia, femur, humerus, and radius. A history of trauma is frequently obtained and there is reason to suspect that local injury influences the site of infection by creating an area of lowered resistance to an already present systemic infection.

Staphylococcus aureus is the infecting microorganism in 70 to 80 per cent of patients. Salmonella osteomyelitis is frequent in patients with sickle cell disease. Less frequently found organisms are streptococcus and pneumococcus. The organism enters the bone through the nutrient or metaphyseal vessels and localizes in the venous sinusoids of the metaphysis. Once established in a bone, infection may spread throughout the entire bone in an adult. In children, infection does not gain direct transport across the growth plate because the epiphyseal cartilage blocks anastomosis between blood vessels in the shaft and those in the epiphysis. If any of the

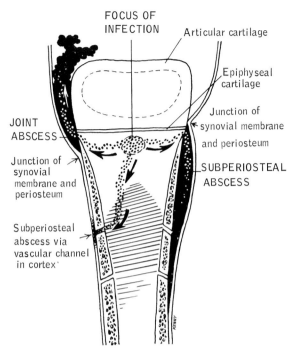

FOCUS OF INFECTION

Articular cartilage

Epiphyseal cartilage

JOINT ABSCESS

Junction of synovial membrane and periosteum

SUBPERIOSTEAL ABSCESS

Junction of synovial membrane and periosteum

Subperiosteal abscess via vascular channel in cortex·

FIGURE 7-1. The possible routes infection may take as it spreads from a focus in the metaphysis. (Redrawn from Shands: Handbook of Orthopaedic Surgery [After Hart]. St. Louis: C. V. Mosby Co., 1971.)

metaphyseal area lies within the capsule, such as in the hip joint, for example, infection can burrow around the growth plate to involve the joint (Fig. 7–1).

Pathology. Initially there is acute exudative inflammation with increased vascularity, edema, and polymorphonuclear leukocytes. Within two to three days, thrombosis and obliteration of the vessels through increased intramedullary pressure produce ischemia and bone necrosis. An intramedullary abscess forms, and edema fluid and purulent exudate are forced through the haversian and Volkmann's canals, stripping periosteum from the bone. This isolates the cortical bone from its blood supply and produces more dead bone. Bacteria and their toxins, pH change, local edema, and vascular occlusion all contribute to the bone necrosis. The pus, following the line of least resistance, may re-enter the medullary canal through the cortex at another point, may form subperiosteal abscesses, may perforate the periosteum and enter soft tissues, or may extend into the neighboring joint. The admixture of dead and viable bone tissue explains the irregular decalcification seen on the radiograph during

FIGURE 7-2.   Acute osteomyelitis of proximal humeral shaft in young child.

the course of acute osteomyelitis (Fig. 7–2). The special pathologic tissue reactions, which are characteristic of suppurative osteomyelitis, are the lysis of bone, the formation of new bone, and the presence of dead bone.

Elevation of the periosteum and vascular thrombosis both contribute to bone necrosis, and portions of the bone die. The body tries to extrude the dead bone by forming granulation tissue beneath it, lifting it out of its bed in the bone. This separated bone is called a *sequestrum*. Small sequestra may revascularize after the infection is controlled, but large ones will persist. The presence of retained sequestra is the chief reason for continued drainage in osteomyelitis (Fig. 7–3).

The elevated periosteum retains its osteogenic capability and starts to lay down new live bone as one of the first steps in the reparative process. This new live enveloping bone is called the *involucrum,* and it is laid down over and around the granulation tissue separating the sequestra. The involucrum may be pitted with sinuses called *cloacae,* which permit the escape of pus. If an early diagnosis is made and if adequate and efficient treatment is carried out, infected bone tissue possesses the capability of reverting to a normal structure and appearance.

Clinical Picture. The patient with acute hematogenous osteomyelitis may develop general and local symptoms. The general symptoms are those of an acute toxic illness with fever. There may be vomiting with subsequent dehydration. Locally the involved area may be swollen, warm, and exquisitely tender to touch. The most valid clinical sign is the presence of localized bone tenderness in a patient exhibiting a febrile course. Since there is pus under pressure in the bone, the patient may complain of severe, constant pulsating pain in the part — usually aggravated by motion. The adjacent joints may be held in a flexed position in an effort to splint the painful part.

FIGURE 7–3. Chronic osteomyelitis with large retained sequestrum.

For the first week or two the radiographic examination may be negative except for soft tissue swelling. An inflammatory process is well established in bone before radiological changes occur because bone is slow to respond to insult and because changes in medullary bone are virtually invisible radiologically. Since medullary bone destruction is radiologically invisible, massive medullary pus collections can occur with minimal radiological signs of bone destruction. Roentgenographic evidence of bone destruction does not appear before the tenth to fourteenth day. As bone tissue dies, the radiograph will reflect spotty irregular areas of decalcification usually in the metaphyseal area of the bone. This type of change may gradually extend to involve the entire shaft. Periosteal new bone formation becomes visible. As sequestra form they may appear as pieces of dead separated bone. Still later, involucrum formation becomes evident.

In the acute stage of the disease, study of the patient's blood

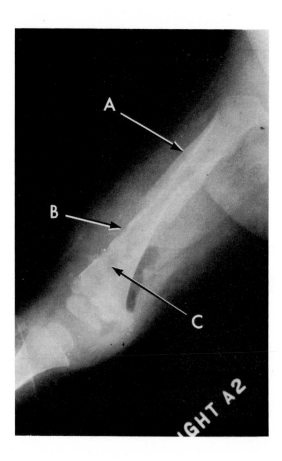

FIGURE 7-4. Acute osteomyelitis of the femur in young child. A, reactive periosteal bone. B, multiple cortical defects. C, area of bone destruction. (Courtesy Dr. Roshen Irani, Thomas Jefferson University Hospital, Philadelphia, Pa.)

may reveal an elevated leukocyte count and sedimentation rate. The blood culture is usually positive.

In a child, the presence of infection near a growth plate may trigger an abnormal growth response (Fig. 7–4). The result might be shortening, lengthening, or directional change in the growth of the bone.

Differential diagnosis should include cellulitis, Ewing's tumor, acute rheumatic fever, pyogenic arthritis, and blood dyscrasias such as leukemia. The diagnosis of acute osteomyelitis ideally requires the identification of the organism from the pus or from blood culture. To obtain valid material for culture, pus and tissue should be obtained deep to the skin and fascia from the site of active osteomyelitis.

Treatment. The object of treatment is to produce a permanent arrest of the infective process and to do so early enough so that there is no permanent impairment of limb function or growth. A successful clinical outcome is completely dependent upon establishing an early clinical and bacteriologic diagnosis. Adequate treatment must be started early. There is usually a two to three day delay from the onset of symptoms to hospitalization. Blood cultures may require an additional two to three days. As soon as the diagnosis is suspected clinically, at least two blood samples from different sites should be drawn for culture and antibiotic sensitivity studies. On examination of the patient, a source of infection may be found on the skin, middle ear, throat, lungs, or urinary tract. Appropriate cultures from these areas may be helpful.

Treatment should be begun as soon as the culture specimens are taken so that valuable time is not lost while waiting for bacteriologic results. The assumption can be made that *Staphylococcus aureus* is the etiologic agent in the majority of patients. At the present time, staphylococci should be presumed resistant to penicillin until proved otherwise. Unless the penicillins are contraindicated, a semisynthetic penicillin that is effective against penicillinase-producing staphylococci should be used in adequate doses. In the United States the vast majority of these organisms are sensitive to nafcillin, methicillin, oxacillin, cephalothin and cefazolin. In addition, crystalline penicillin G in a dose of two million units every four hours is usually added to the antibiotic coverage. Appropriate adjustments in the antibiotic program can be made when the results of the culture and sensitivity studies are known. As the disease is controlled, a corresponding reduction in dosage should follow. It appears that once acute hematogenous staphylococcal osteomyelitis is controlled with parenteral therapy, oral therapy should suffice. It is important not to give oral antibiotics with food because this markedly reduces absorption from the gastrointestinal tract and seriously diminishes the drug level in the blood. Antibiotics should be continued for three to four weeks after the patient becomes afebrile.

The body's resistance is supported by the use of small blood transfusions and intravenous fluids to maintain electrolyte balance. Local treatment consists of plaster immobilization of the infected part.

The availability of effective antibiotic therapy has relegated surgery to a secondary position in the treatment of acute hematogenous osteomyelitis. Operative intervention is usually not necessary if effective medical treatment is instituted within 72 hours after onset of the disease. Bone is a highly vascular tissue and thus, until the infection progresses to the state of producing vascular thrombosis and pus with increased marrow pressure, antibiotic treatment will be effective.

Surgical intervention is reserved mainly for the drainage of subperiosteal abscesses and the removal of sequestra. Early surgical decompression of the bone would be indicated if antibiotic treatment had not been instituted within 72 hours of onset or if it fails to control the infection completely.

With early diagnosis and effective treatment, a good result can usually be expected with the infection eradicated and bone substance returned to a normal state. A breakdown in either diagnosis or treatment may lead to chronic osteomyelitis or to a localized bone infection known as *Brodie's abscess.*

ACUTE OSTEOMYELITIS IN THE ADULT

Acute osteomyelitis is rare in the adult, whereas the chronic form is not. It may begin by hematogenous origin or by local implantation of bacteria associated with open fractures or gunshot wounds. Osteomyelitis in the foot is usually associated with occlusive vascular disease or diabetes mellitus or both.

Unlike the situation in children, acute hematogenous osteomyelitis in the adult rarely affects the long bone. In adult patients, acute osteomyelitis occurs most common in the spine. Vertebral osteomyelitis usually occurs in elderly patients, with *Staphylococcus aureus* being the most frequently encountered organism. Recently, acute vertebral osteomyelitis has beeen identified in drug addicts, with gram negative rods or even fungi such as Candida being recovered.

Osteomyelitis associated with nonunion of fractures is seen fairly frequently. Both the infection and the nonunion of the fracture may follow unsuccessful open reduction of the fracture. Polymicrobic infections and cultures of resistant forms of *Staphylococcus aureus* are indicative of the nosocomial nature of the infecting organism. An increasing number of anaerobic organisms are now being noted on culture. The combination of bone infection and fracture nonunion poses a very complex therapeutic problem. A totally successful clinical outcome has been possible to date in only a limited number of patients.

CHRONIC OSTEOMYELITIS

The progression from acute to chronic osteomyelitis is graded and is characterized by the accumulation of pus under pressure, causing bone ischemia and forcing bacteria into the vascular channels and bone lacunae. As the chronic infection continues, proliferative granulation tissue, once highly vascular, turns to dense scar. This avascular scar forms an impenetrable barrier around the infected area. New bone may be laid down adjacent to the old bone spicules and may further isolate dead infected bone. Chronic osteomyelitis, therefore, is a disease of ischemia more than of infection and is seen mostly in adult patients. Organisms thrive in avascular bone, and scar tissue acts as an impenetrable membrane to antibiotic therapy. Over the past decade, there has been a significant shift to a preponderance of gram negative bacillary organisms cultured from patients with chronic osteomyelitis. This has been associated with a lower success rate in treatment of these patients.

Clinical Picture. The patient with chronic osteomyelitis may present in one of two clinical situations:

1. The infection may remain persistent and active and may be characterized by recurring sequestration of bone and continuous drainage of pus from sinuses (Fig. 7-5). Chronic drainage over a long period of time may lead to nephritis, amyloid disease, or squamous cell carcinoma in sinus tracts.

2. The process may seemingly quiet down and the sinuses close. However, residual infection may lurk within the bone substance ready to flare up intermittently. When this occurs, the part becomes painful, swollen, and inflamed. The closed sinus tracts may open to discharge pus and occasionally pieces of dead bone. A pocket of infection may be present within the bone and give no indication of its presence for years.

On radiographic examination, chronic osteomyelitis is characterized by an enlarged irregular and dense bone structure with involucrum formation. Cavities and sequestra within the bone substance are frequently noted (Fig. 7-6).

Treatment. Effective treatment of chronic osteomyelitis de-

FIGURE 7–5. Chronic osteomyelitis of the tibia. Leg exhibits marked scarring of the skin and draining sinuses.

FIGURE 7–6. Chronic osteomyelitis of the tibia in an adult.

pends first and foremost on radical surgical debridement of the bone with excision of all sinuses, dead bone, and scar and grossly necrotic tissue in order to mechanically eradicate the infection. The role of antibiotics at this stage is more supportive than curative. They aid in preventing septicemia and fulminating local infection. Culture specimens are taken preoperatively from the depth of the wound or sinus, and the appropriate antibiotic is started a few hours before surgery to insure an adequate level of antibiotic in any small hematoma that might form postoperatively. Fresh culture material should also be taken from the depths of the wound at the time of operation. A large bolus of antibiotic should be given intravenously during the operative procedure to aid in sterilizing the hematoma. The wound should be closed, if possible, with stainless steel wire and as much dead space as possible obliterated by tight closure if the local skin condition permits. A closed system of suction irrigation may be incorporated into the wound at the time of closure.

Suction-irrigation is a popular method for managing problems of dead space, but much early enthusiasm for its promise has waned. The technique appears useful, but the data supporting its use are empiric. The method can be disappointing and, in fact, provides an entryway for superinfection. Recent data contraindicate its use in acute osteomyelitis in children. Furthermore, adding antibiotics to the solution can be questioned, particularly the potentially toxic forms that will be absorbed in large quantities from the freshly granulating surface. The method is probably best used as an adjunct to primary or delayed closure, but as a mechanism to control hematoma formation after closure and not as a means to deliver a drug. The technique requires soft tissue of good enough quality to insure a firm closure. Preliminary data suggest that suction-irrigation should not be used longer than seven to eight days and that only physiologic saline solution be used as the irrigant.

Appropriate antibiotics are given orally or intramuscularly during the period of hospital treatment. All antibiotic treatment should be continued for at least six weeks in the postoperative period in an attempt to reduce the incidence of recurrent infection.

In some patients it will prove impossible to obtain closure of the soft tissue. In that situation, the surgeon may choose to pack the wound open with gauze to be followed later by delayed closure or skin grafting. The use of a muscle pedicle flap has been reported to be an excellent method for obliterating dead space, but may fail if the blood supply to the pedicle has been damaged. Inserting bone grafts to obliterate dead space is no longer an acceptable technique except as a delayed procedure in patients with fracture nonunion after the infection has been arrested.

BRODIE'S ABSCESS

Brodie's abscess is a chronic localized form of osteomyelitis due frequently to a staphylococcus of low virulence. The infection causes localized bone destruction that becomes sealed off by fibrous tissue and sclerotic bone formation, resulting in a sharply demarcated lytic lesion in the bone. This localized bone abscess is frequently found at the lower end of the tibia.

The patient complains of bone pain of gradual onset which is frequently worse at night. There may be tenderness to palpation at the site of the abscess. Many of these patients may have normal temperatures, normal white blood counts, and normal sedimentation rates.

Radiographic examination reveals a well-circumscribed lytic lesion surrounded by an area of dense sclerotic bone (Fig. 7–7). Differential diagnosis includes unicameral bone cyst, osteoid osteoma, fibrous dysplasia, and eosinophilic granuloma.

FIGURE 7-7. Brodie's abscess of os calcis.

Treatment consists of draining the abscess at operation and scraping the inside of the bone cavity clean. Occasionally it is possible to expedite healing by filling the empty cavity with bone chip grafts taken from the ilium.

PYOGENIC ARTHRITIS

Infection of a joint with pus-forming organisms is called pyogenic arthritis, infectious arthritis, or septic arthritis. It is more common in infants and children than in adults and has an affinity for the hip and knee joints. *Staphylococcus aureus* is the infecting agent in 40 to 60 per cent of these patients; streptococcus is next in frequency. Pyogenic arthritis ·may be the result of metastatic infection arising from a primary infection source, such as pneumonia, gonorrhea, meningitis, upper respiratory infection, otitis media, furuncle, infected abrasion, or umbilical vein infection. Osteomyelitis localized in a bone may spread to involve an adjacent joint, or direct inoculation of the joint with organisms may follow trauma, penetrating wounds, or joint aspiration. In the infant below one year of age and in adults, metaphyseal capillaries perforate the growth plate, allowing metaphyseal infection to spread into the epiphysis and adjacent joints, producing pyogenic arthritis. Between the age of one year and puberty, infection in the metaphysis is contained by the growth plate and must spread laterally, perforating the periosteum and gaining entry to the joint by a subperiosteal route.

The hematogenous form of pyogenic arthritis is uncommon in the adult patient. When it is encountered, *Staphylococcus aureus* is the offending organism in about 75 per cent of patients and the. most frequently involved joints are the knee, hip and shoulder. The not uncommon association of pyogenic arthritis with other medical conditions such as rheumatoid arthritis, malignant disease, or bowel disorders has been noted. It has been suggested that invasion of the synovial membrane by bacteria is a result of lowering of immune defense mechanisms in appropriate patient types.

Regardless of how the organisms find their way into a joint, pyogenic arthritis, once established, is a grave problem in any age group and requires immediate recognition and vigorous treatment for its control. Militant attention to every suspected joint infection is demanded to prevent irreparable joint damage. Articular hyaline cartilage is digested by pyogenic exudates; if this occurs, the joint will be damaged beyond repair. A nonvascular tissue such as articular cartilage is defenseless in the face of microorganism invasion. It has been shown experimentally that under certain conditions hyaline cartilage can be completely digested within 24 hours by action of the proteolytic enzymes in the pyogenic exudate.

Pathologic Features. The organisms gain entrance to the joint by several routes. They may be blood-borne from some distant focus of infection. This is the usual mechanism in the infant or when pyogenic arthritis complicates an infectious disease such as gonorrhea. They may erode into the joint from an adjacent focus of osteomyelitis, or they may be inserted directly into the joint from outside. The pathologic changes in the joint once microorganisms have gained entrance are those changes initiated by infection. Inflammation begins in the synovial membrane, which becomes swollen, reddened, and hyperemic. The joint distends with cloudy fluid that becomes frank pus in a few days. If the pus is allowed to remain in the joint, it will destroy the articular cartilage through chondrolysis. This destruction occurs first and most extensively at points of joint contact. The process allows raw bone surfaces to be bathed by infection, potentially leading to fibrous or bone ankylosis of the joint, or if the infection has invaded the substance of the bone, to the development of osteomyelitis as a complication of the pyogenic arthritis.

Clinical Picture. The acute onset of painful and hot joint swelling, associated with the systemic signs of infection, particularly after trauma or during the treatment of some primary source of infection, should immediately signal the possibility of pyogenic arthritis. The patient is sick, febrile and irritable, and shows a marked unwillingness to move the affected joint or bear weight on it because of pain. The joint will be maintained in a flexed position, which is the position of comfort. If the joint involved can be palpated, it usually feels hot and, to the patient, exquisitely tender.

Laboratory studies reveal an increased leukocytosis and an elevated erythrocyte sedimentation rate. Except for signs of capsular swelling and widening of the joint space, the radiographic examination should be negative. If bone destruction is seen on the radiograph, it means that osteomyelitis has already complicated the problem.

The diagnosis is made by inserting a needle into the joint and withdrawing pus. This immediately differentiates pyogenic arthritis from hemarthrosis, rheumatoid arthritis, joint tuberculosis, and any other condition causing joint symptoms.

HIP JOINT INVOLVEMENT. Involvement of the hip joint, particularly in the infant, can easily be overlooked because the joint is deeply placed, causing the local signs of infection to be less readily apparent. The patient holds the leg in a flexed position at the hip and resists all efforts to move the joint either actively or passively. There may be swelling over the hip and trochanteric area. In children a mechanical complication of pyogenic arthritis of the hip may be pathologic dislocation of the joint. This has been reported to occur in as many as 40 per cent of children with pyogenic arthritis of the hip.

KNEE JOINT INVOLVEMENT. Involvement of the knee joint is more obvious because of its exposed position in the body. The joint and suprapatellar pouch may distend with fluid and the joint is usually held in a flexed position by hamstring muscle tightness and spasm. The joint will feel hot and the overlying tissue will appear red and inflamed. The joint will be markedly tender to palpation and the patient will resist movement of the joint. Because of the severe penalties attached to delay, there should never be any hesitation about aspirating a joint for verification if suppuration is suspected.

Treatment. Treatment must be immediate and vigorous, considering the time limitations imposed by the defenselessness of the articular cartilage. Infected joints should be protected by traction or splinting during the treatment period.

Accurate bacteriologic diagnosis is essential, since antibacterial agents and adequate surgical drainage complement each other in the treatment of pyogenic arthritis. Direct smear of the articular fluid frequently will give immediate valuable information concerning the involved microorganism. Organisms cannot always be cultured, even from purulent articular fluid, but often a presumptive etiologic diagnosis can be made from culture of other sources such as blood, spinal fluid, and throat.

Owing to its relative depth, the hip joint should be surgically drained of pus and all infected joint material and clots as soon as the diagnosis has been verified. A suction-irrigation system may be closed into the joint for the purpose of irrigation with physiologic saline solution for a four to six day period. Antibiotics are no longer introduced into the joint by means of the suction system, but rather given systemically in sufficently high doses. There is convincing evidence in the literature to indicate that whenever surgical drainage has been neglected, usually in favor of a new and promising antibiotic, the incidence of complications increased and when surgical evacuation was emphasized, the results of treatment improved.

Some of the smaller and more superficially placed joints may be treated by aspiration with a large bore needle and irrigation with physiologic saline solution. Unless penicillin is contraindicated, a semisynthetic penicillin that is effective against penicillinase-producing staphylococci should be used systemically in adequate doses. Appropriate adjustment in the antibiotic program should be made if the results of culture and sensitivity tests warrant it. The joint should be reaspirated and irrigated as often as effusion recurs during the initial 36 to 48 hours of treatment. Failure of the infection to subside promptly usually indicates the presence of walled off collections of pus within the joint and signals failure of aspiration treatment. Surgical drainage of the infected joint should then be carried out without delay. The appropriate antibiotic should be continued for a two to three week period after the patient becomes afebrile and joint effusion ceases.

It is no longer considered appropriate or necessary to inject antibiotics intra-articularly or add them to suction-irrigation systems. There is now convincing evidence that antibacterial drugs cross the synovial membrane when given in sufficiently high doses parenterally. Inflamed synovial tissue seems to allow easy passage of antimicrobials into the joint cavity and almost all antibiotics appear to enter inflamed joints and produce bactericidal concentrations within them, both in adults and in children.

Prognosis. With early diagnosis and rapid effective treatment, the prognosis for joint function is good. Delay in diagnosis will lead to joint damage and possibly fibrous or bony ankylosis of the joint. If minimal or moderate damage is sustained in childhood, progressive joint deformity in adult life is possible with the subsequent development of degenerative arthritis. Pathologic dislocation of the hip, occurring as a complication of the sepsis, may seriously impair the future function of the joint. With delay in diagnosis or ineffective treatment, the infection will progress in some patients to osteomyelitis.

TUBERCULOUS INFECTION

Tuberculosis is a constitutional infection caused by the tubercle bacillus and resulting in focal lesions in the respiratory or alimentary organs with involvement of the regional lymph nodes. Infection produces metastatic lesions in other tissues and organs, notably the urogenital and skeletal systems, by means of lymphatic spread and arteriolar infarction. In the involved tissue or organ, the characteristic granulation tissue and spreading avascularity lead to necrosis, caseation, and abscess formation. The abscesses may spread along tissue planes, particularly along neurovascular pathways, for a great distance.

INCIDENCE

During the early years of the present century, skeletal tuberculosis constituted the most common single cause of childhood crippling in the world. Today skeletal tuberculosis is relatively uncommon except in underdeveloped countries. This dramatic change has been produced by rigid inspection of dairy herds, pasteurization of milk, sufficient public health measures, and effective chemotherapeutic agents. In the countries where these measures are enforced, human contact is the most common form of transmission. Bovine tuberculosis is seen in those countries where the practice of drinking raw milk is allowed. Although tuberculosis is now a relatively rare disease in Europe, North America, and Australia, it may still be fairly described as a worldwide scourge. It is estimated that there may be as many as 20 million infectious cases centered mainly throughout Asia and Africa. Skeletal tuberculosis, though only a small part of the problem as a whole, still imposes a great strain on medical services in many parts of the world. Of bone involvement, tuberculosis of the spine is the most common and most dangerous form.

Although it is difficult to be certain of this, skeletal tuberculosis is thought to constitute about 3 per cent of total tuberculous infection. It is believed that most bone and joint lesions appear within two years of the onset of the primary lesion. Because their immunity is less developed than that of adults, about 85 per cent of patients with skeletal tuberculosis are children, the peak incidence occuring at about five years of age. Skeletal tuberculosis affects the spine, hip joint, or knee joint in about 95 per cent of patients. The joints of the upper extremity are affected relatively more frequently in adults than in children.

GENERAL CONSIDERATIONS

Since tuberculosis is a constitutional infection of which the skeletal focus is but a metastatic manifestation, a search must be made for the primary focus. If the focus is located, it must be determined whether it is healed, quiescent, or active.

The pathologic response of bone tissue to the tubercle bacillus is rather characteristic, although influenced to a certain extent by the anatomy of the area involved. The infection causes local death of bone, with caseation necrosis and destruction of bone structure. Endarteritis occurs with further necrosis, and the ever-widening circle of destruction continues. The necrotic caseous material may burst through joint capsules and tissue planes and present under the skin as an abscess. This type of abscess, filled with necrotic debris, is called a "cold" abscess, in contrast to a "hot" abscess, which is filled with pyogenic pus. A "cold" abscess may burst through the skin to become a draining tuberculous sinus.

Unlike bone tissue involved with pyogenic organisms, bone tissue infected with tuberculosis makes little or no attempt to defend or protect itself and as a consequence, no new bone formation is usually noted on the radiograph. It is the presence of bone destruction, associated with the absence of bone repair, that is characteristic of the tuberculous skeletal lesion as seen on the radiograph (Fig. 7–8)

When tuberculosis invades a joint, the synovial membrane becomes thickened, secretes excessive fluid, and becomes sprinkled with tubercles. A pannus of tuberculous granulation tissue slowly covers the articular hyaline cartilage, gradually destroying it and the underlying subchondral bone.

The radiograph reflects the pathologic changes brought about by tuberculosis. The presence of bone destruction and the absence

FIGURE 7–8. Tuberculosis involving body of fifth lumbar vertebra. Note narrowing of intervertebral disc space, destruction and collapse of vertebral body, and absence of a bony reparative process.

of new bone formation are noted. Gradual destruction of the joint cartilage leads to joint narrowing. Continued weight bearing results in collapse of the involved joint.

The symptoms of tuberculous involvement of the musculoskeletal system may be general and local. The general symptoms can include malaise, loss of appetite, loss of weight, and intermittent fever. The local presenting symptoms can include pain, swelling, and limitation of motion, and possibly deformity of the affected part.

Even through the clinical picture presented by the patient and the changes noted on the radiograph may seem typical of skeletal tuberculosis, experience has shown that dependence on these alone will lead to a wrong diagnosis in about 25 per cent of patients. Laboratory substantiation of the diagnosis must be obtained.

The tuberculin test is of value when negative, but gives no specific information when positive. Unfortunately, culture of aspirated material and guinea pig inoculation gives a negative result in a large number of patients who actually have tuberculosis. Synovial biopsy may prove to be the important diagnostic test in many patients.

For many years it was recognized that the cornerstone of treatment of tuberculosis was rest of the involved part. When the skeleton was involved, this treatment was carried out by prolonged plaster immobilization in a tuberculosis sanitarium in association with nourishing food and exposure to sunlight. In 1911 Hibbs performed the first spinal fusion for tuberculosis and introduced the concept of total and complete rest of the joint by arthrodesis.

The next major advance in the treatment of skeletal tuberculosis came with the introduction of the chemotherapeutic drugs: streptomycin, para-aminosalicylic acid (PAS), and isonicotinic acid hydrazide (I.N.H.). The use of these agents has resulted in a reduction of the primary mortality in bone and joint tuberculosis. Because of these drugs, normal function has been restored to many joints that formerly would have gone on to destruction and ultimate fusion. These agents have also made it possible to gain adequate control over abscesses and sinus tracts. With adequate blood drug levels, it is now possible to operate on skeletal tuberculosis without fear of hematogenous spreading of the disease or postoperative abscess or sinus formation as was formerly the case.

TUBERCULOSIS OF THE SPINE

Tuberculous infection of the spine, by far the most common form of skeletal tuberculosis, is known as Pott's disease (Sir Percival Pott, 1779). It commonly affects the segment from the tenth thoracic to the first lumbar vertebra, called the thoracolumbar junction, since this is the segment possessing the greatest mobility. Although spinal tuberculosis may strike any age group, about half of the patients are between three and five years of age at the time of onset. In general, spinal lesions can be much more serious than those in peripheral joints because of the possibility of implicating the spinal cord. Other factors that might add to the seriousness of the problem are the presence of multiple lesions, the degree of activity of the primary focus, the extreme youth or old age of the patient, and associated debilitating conditions, such as diabetes, nephritis, and anemia.

Pathology. The skeletal focus begins in the vertebral body, usually along the anterior aspect of the bone. In a way this is fortunate, for it is infection in the posterior aspect of the vertebra that is most likely to cause compression of the spinal cord. The disease causes destruction of bone, which leads to collapse of the vertebral body. As the vertebral body collapses, caseous necrotic material may be squeezed out into the soft tissues to form paravertebral abscesses. Infection may spread beneath the anterior longitudinal spinal ligament to involve several vertebrae.

Compression of the spinal cord may occur at any level from the foramen magnum to the upper lumbar region, but it is most common in the thoracic spine area. Here the spinal canal is narrow and the cord occupies most of the space so that even a small abscess or bone sequestrum may produce cord pressure and paraplegia. In the cervical region, infected material can track sideways along the fascial plane and in the lumbar region along the psoas muscle sheath of the groin. In the thoracic region, pus tends to collect beneath the anterior and posterior longitudinal ligaments under tension, possibly spreading upward and downward to form a paravertebral abscess.

Clinical Picture. The patient complains of back pain that restricts spinal movement. Characteristically, a patient will squat rather than bend to retrieve an object from the floor. Because of pain, all spinal movements are guarded and the patient tends to walk with a protective gait. With marked anterior collapse of several vertebral bodies in the thoracic spine region, the patient may develop a sharp angular deformity of the spine called a *gibbus*. In the days when spinal tuberculosis was common, this was one of the chief causes of "hunchback" deformity.

The earliest sign on the radiograph of tuberculous infection of the spine is deossification of the vertebral bodies associated with thinning of the involved disc space. As the disease progresses, bone destruction leads to progressive anterior wedging of the vertebral bodies and ultimate vertebral collapse. The psoas muscle shadow may appear enlarged on the radiograph because of the presence of a paravertebral abscess. The radiograph is then said to show the presence of a "psoas abscess."

Complications. The chief complications of spinal tuberculosis are psoas abscess, paraplegia, and tuberculous meningitis.

A psoas abscess is a paravertebral abscess composed of necrotic debris that pushes out against the psoas muscle, causing its shadow to appear enlarged on the radiograph. This abscess may spread down tissue planes, point in the thigh, or spread backward through the lumbar triangle to form a lumbar abscess. If the abscesses drain out to the skin surface, tuberculous sinuses are formed.

Paraplegia is one of the most disabling and distressing complications of spinal tuberculosis. The type of paraplegia seen with tuberculous cord compression may vary from a slightly spastic gait to complete paralysis and is encountered in about 10 per cent of patients with spinal tuberculosis. Partial or complete paralysis of the legs results from spinal cord compression secondary to pressure from abscess, tuberculous granulation tissue, a tuberculoma, or extreme gibbus formation. This complication is more common with involvement of the posterior aspect of the vertebral body, laminae, pedicles, or transverse processes, because of the close proximity of the spinal cord.

If a patient with spinal tuberculosis shows any evidence of incipient or actual paralysis, total and complete bed rest with adequate antibiotic coverage should be ordered. When indicated, abscesses are drained surgically and diseased tissue is removed as early and as thoroughly as possible.

Tuberculous meningitis is an extremely grave complication resulting from the rupture of a tuberculous abscess through the dura. Before antituberculosis drugs were available for treatment, tuberculous meningitis frequently had a fatal outcome.

Treatment. Although all treating physicians are agreed on the value of immobilization and chemotherapy for the treatment of spinal tuberculosis, no standard treatment program exists throughout the world. In many American and European centers, immobilization of the spine by bed rest, plaster cast, or spinal brace, coupled with prolonged chemotherapy, is considered adequate treatment for most patients. At other centers in the same countries, posterior spinal fusion of the involved segment is carried out to obtain complete immobilization of the joint.

The disease appears to be more destructive in Asia and Africa, and physicians in these areas believe surgery is needed much earlier than formerly was thought desirable. Most of these physicians favor a direct attack on the lesion through an anterior surgical approach. This allows removal of diseased tissue by extensive vertebral body curettage. Bone grafts are used to fill the large intervertebral defect created by the removal of diseased tissue. This gives spinal stabilization by anterior spinal fusion.

Regardless of whether or not surgery is used, all are agreed that the introduction of chemotherapy has led to better results in all forms of treatment.

TUBERCULOSIS OF THE HIP JOINT

The second most common skeletal area for tuberculosis infection is the hip joint. Here again the majority of patients are young children.

The disease may begin in the synovial membrane, in the metaphyseal portion of the bone adjacent to the capital femoral epiphysis, or in the acetabulum, but it eventually progresses to involve the entire joint. The disease usually does not spread across the growth plate to involve the capital epiphysis, and early in the process this may differentiate the radiograph from those showing evidence of Legg-Calvé-Perthes disease. Tuberculous granulation tissue spreads over the articular cartilage of the joint like a pannus, ultimately destroying the cartilage and subchondral bone. Gradual collapse of the joint occurs with weight bearing. Abscesses formed within the joint space may eventually rupture through the joint capsule to cause draining sinuses.

A painful limp is often the first sign produced by tuberculous infection of the hip joint. The pain may radiate to the knee area. Examination usually discloses obvious muscle atrophy of the leg and limitation of hip joint motion. There may be a flexion-adduction contracture of the leg at the hip joint.

Radiographic examination may show demineralization of the bone structure with joint narrowing and some local bone destruction. There may be capsular swelling. As the disease progresses, gross destruction of the bone and collapse of the joint may be seen on radiographs.

Treatment. The patient is put to bed, and traction is used in the early stages to combat muscle spasm and pain. If the diagnosis is made early in the course of the disease before joint destruction occurs, immobilization and chemotherapy may induce healing and preserve joint mobility.

If there is irreparable joint destruction, operative fusion of the hip joint will be required for control of the infection and relief of pain. In this instance the joint is surgically cleaned of all tuberculous tissue and articular cartilage and the denuded cancellous bone of the femoral head and acetabulum are placed in contact. An iliac bone graft is usually placed between ilium and femur to promote osteogenesis. Immobilization is obtained in a plaster hip spica cast.

In the event the hip joint is the site of abscess formation or if draining skin sinuses exist about the hip joint, fusion can be obtained by bypassing the hip joint proper and running an iliac graft from the trochanteric area of the femur to the ischium. This is called an *extra-articular fusion*.

TUBERCULOSIS OF THE KNEE JOINT

The third most common locus for skeletal tuberculosis is the knee joint. The distinguishing characteristic of this form of tuberculosis is that the major involvement is initially in the synovium. The synovial membrane responds to tuberculous infection by villous hypertrophy and an effusion with a resultant distention of the joint capsule. Small tubercles may be seen on the inflamed synovial surface. Early diagnosis is necessary to save the joint from destruction and eventual fusion (Fig. 7–9).

FIGURE 7–9. Extensive destruction of knee joint secondary to tuberculosis.

The patient with a tuberculous infection of the knee joint may develop a painful swollen boggy knee. The suprapatellar pouch may be filled with fluid and a thickened synovial membrane. There may be a flexion contracture of the knee joint and marked quadriceps muscle atrophy at the thigh.

Immobilization and chemotherapy, if started before joint destruction appears, often arrest the process and preserve a well-functioning joint. Some authorities recommend surgical excision of the synovial membrane (synovectomy) and others do not. If bone destruction is severe, joint fusion will be necessary to control the infection and provide pain relief.

References

Curtis, P. H., Jr., and Klein, L.: Destruction of articular cartilage in septic arthritis. J. Bone and Joint Surg., 45-A:797, 1963.

Gillespie, R.: Septic arthritis of childhood. Clin. Ortho. and Rel. Res., 96:152, 1973.

Gustilo, R. B., and Anderson, J. T.: Prevention of infection in treatment of 1,025 open fractures of long bones. Retrospective and prospective analysis. J. Bone and Joint Surg., 58-A:453, 1976.

Hibbs, R. A.: An operation for progessive spinal deformities. A preliminary report of three cases from the service of the orthopaedic hospital. N.Y. Med. J., 93:1013, 1911.

Kelly, P. J., and Fitzgerald, R. H., Jr. (Ed.): Infections in orthopaedics. The Ortho. Clinics of N. A., Vol. VI, No. 4, 1975.

Medical Research Council Working Party on Tuberculosis of the Spine: A five-year assessment of controlled trials of in-patient and out-patient treatment and of plaster of paris jackets for tuberculosis of the spine in children on standard chemotherapy. Studies in Masan and Pusan, Korea. J. Bone and Joint Surg., 58-B:399, 1976.

Orthopaedic sepsis. American Academy of Orthopaedic Surgeons Instructional Course Lectures, Vol. XXVI. St. Louis: C. V. Mosby Co., 1977.

Pott, P.: Remarks on the kind of palsy of the lower limbs which is frequently found to accompany curvature of the spine. London: Johnson, 1779. Also in: Medical Classics, 1:218, 1936.

Waldvogel, F. A., Medoff, G., and Swartz, M. N.: Osteomyelitis, a review of clinical features, therapeutic considerations, and unusual aspects. Part I. N. Engl. J. Med., 282:198, Jan. 22, 1970.

Waldvogel, F. A., Medoff, G., and Swartz, M. N.: Osteomyelitis, a review of clinical features, therapeutic considerations, and unusual aspects. Part II. N. Engl. J. Med., 282:260, Jan. 29, 1970.

Waldvogel, F. A., Medoff, G., and Swartz, M. N.: Osteomyelitis, a review of clinical features, therapeutic considerations, and unusual aspects. Part III. N. Engl. J. Med., 282:316, Feb. 5, 1970.

CHAPTER 8

NEUROMUSCULAR DISORDERS

John J. Dowling, M.D.*

A variety of musculoskeletal problems are caused by lesions of various portions of the nervous system or intrinsic disease of the muscular apparatus itself. In general, the symptoms and signs produced by a disorder of this type will depend upon the level of the involvement within the neuromuscular system. Most of these disorders become clinically evident in infancy or childhood. Some of the causative lesions are static, such as the cerebral palsies and myelomeningocele, though their effects may change with time and particularly with growth. Some few, such as the muscular dystrophies and "degenerative" central nervous system diseases are progressive. Recent study and research into these conditions has resulted in earlier identification, more aggressive treatment, and a new appreciation of more accurate prognostic factors as a guide to appropriate management.

INVOLVEMENT AT BRAIN LEVEL

CEREBRAL PALSY (LITTLE'S DISEASE)

Cerebral palsy is a condition in which the major expression of dysfunction is in the voluntary muscular apparatus, but secondary to

*Chief of Orthopaedic Surgery, Lankenau Hospital, Philadelphia, Pa.; Orthopaedist-in-Chief, St. Edmund's Home for Crippled Children, Rosemont, Pa.; Clinical Professor of Orthopaedic Surgery, Jefferson Medical College of Thomas Jefferson University, Philadelphia, Pa.

a lesion of the brain that is sustained in infancy or early childhood, thus before motor functions have been developed or learned and affected by growth. The brain lesions are nonprogressive, but not necessarily confined to the motor cortex, basal ganglia, cerebellum, or areas exclusively in control of muscular action, so that associated mental impairment, convulsions, speech problems, hearing loss, visual defects, and perceptual deficiencies are not uncommon and may affect prognosis. The incidence of cerebral palsy has been estimated to vary between 0.6 and 5.9 per 1000 births.

Classification of cerebral palsy into types is helpful in planning appropriate treatment and is based on the physiologic motor abnormality presented and is usually referable to the major area of brain damage: spastic, dyskinetic, ataxic, rigidity, and mixed. Though each type presents a different clinical muscular dysfunction, all share a delay in development of milestones achieved by children of comparable age. In fact, this delay is the commonest presenting complaint in a great majority of patients. The incidence of associated physical handicaps tends to increase in proportion to the severity of the motor and mental deficits.

SPASTIC TYPE. Patients with the spastic type of cerebral palsy exhibit hypertonus of the clasp-knife type giving rise to the "stretch reflex," hyperactive deep tendon reflexes, a loss of control of refined voluntary movements, and pathologic reflexes referable to the pyramidial pathway, such as the Babinski response. Involvement may be monoplegic (one limb involvement is rare), hemiplegic (one side only affected), paraplegic (legs only), quadriplegic (all four extremities), or diplegic (a specific term used to indicate a greater spasticity in the lower extremities than in the uppers). There may be spasticity of the trunk musculature also, especially in hemiplegics and quadriplegics, with the threat of paralytic scoliosis. Mental retardation and seizures are more common in patients with spasticity.

The typical patient deformities in spastic cerebral palsy result from the fact that flexor muscle tone tends to be greater than extensor muscle tone and that certain muscle groups have an inherent mechanical advantage (the hip adductors over abductors for instance). Thus, in the upper extremities, the posture typically is internal rotation of the shoulders, flexion of elbows, palmar flexion and pronation of wrists, flexed fingers, and adducted thumbs. In the lower extremities there is almost invariably hip flexion, adduction and internal rotation, knee flexion, and plantar flexed ankles with inversion of feet more common than eversion. The lower extremity posture frequently gives rise to a "scissors gait" and toe-walking. Because of the constant contraction of the spastic muscles, second-

FIGURE 8–1. Spastic form of cerebral palsy, illustrating the typical positional deformities of the upper and lower extremities.

ary contractures of the joints in these abnormal postures are an ever present threat (Fig. 8–1).

DYSKINETIC TYPE. The dyskinetic type of cerebral palsy includes abnormalities of movement and alterations in postural tone, with extensor tone tending to predominate. The brain lesion is in the extra-pyramidial system (basal ganglia). There are several different types of unwanted movements that may present. The most common manifestation is athetoid movements, which can be described as involuntary, uncoordinate, uncontrollable, purposeless movements with no pattern. More rare are dystonic movements (torsion spasms) that tend to involve larger portions of the body and the trunk, large scale violent tossing or flinging movements, and tremors that are much the same as athetoid movements but have a more predictable pattern, varying between agonist-antagonist muscle groups. All of the dyskinetic types exhibit a certain amount of overlying "tension" in the muscles at times. Whether this is a voluntary or involuntary attempt to control unwanted motions, it creates the major problem of relaxation necessary to initiate purposeful action.

LESS COMMON TYPES. The *ataxic* type, in which damage is almost exclusively confined to the cerebellar apparatus, is fairly rare. These children tend to be hypotonic, with loss of balance, slurring speech, and all the stigmata on physical examination of the ataxic cerebellar patient.

Also rare is the clinical type called *rigidity* in which there is a "lead-pipe" resistance to slow passive motion, rather than the stretch-reflex of the spastic. Mental retardation is often found, and prognosis is invariably poor.

A *mixed* type, usually with elements of spasticity and athetosis, is also encountered. Judgment in its management, particularly with regard to surgical intervention, is critical.

Diagnosis. A suspicion that brain damage has resulted in muscular disturbance may be entertained when any perinatal or infantile situation might have led to hemorrhage or cerebral anoxia. Premature infants are undoubtedly more vulnerable, and many "floppy babies" eventually exhibit permanent muscular disturbance. Suspicion may also be alerted by early afebrile convulsions and disturbances in the sleep pattern or feeding habits. However, it is from a knowledge of the normal orderly development of the central nervous system control over the muscular system that diagnosis is facilitated. Normal neurophysiologic maturation has been characterized as a progression of dominance from the spinal cord to the brain stem to the mid-brain and finally to cortical control. These phases occupy roughly the first year of an infant's development and are characterized by the achievement of certain "milestones" in the ability to utilize muscular control and by the presence of primitive reflexes that later disappear to be replaced by more mature ones. The delay in achievement of motor milestones is the most common presenting complaint in cerebral palsy, and the physical examination must include testing for these, as well as for the primitive reflexes of spasticity, dyskinesia, ataxia, or rigidity described in the preceding paragraphs on types of cerebral palsy and observation for associated non-muscular physical defects.

Serial examinations provide much more useful information than single examinations and require great patience on the part of the physician and forbearance on the part of parents.

Differential diagnosis must include the myopathies, progressive degenerative disorders, and tumors of the nervous system, metabolic syndromes, congenital malformations of the skeleton (Arnold-Chiari syndrome, diastematomyelia), toxic effects (lead poisoning), and genetic defects (Down's syndrome).

Treatment. Once the diagnosis is established, treatment for the cerebral palsied child will depend upon the type and upon the potential of the individual child. The aim of treatment is to make the child as independent and self-sufficient as the inherent disabilities will allow.

Physical therapy modalities are the mainstay of management. Major efforts are in relaxation, appropriate stimulation, and teaching the coordinated motor activities that normal children instinctively develop. Unusual patience on the part of the therapist is required and the use of aids, such as the adjustable reclining chair, the standing table, wheeled and weighted vehicles, parallel bars with a median strip to prevent scissoring of legs, and various kinds of crutches and other external supports, is almost indispensable. A therapeutic pool in which the buoyancy of the water helps is a valuable adjunct. Passive stretching is of very questionable merit. Constant re-evaluation and adjustment of goals is necessary (Fig. 8–2).

Although the current tendency is to avoid braces and a concert-

FIGURE 8–2. Patient in a standing table.

FIGURE 8–3.   Type of braces used to support weak lower extremities.

ed aim is to rid the child of them by the time school starts, they occasionally are indicated for a specific reason. It is generally unrealistic to use braces to correct deformities, but they may be helpful to prevent deformity, to hold a corrected deformity post-operatively for a time, to support very weak extremities, or sporadically as "control" braces to dampen the movements of the dyskinetic child. Splints worn only at night to help prevent contractures may be advisable for prolonged periods (Fig. 8–3).

Drugs other than those used for specific control of seizure disorders have proven of very limited benefit. Speech therapy is frequently needed and prolonged.

Surgery.   Operative intervention is used when a specific condition is limiting progress in therapy. The types of operations that have proven useful are:

1. Release of contractures of tendons or joint capsules, with the tendo-achilles lengthening procedure probably the commonest performed.

2. Neurectomies (usually partial) to inhibit excessive muscular spasticity.

3. Tendon transfers (to convert a deforming force to a corrective one).

4. Osteotomies (particularly varus-derotation osteotomy of the femur) for correction of angular bony deformities.

5. Arthrodesis of poorly controlled or degenerated joints.

Experience with surgery in dyskinetic children has been very poor and is confined mostly to arthrodeses, so that for the most part, operations are confined to the spastic type of cerebral palsy.

ADULT SPASTIC PARALYSIS

Spastic hemiplegia in the adult may follow cerebral vascular disorders, such as hemorrhage, thrombosis, or embolus formation. As in cerebral palsy, treatment involves muscular re-education through therapy and exercise and the use of splints or braces if necessary. Nerve blocks may be used to relieve spasticity. Surgical correction of joint contractures or tendon transfer operations may be useful to restore muscle balance and improve function.

INVOLVEMENT AT SPINAL CORD LEVEL

ANTERIOR POLIOMYELITIS (INFANTILE PARALYSIS)

Until recently, anterior poliomyelitis ranked as the most frequent cause of childhood crippling in this country, supplying large numbers of paralytic patients to orthopaedic services for rehabilitation and reconstruction. The widespread use of polio vaccines since 1955 has resulted in the virtual elimination of paralytic poliomyelitis in the United States, with only eight cases having been reported in 1976. However, sporadic cases, requiring orthopaedic care, will undoubtedly continue to appear.

This viral disease attacks the anterior horn cells of the spinal cord and brain stem, destroying some of these, and leads to an irregular pattern of flaccid paralysis or weakness of limb or trunk musculature of a permanent nature. The random distribution of paralysis could lead to static or dynamic deformities. Frequently, permanent brace support is necessary. Many surgical procedures, such as tendon transfers and arthrodeses, are helpful in combating the effects of residual paralysis.

FRIEDREICH'S ATAXIA

Friedreich's ataxia or hereditary spinal ataxia is a heredofamilial disorder exhibiting both dominant and recessive inheritance

FIGURE 8–4. *A*, positional foot deformity in Friedreich's ataxia. *B*, appearance after surgical correction.

patterns and involving chiefly the posterior columns of the spinal cord. The disease manifests itself sometime between 5 and 20 years of age with the highest incidence at puberty. The course of the disease is generally slow with frequent periods of remission. Affected patients develop a lurching ataxic gait that may progress to a severe disability. Intention tremors and scanning speech are noted with progression of the disease. As a result of muscle weakness and deformity, the patient is often unable to walk by the fourth decade, and death from intercurrent disease frequently occurs by the age of 40 years.

This disease is of orthopaedic interest because the resulting muscle imbalance may allow the development of a particular foot deformity known as cavus or "claw foot," characterized by a high curved longitudinal arch, prominence of the metatarsal heads, and clawing of the toes. "Claw foot" is frequently a painful deformity because of malalignment of the weight bearing surfaces of the foot (Fig. 8–4).

For many patients progress of the neurologic disease is slow and operative correction of this deformity is indicated to bring about a more functional alignment of the weight bearing surface of the foot.

CHARCOT-MARIE-TOOTH DISEASE

Charcot-Marie-Tooth disease or progressive muscular atrophy of the peroneal type is a heredofamilial disease transmitted either as an autosomal dominant, X-linked recessive, or autosomal recessive trait. The disease — affecting males more often than females — is associated with degenerative changes in the posterior column of the spinal cord, the spinal roots, and the peripheral nerves.

When dominant, the disease manifests itself at about 30 years of age and tends to run a prolonged course with only moderate atrophy. The X-linked variety is usually manifested during the second decade of life and tends to run a more severe course with marked disability by about 30 years of age. The most severe form, the autosomal recessive, has its onset at about eight years of age and usually produces profound weakness by the second decade.

Orthopaedic attention focuses upon the peripheral deformity brought about by the neurologic changes. The characteristic changes seen in the upper extremity are intrinsic atrophy and weakness of the radially innervated forearm muscles, and in the lower extremity paralysis of the peroneal and toe extensor muscles may allow the foot to assume a clubfoot appearance resulting from overpull of the unaffected foot muscles (Fig. 8–5).

FIGURE 8–5. *A*, positional foot deformity in Charcot-Marie-Tooth disease. *B*, appearance after surgical correction.

Deformity in the lower extremity may be lessened by supporting the foot in a brace. If the disease is not rapidly progressive, operative correction of the foot deformity by removal of bone wedges, followed by triple arthrodesis, will provide a better functioning extremity for the patient.

SYRINGOMYELIA

Syringomyelia is a chronic, slowly progressive disease of the cervical portion of the spinal cord characterized by cavity formation within the substance of the spinal cord tissue. The disease chiefly affects young people and causes a variety of motor, sensory, and trophic disturbances.

Orthopaedic interest in this neurologic disease centers about the possible development of a neuropathic joint deformity in the upper extremity. Syringomyelia usually results in a segmental loss of pain and temperature sensation and a loss of position and vibration senses. In 10 to 40 per cent of patients these sensory and trophic disturbances will allow the formation of a neuropathic or Charcot joint deformity in the upper extremity, most frequently the shoulder joint.

TRAUMATIC PARAPLEGIA AND QUADRIPLEGIA

Severe injuries to the spine, such as fracture-dislocations and gunshot wounds, may damage the spinal cord and result in traumatic paraplegia or quadriplegia. Injuries below the level of the first thoracic vertebra produce a paralysis of both lower limbs (paraplegia); those above that level produce a paralysis of all four limbs (quadriplegia). Complete transection of the spinal cord results in permanent paralysis of all muscles supplied by motor neurons below the level of the lesion and permanent loss of skin sensation in all areas supplied by sensory neurons below the lesion.

Initially after injury, the patient exhibits a state of spinal shock characterized by flaccid paralysis and complete loss of skin sensation. After a few weeks, the affected muscles develop permanent spasticity and the skin sensibility may drop to a slightly lower permanent level. Among the serious complications of spinal cord injury are paralytic incontinence of the bladder and rectum, urinary tract infections, and decubitus ulcers.

Surgical decompression of the spinal cord may be indicated if the paraplegia is incomplete at the beginning or there is evidence of progression in the neurologic deficit. If the paraplegia is complete from the beginning, there is no value in surgical decompression. If an unstable fracture-dislocation of the spine is present, operative reduction and stabilization by fusion facilitates nursing care and enables the patient to get up with safety and comfort at an early stage in the rehabilitation period.

As soon as the patient's condition will permit, transfer to a spinal paraplegic center or center for long-term care and rehabilitation should be effected. The overall management of paraplegic patients requires the combined skills of a large team. With wheelchair transfer, long leg braces, and gait training, the strongly motivated paraplegic, whose cord lesion is not at too high a level, may return to walking and may become self-supporting.

REFLEX SYMPATHETIC DYSTROPHIES

Though relatively uncommon and enigmatic, but all too often unrecognized and poorly managed, the collection of related entities that should be grouped under this heading can be devastating and tragically disabling. The conditions that in the past have been described as causalgia, Sudeck's atrophy, shoulder-hand syndrome, traumatic dystrophy, and sympathalgia belong in this category because they all have a common pathophysiologic mechanism, certain common clinical manifestations, and a response to the same appropriate treatment. Though the details of clinical presentation may differ among the conditions, they all manifest excessive or unduly prolonged pain, hypersensitivity, vasomotor and trophic changes, and can occur in either upper or lower extremities.

It would appear that three conditions must be present for reflex sympathetic dystrophy to occur in a patient. A painful lesion is the first. This may be traumatic or visceral (heart attack, peptic ulcer) and may seem very minor in contrast to the symptoms and signs evoked. The second condition is susceptibility or "diathesis." The person who develops reflex sympathetic dystrophy tends to be insecure, fearful, emotionally labile, worrisome with a dependent personality, sometimes hostile, but not a malingerer. The third condition is an abnormal autonomic reflex. The exact mechanism which produces this is unclear, but it seems to be an abnormality centered at the spinal cord level with disturbance in the "internuncial pool" of neurons or in special cells in the substantia gelatinosa of the dorsal horn, but leading to sympathetic hyperactivity.

Typically, the condition progresses through recognizable stages if untreated. Early there is swelling of a soft puffy type, increased warmth and redness, hyperesthesia, and hyperhidrosis (Fig. 8–6). Radiographic changes of osteoporosis, especially at the ends of long bones, appear about the third or fourth week. If unrecognized or

FIGURE 8-6. The puffy hand of reflex sympathetic dystrophy.

untreated, the swelling becomes brawny and fusiform. The skin becomes shiny and tight. Limitation of joint motion becomes increasingly worse and pain persists. If still uninterrupted, cold pallor or cyanosis ensues and contractures of joints become fixed. Muscle atrophy and weakness become marked. Ankylosis or even subluxation of joints may occur. Radiographic examination reveals diffuse bone atrophy.

A high index of suspicion is necessary to identify reflex sympathetic dystrophy early when it is still treatable. When it is noted that a patient's complaints are out of proportion to the degree of trauma or disease, the examiner should watch for color, temperature or sweat changes. The most effective treatment is sympathetic ganglionic block with local anesthesia. A successful block with a good response is also helpful diagnostically to verify the diagnosis. Surgical sympathectomy may become necessary for especially stubborn or neglected cases. Adjunctive therapy is also very important, consisting of appropriate protective splinting, super-gentle physical therapy, judicious use of tranquilizers, and most importantly, plenty of supportive reassurance.

INVOLVEMENT AT NERVE ROOT LEVEL

MYELOMENINGOCELE (See p. 74.)

With the declining incidence of poliomyelitis and tuberculous bone and joint disease, myelomeningocele now stands second in importance to cerebral palsy as a cause of locomotor disability in children. This condition is caused by the unfused state of vertebral arches with cystic distention of the meninges and associated myelodysplasia of the spinal cord causing neurologic signs. The current incidence has been reported at about 2.5 per 1000 live births. Studies have shown that about 20 children with severe neurologic disability are expected to survive to school age and onwards annually in a community of two and one-half million people. Another eight patients will survive annually with minimal or no disability (Fig 8–7).

The etiology is not known. However, as stated by authorities in

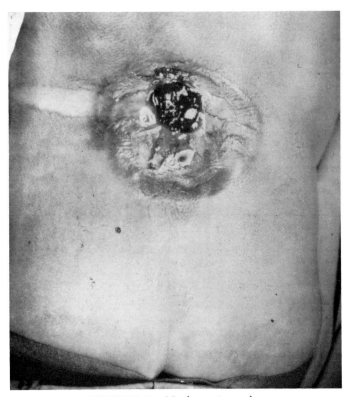

FIGURE 8-7. Myelomeningocele.

the field, "there can be few diseases in which the clinical state is so desolate and diverse, the outlook so poor, and in which so many of the survivors are so tragically afflicted." Nevertheless, since 1959 there has been a radical change in the future of these children dating from the introduction of the ventriculoatrial shunts for the frequently accompanying hydrocephalus, which previously accounted for a high early mortality rate and for destruction of brain tissue.

With the salvage of these children beyond the first year, urinary tract complications become the next important problem to be solved in order to preserve renal function and sustain life. Because of the predominance of myelomeningocele in the lumbosacral region (90 per cent below the second lumbar vertebra), an enormous number of the patients have lack of bladder or bowel control (90 to 97 per cent). The myelomeningocele bladder is nearly always of the lower motor neuron type with a flaccid bladder barely amenable to conservative training. Apart from the neurogenic state, spina bifida cystica patients exhibit a high incidence of congenital urinary abnormalities. Apart from the embarrassment of constant wetness with its concomitant irritation and odor, there is the constant threat of stasis and obstruction with infection and destruction of renal tissue. Intensive training programs for control may fail and various urologic surgical procedures, including permanent urinary diversion by one of several methods, may become necessary at some time.

The locomotor disability is related to the level of spinal cord dysplasia, which is not always the same level as the vertebral bony defect. The paralysis is almost always a flaccid paralysis of lower motor neuron type and complicated by sensory loss which, however, does not always correspond completely with the motor level. It is of little clinical significance to know the exact spinal segment involved since treatment, for practical purposes, is based upon what joint movements the child can or cannot perform, and in young infants it is almost impossible to carry out examination of individual muscle action.

With a grading of disability roughly according to spinal segments, it is possible to establish four groups of varying severity, each with a different therapeutic and prognostic significance.

Group I — Level above L-3 with total paraplegia and the necessity for total support of the lower limbs.

Group II — Level L-4 and below in which hip extensors and abductors, knee flexors, and all the motors to the feet are paralyzed, but action remains in knee extensors and hip flexors and adductors. Major support must be given to hips and feet by bracing or surgical procedures.

Group III — Level S-1 and below in which hip extensors and knee flexors are weak, as are invertors and evertors of the feet, but plantar flexors of feet are paralyzed. Knee extensors, hip flexors and adductors, and dorsiflexors of the feet are retained. There may be adequate function of the hips and knees, but the feet need support because of lack of push-off.

Group IV — Level S-3 and below in which the lower limbs are normal and require no support.

It should be pointed out also that the disability of the muscular system secondary to neurologic deficit may be complicated by any of a number of associated skeletal anomalies, including congenital dysplasia of the hip, clubfoot, and vertebral defects aside from the spina bifida. Their treatment may be hindered by the skin insensitivity.

Orthopaedic management early in life is directed mainly to the prevention of joint contractures, particularly of the hips and feet, occasioned by muscle imbalance and is accomplished by the use of splints of various materials, always remembering the treacherous nature of the anesthetic limb in developing pressure ulceration. When the child becomes old enough to cooperate, physical therapy is indicated to encourage and develop every active muscle group in anticipation of upright stance ambulation. Attention at this time may also be directed at the upper extremities for strengthening musculature that will be needed in the face of lower extremity weakness. When the child is two or three years of age, attempts may be made to train in ambulation, most often necessitating leg braces for support, the extent of bracing being determined by the observed muscle paralysis or weakness (Fig. 8–8).

Surgical treatment may be indicated as the child's progress is noted. The defective spine may require correction and fusion for unstable lumbar lordosis or scoliosis. The hips may necessitate soft tissue releases for flexion or abduction contractures, and if paralytic subluxation or dislocation of the hips becomes a problem, as in Group II, transfer of the iliopsoas muscle insertion from the lesser to the greater trochanter (Sharrard procedure), femoral osteotomy, or pelvic osteotomy may need to be done. Foot deformities are often static in nature, but may require metatarsal osteotomies to correct forefoot varus or triple arthrodesis for stabilization. Occasionally, neglected pressure ulcers, particularly over the sacrum, ischial tuberosities, or the greater trochanters, must be handled by resection of underlying bony prominences and secondary closure or skin graft.

FIGURE 8–8. Ambulatory training often requires bracing and walking aids.

OBSTETRICAL PALSY

Obstetrical palsy is the name given to a traction injury of the infant's brachial plexus caused by pulling on the arm during a difficult delivery. Injury to the nerve roots contributing to the brachial plexus may cause a muscular paralysis involving either the entire arm, the upper arm and shoulder only, or just the lower arm and hand. The most common injury, called *Erb's palsy,* involves the fifth and sixth cervical nerve roots and is associated with paralysis of the upper arm and shoulder region.

Following traction injury to the fifth and sixth cervical nerve roots, paralysis involves mainly abductors and external rotators of the upper arm and shoulder. As a result, the infant will be noticed to lie with the shoulder and arm in adduction and internal rotation and the forearm pronated. If the limb is allowed to remain in this position, the deformities will become fixed because of contracture of the unopposed normal muscles. If this occurs, the child will be unable to abduct the arm well or to elevate it beyond the shoulder level (Fig. 8–9).

The majority of patients suffering traction injuries to the brachial plexus recover spontaneously. During this time, all joints of
the involved limb must be put through a full range of motion in an
attempt to prevent contractures. The affected upper extremity may
be supported in a brace with the arm held in a position opposite to
that assumed by the deformity. The brace supports the weakened
musculature while it regains strength and also helps prevent the
formation of joint contractures.

Operative treatment may be indicated in older children in
whom complete spontaneous recovery has not occurred. Cutting
through contracted tendons and muscles may allow better positioning of the arm. Transplantation of normal muscles to replace the
paralyzed ones may effectively increase the muscular strength and
function of the arm and shoulder. In some patients, osteotomy
through the shaft of the humerus is performed to allow rotation of
the deformed upper extremity into a more functional position.

FIGURE 8–9. Internal rotation contracture of left upper extremity in adolescent boy
with untreated obstetrical palsy.

NERVE ROOT COMPRESSION

Abnormal conditions arising in the spine may be associated with mechanical compression of the adjacent spinal nerve roots. Herniated intervertebral disc, bony compression of the intervertebral foramen, tumor, or an osteoarthritic spur projecting posteriorly into the nerve root may give rise to rather characteristic signs and symptoms that would indicate compression at the nerve root level.

Abnormalities associated with nerve root compression occur most frequently in the cervical and lumbar segments of the spine.

The cervical nerve root compression syndrome is discussed on page 320. The lumbosacral nerve root compression syndrome is discussed on page 350.

INVOLVEMENT AT PERIPHERAL NERVE LEVEL

POLYNEURITIS

The term polyneuritis may be applied to any condition associated with irritation of multiple peripheral nerves. In general, the condition is characterized by pain and tenderness along the affected nerve trunks and associated musculature. Paresthesias are common. Examination may disclose decreased or absent tendon reflexes along with motor and sensory disturbances.

Polyneuritis commonly has a nutritional, metabolic, or infectious basis. Nutritional polyneuritis may be seen in the alcoholic and is thought to be due largely to avitaminosis. Polyneuritis may also be seen in the true vitamin deficiency diseases, such as beriberi and pellagra, and in leprosy.

Diabetes is the most frequent metabolic cause of polyneuritis. Polyneuritis is more likely to affect those patients whose diabetes is not under adequate control. It has been estimated that it occurs at one time or another in about 5 per cent of all patients with diabetes.

Infectious polyneuritis (Guillain-Barré syndrome) is an acute process characterized by an ascending progressive symmetrical paralysis. The onset of this disorder frequently follows an upper respiratory infection. There is usually no associated sensory change. The process is differentiated from anterior poliomyelitis by the fact the patient is afebrile and by the presence of an abnormally elevated spinal fluid protein content. Most patients make a spontaneous recovery following symptomatic and supportive treatment.

TRAUMA TO PERIPHERAL NERVES

Certain specific orthopaedic lesions carry with them the potential for damage to adjacent peripheral nerves. The examiner must be aware of this possibility so that the status of the peripheral nerve can be determined at the time of the initial examination. The radial, median, ulnar, and sciatic nerves are injured more frequently than other peripheral nerves in the body.

Radial Nerve. The radial nerve may be damaged in association with fractures through the midshaft of the humerus (see p. 271). Trauma to the radial nerve at this level may result in "wrist drop" deformity in which the patient loses the ability to actively raise the wrist and thumb and the metacarpophalangeal joints of the hand. Improper use of crutches by taking weight through the axilla rather than on the hand may also, in time, produce a radial palsy with a "wrist drop."

Median Nerve. The median nerve may be damaged by dislocation of the lunate bone at the wrist and may be implicated in the carpal tunnel syndrome (see p. 294). Trauma to the median nerve at this level may result in paralysis of the opponens pollicis muscle. If this occurs, the patient loses the ability to actively oppose the thumb to the remaining fingers.

Ulnar Nerve. The ulnar nerve may be damaged by trauma or fracture involving the medial epicondyle of the humerus at the elbow (see p. 284). Trauma to the ulnar nerve may result in paralysis of intrinsic hand muscles, and the patient may lose the power to spread and bring together all the fingers. Clawing of the fourth and fifth fingers may develop.

Sciatic Nerve. The sciatic nerve may be damaged in association with a fracture through the midshaft of the femur (see p. 402), or it may be damaged by the femoral head following traumatic posterior dislocation of the hip joint (see p. 393). Trauma to the sciatic nerve may result in complete paralysis of all the muscles of the lower leg and foot and partial paralysis of the thigh muscles.

Axillary Nerve. The axillary nerve may be damaged in association with anterior dislocation of the shoulder joint. Trauma to the axillary nerve may result in paralysis of the deltoid muscle and the patient may lose the ability to actively abduct the arm at the shoulder joint.

Common Peroneal Nerve. The common peroneal nerve may be damaged by excessive pressure or injury to the head and neck region of the fibula. The most frequent orthopaedic cause of this involvement is a tight or inadequately padded plaster leg cast. Trauma to the common peroneal nerve may result in paralysis of the long toe extensor muscles, the anterior tibial muscle, and the peroneals. The patient may note a "foot drop" with loss of the ability to actively dorsiflex or evert the foot.

INVOLVEMENT AT MUSCLE LEVEL

MUSCULAR DYSTROPHIES

The muscular dystrophies, like the cerebral palsies, are a group of syndromes in which there is primary myopathy, genetically determined, but with diverse clinical presentations. They have in common various degrees of muscle wasting and weakness, elevated serum enzyme levels (creatine phosphokinase, aldolase), a characteristic pattern on electromyography, and fairly typical findings on muscle biopsy. The laboratory studies have become critical for differentiation from other, very similar diseases of neurogenic origin (Werdnig-Hoffmann, etc.). Electron microscopy or histochemical studies of the muscle biopsy may be advisable in some patients to validate the diagnosis. Particularly troublesome and critical is the differentiation from polymyositis, which may mimic the dystrophies even to the elevation of CPK but which is amenable to steroid therapy while the dystrophies are not.

The muscular dystrophies differ from one another in the pattern of inheritance, age and onset, muscle groups involved, and the severity and rate of progression. The most common and most disabling type is pseudohypertrophic muscular dystrophy of Duchenne, which appears early, progresses rapidly, and leads to an early death. The enlargement of the calves which occurs in 80 per cent of patients is a pseudohypertrophy brought about by replacement of the bulk of muscle fibers by fat and fibrous tissue. Major weakness is found symmetrically in the pelvic girdle muscles, mainly the quadriceps, iliopsoas and gluteals, followed by the tibialis anterior and, later, shoulder girdle and arm musculature. Other types are facioscapulohumeral (Landouzy-Déjerine) and limb girdle muscular dystrophy.

Although the ultimate outlook may be discouraging, the present attitude is that every attempt should be made to keep the child ambulatory and independent as long as possible. The better preservation of the child's physical and emotional status should increase the chance for benefit from any future pharmacologic advance in therapy that may result from research in these diseases. It has been shown that the duration of ambulation can be increased if a helpful, comprehensive, and vigorous approach is maintained. In the early phase, muscle strength is preserved by regular exercises. Swimming is particularly helpful for general strength and endurance. The development of joint contractures is delayed by passive stretching and the use of night splints. Maintenance of ambulation can be prolonged by several years by the use of support braces. Surgical release of contractures or joint stabilizations are occasionally helpful.

INVOLVEMENT AT MYONEURAL JUNCTION LEVEL

MYASTHENIA GRAVIS

Myasthenia gravis is a disease characterized by excessive fatigability of voluntary muscles. The disease is thought to be due to an abnormality at the myoneural junction and may affect a single muscle, a group of muscles, or all the muscles. Characteristically, muscle fatigue and weakness are aggravated by exertion and are typically worse towards the end of the day. A degree of muscle strength can usually be restored by rest.

The disease affects adult females most commonly. Most patients note facial symptoms due to fatigue of ocular, facial, jaw, and tongue muscles. Symptoms due to weakness of the upper and lower extremity muscles may also be noted. The muscles of the abdomen and the back may be affected. As a rule, myasthenia gravis is not progressive and may be characterized by long periods of remission.

Muscles fatigued as a result of myasthenia gravis show a dramatic return of strength following administration of neostigmine bromide, which is a parasympathetic stimulant. Treatment of this disorder consists of a properly adjusted dose of neostigmine bromide usually given daily in three oral doses of 15 mg each, or the use of other indicated parasympathomimetic drugs.

References

Adams, R. D.: Diseases of Muscle. New York: Harper and Row, 1975.

Bleck, E. F.: Locomotor prognosis in cerebral palsy. Paper presented at the Annual Meeting American Academy of Cerebral Palsy, Cleveland, 1965.

Bonica, J.: Causalgia and other reflex sympathetic dystrophies. Postgrad. Med., 53 (6): May 1973.

Egan, D. F., Illingworth, R. S., and MacKeith, R. C.: Developmental screening 0–5 years. Clin. Dev. Med., Vol. 30, 1969.

Fiorentino, M. R., Gesell, A., and Amatruda, C. S.: Developmental Diagnosis. New York: Hoeber, 1947.

Frankenburg, W. K., and Dodds, J. B.: The Denver developmental screening test. J. Pediatrics, 71, No. 2, Aug. 1967.

Furukawa, T. and Peter, J. B.: I. The Muscular Dystrophies, April 14, 1978. II. Diseases simulating muscular dystrophies, April 21, 1978. JAMA, Vol. 239, April 1978.

Gillette, H. E.: Systems of Therapy in Cerebral Palsy. Springfield, Illinois: Charles C Thomas, 1969.

Hoffer, M. M.: Basic considerations and classifications of cerebral palsy. Am. Academy of Orthopaedic Surgeons Instructional Course Lectures, Vol. V, XXV. St. Louis: C. V. Mosby Co., 1976.

Ketenjian, A. Y.: Muscular dystrophy: diagnosis and treatment. Orthop. Clin. North Am., Vol. 9, #1, Jan. 1978.

Kupka, J., Geddes, N., and Carrol, N. C.: Comprehensive management in the child with spina bifida. Orthop. Clin. of North Am., Vol. 9, #1, Jan. 1978.

Lankford, L. L., and Thompson, J. E.: Reflex Sympathetic Dystrophy, Upper and Lower Extremity: Diagnosis and Management. Am. Academy of Orthopaedic Surgeons Instructional Course Lectures, Vol. V, XXVI. St. Louis: C. V. Mosby Co., 1977.

Leach, R. E., and Clawson, D. K.: Continuous elevation by spica cast in treatment of reflex sympathetic dystrophy. J. Bone and Joint Surg., 56A, March, 1974.

Payne, R. S.: Cerebral Palsy: Symptoms and Signs of Diagnostic and Prognostic Importance. *In* Current Practice in Orthopaedic Surgery. St. Louis: C. V. Mosby Co., Chapter 3, Vol. 3, 1966.

Samilson, R. L.: Orthopaedic Aspects of Cerebral Palsy. Philadelphia: J. B. Lippincott Co., 1975.

Sammons, J. H.: Editorial: Polio — out of sight, out of mind. JAMA, 238, No. 22, 1977.

Sharrard, W. J. W.: Posterior iliopsoas transplantation in the treatment of paralytic dislocation of the hip. J. Bone and Joint Surg. 46B: Aug. 1964.

Smith, E. D.: Spina Bifida and the Total Care of Spinal Myelomeningocele. Springfield, Illinois: Charles C Thomas, 1965.

Vignos, P. J., Jr., Spencer, G. E., Jr., and Archibald, K. C.: Management of progressive muscular dystrophy in childhood. JAMA, Vol. 184, April 13, 1963.

Walton, J. N., and Adams, R. D.: Polymyositis. Edinburgh: E. & S. Livingstone, 1958.

CHAPTER 9

BONE TUMORS

INTRODUCTION

As in other organ systems of the body, tumor formation may take place in the tissue of the skeletal system. These tumors may arise within the skeletal system as primary growths or may spread secondarily to the skeleton from some distant primary location. Some of these tumors are relatively common; others are quite rare. Some pose no particular threat to the patient's life or function; others are rapidly debilitating and often fatal. It is imperative that the diagnosis of a bone tumor be made with absolute accuracy and that the treatment be planned with extreme care. Diagnosis is best established by a searching history and physical examination, close scrutiny of all essential radiographic views, including tomograms, bone scans, and arteriography if indicated, careful biochemical investigation of the patient's blood and urine, and surgical biopsy with ultimate histologic tissue identification. Few immediate diagnoses of malignant tumors can be made on frozen section examination. It is generally better to await permanent paraffin sections.

Accurate tissue identification may prove quite difficult. Some tumors are classic and identification proves easy while others may be borderline, rendering the difference between a benign and a malignant state unclear. This difficulty frequently arises with cartilage tumors and giant cell tumors. Another problem occasionally encountered in planning appropriate tumor treatment is the erratic biological behavior of some tumors. A tumor that appears benign by most criteria may occasionally behave in an aggressive or malignant manner while a tumor identified as malignant may be quite limited in its progression.

Primary bone tumors may be benign or malignant. Benign bone tumors generally are slow-growing, well-circumscribed, noninvading tumors that cause few symptoms, do not spread or metastasize, and do not cause the death of the patient. The radiographic appearance suggests a benign tumor if the lesion is limited to the confines of the bone, if it has a well-demarcated border surrounded by a thin rim of sclerotic bone, and if it has not broken through the overlying cortex. A few benign tumors, however, apparently possess the capability of malignant transformation.

Primary malignant bone tumors are rare, with the incidence believed to be in the ratio of approximately five per one million population. These tumors grow rapidly, spread, expand and invade irregularly, and are associated with pain and disability. They tend to affect children and young adults most frequently. They spread or metastasize to the lungs and other tissues, bringing about a rapid, fatal outcome. Any hope for survival depends upon early diagnosis, usually best established by biopsy. The radiographic appearance suggests a malignant lesion if the tumor boundaries are ill-defined with no sharp borders, if the lesion has a mottled appearance, and if it has broken out of the confines of the bone and destroyed the overlying cortex. Since the cells of the skeletal system are derived from mesoderm, primary malignant bone tumors are called sarcomas.

Tumors that spread secondarily to the skeleton from some distant primary location are malignant, and are called *metastatic tumors*. They are generally carcinomas arising originally in tissues such as breast, prostate, kidney, thyroid, and lung. As they grow and invade within their tissue of origin, clumps of tumor cells may be carried off by the blood stream or lymph channels to lodge and grow within bone, but they continue to maintain the microscopic characteristics of the original tumor. Since most metastatic tumors to bone originate in tissue of ectodermal origin, these tumors are known as *metastatic carcinomas.*

It is very important to determine whether bone formed in a tumor is being produced by the actual tumor cells or by normal osteoblasts reacting to the tumor. In most situations the host bone responds to a tumor by a combination of resorption and bone formation. Tumor cells in bone generally do not destroy bone tissue, but their presence can evoke several types of host response helpful in identification and diagnosis on the roentgenogram. Tumor cells in bone may incite local osteoclastic resorption of bone with the formation of radiolucent areas on the radiograph. Some tumor cells may evoke the opposite response and cause an osteoblastic response in the host, with the production of a protective wall of dense normal bone around the lesion. This response is known as *reactive bone formation*. Certain tumors, such as osteosarcomas, are capable of producing osteoid and bone by their own aberrant growth pattern. This bone production within a tumor is called *tumor bone* or *neoplastic bone*.

Several types of periosteal response may also be seen. A tumor that causes expansion of a segment of bone does this by slowly eroding bone from the inside, while at the same time stimulating the periosteum to deposit bone on the outside.

If the periosteum is elevated by a tumor that has broken through the cortex, it is stimulated to produce reactive bone at its remaining point of attachment to the cortex. This produces a triangular-shaped piece of reactive bone on the radiograph known as *Codman's triangle*.

Elevation of the periosteum in progressive stages stimulates the formation of layers of reactive periosteal bone, giving the so-called "onion-skin" appearance on the radiographs.

Treatment of tumors of the skeletal system utilizes surgery — occasionally cryosurgery — radiation therapy, and chemotherapeutic drugs. A new approach in controlling certain types of locally destructive tumors is cryosurgery utilizing liquid nitrogen. These modalities may be used singly or in thoughtful combination, depending upon the situation presented by each tumor.

The surgical techniques used for tumor surgery include local excision, local excision with restoration of continuity by bone grafting, wide block excision with restoration of continuity by bone grafting, wide block excisions, amputations, and limb disarticulations including hemipelvectomy and interscapulothoracic amputations.

Generally, benign bone tumors are treated by surgical excision, with no need for the use of radiation therapy or chemotherapy. If a large defect remains in the host bone after excision of a benign tumor, it is considered wise to pack the defect with bone chips taken from the ilium in order to accelerate healing of the defect and restore structural integrity to the host bone. The recurrence rate for most surgically excised benign bone tumors is low.

The treatment of malignant bone tumors remains unsatisfactory from the standpoint of long-term patient survival, but the picture is gradually brightening owing to the use of aggressive adjuvant chemotherapy following surgical ablation of the tumor. Surgery, as utilized in the treatment of primary malignant bone tumors, ranges from wide block excisions to amputation and limb disarticulation. Radiation therapy is employed for its local effect on micrometastases if the tumor cells are radiosensitive. The cytotoxic drugs are used as adjuvant chemotherapy for their systemic effect on micro- and distant metastases in responsive tumors.

Immunotherapy has had sporadic trials in the past in the treatment of malignant tumors. Recently, great strides have been made in the basic understanding of the immunologic host-tumor relationship, mostly based on animal studies. It now seems clear that malignant tumors shed identifiable immunogenic substances that are different for various tumor classes, but it has not yet been established whether these immunogens are common to all sarcomas or specific to individual tumors. Also there is as yet no clear understanding of the role of sensitized lymphocytes, blocking factor, cytotoxic antibody, transfer factor, and other mechanisms that are known to play some part in this interaction. Immunotherapy remains a field of unrealized potential value and great investigative activity at the present time.

Knowledge of the origin, biological behavior, and treatment of

TABLE 9–1. Classification of Bone Tumors

TISSUE	BENIGN	MALIGNANT
Cartilage	Osteochondroma Enchondroma Chondroblastoma Chondromyxoid fibroma	Chondrosarcoma a. primary b. secondary
Bone	Osteoid osteoma Osteoblastoma	Osteosarcoma
Marrow elements	None	Ewing's sarcoma Reticulum cell sarcoma Plasma cell myeloma
Fat	Lipoma	Liposarcoma
Blood vessels	Hemangioma	Angiosarcoma
Fibrous and connective tissue	Subperiosteal cortical defect Nonossifying fibroma Aneurysmal bone cyst Unicameral bone cyst Giant cell tumor	Fibrosarcoma
Notochord	None	Chordoma
Primary carcinoma (breast, lung, prostate, kidney, etc.)	None	Metastatic carcinoma

bone tumors is quite incomplete at the present time, and much of the present information is conflicting and controversial. It is known, however, that various cell types comprising the skeletal system may give origin to tumors that vary considerably in their clinical course. The cells of the musculoskeletal tissue all share a common mesodermal origin, but have differentiated along a variety of lines to become osteoblasts, osteoclasts, chondroblasts, fibroblasts, and myeloblasts. This information is of some help in classifying bone tumors. One group of bone tumors is produced by cells characterized by their ability to synthesize collagen. These are the osteogenic, the chondrogenic, and the fibrogenic tumors. Another group of lesions probably originates from the marrow reticulum and includes the various round cell tumors of bone such as Ewing's sarcoma and reticulum cell sarcoma. Tumors of neurogenic, vascular, muscular, or fatty tissue origin may also arise within bone.

Authoritative bone tumor texts offer detailed classifications containing all types of tumors affecting the skeletal system. Only the more commonly encountered tumors are described in this chapter. A partial classification of these tumors based on origin is presented in Table 9–1.

BENIGN BONE TUMORS

I. Cartilage Origin

OSTEOCHONDROMA

Osteochondroma is the most common of the benign bone tumors and consists of a relatively large sessile or stalked spur or projection of adult bone topped by a cartilage cap and covered by periosteum (Fig. 9–1). This bone projection may spring from flat bones but usually arises at the joint end of a long bone, and characteristically points away from the joint toward the midpoint of the shaft of the bone (Fig. 9–2). Frequently a bursal sac develops overlying the projecting bone mass.

The lesion begins during the growth period and is found most frequently at the knee end of the femur and tibia and at the shoulder end of the humerus. The cartilage cap is most prominent in young patients and tends to involute with age. An osteochondroma ceases to grow at about the same time as the nearest growth line closes and tends to remain static unless disturbed by trauma. The presence of a single osteochondroma is a different, although possibly related, problem from that posed by the condition known as hereditary multiple exostoses (see p. 64).

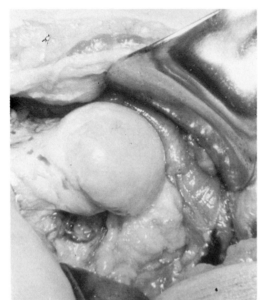

FIGURE 9–1. Gross appearance of an osteochondroma of distal femur exposed at surgery.

FIGURE 9–2. Osteochondroma of the distal femur.

Osteochondromas arise during childhood and 80 per cent are noted in patients under 21 years of age. Unless impinging on sensitive tissues, they are usually painless and asymptomatic. Most commonly the osteochondroma will be discovered quite casually when the patient notices a hard lump near a joint.

The cartilage cap possesses a latent capacity for malignant change, and on occasion, an osteochondroma has been known to undergo malignant transformation to a chondrosarcoma. The catalyst for the transformation is believed to be trauma, which could be delivered during physical activity or following inadequate surgical attempts to remove the bone mass. The incidence of chondrosarcomatous change in a solitary osteochondroma is substantially lower than it is in hereditary multiple exostoses.

Treatment consists of complete operative excision of the entire osteochondroma and overlying periosteum. Incomplete removal may result in recurrence or malignant transformation.

ENCHONDROMA

Enchondroma is a common benign tumor that is composed of facets of mature hyaline cartilage and appears as a single lesion within the confines of a bone. Enchondroma is the most common bone tumor found in the hand but is not infrequently discovered in other locations, such as ribs, femur, tibia, humerus, and pelvis. It seems to favor the distal rather than the proximal part of the shaft of the affected bone. The presence of a single enchondroma is a different, although possibly related, problem from that posed by the condition known as enchondromatosis or Ollier's disease. (see p. 126).

Enchondroma is believed to develop during the growth period, lie undetected for years, and come to clinical attention during adult life. Although some patients may notice mild ache or pain, the majority have no symptoms relative to the enchondroma for long periods of time. Most of these tumors are discovered after pathologic fracture has occurred, often following trivial injury.

Radiographic examination reveals a well-circumscribed round or oval lytic area in the end of the bone (Fig. 9–3). Frequently, radiographic evidence of calcification is noted within the tumor. Differential diagnosis includes small inclusion cysts lined by squamous epithelium, fibrous dysplasia, and bone cyst.

Although enchondromas of long bones may undergo malignant transformation to chondrosarcoma, chondrosarcomatous degeneration is considered more common in multiple enchondromatosis than in solitary enchondroma.

FIGURE 9–3. Enchondroma lying in proximal end of proximal phalanx of fourth finger. Note pathologic fracture.

Treatment of choice consists of opening into the cavity and thoroughly scraping out the cartilaginous contents. The resulting bone defect is packed with bone chips taken from the iliac crest.

BENIGN CHONDROBLASTOMA

Benign chondroblastoma is a relatively rare tumor believed to arise from cartilage cells or cartilage-forming connective tissue. The tumor has a curious predilection for young patients, particularly males in the second decade of life. The tumor regularly involves the epiphyseal end of a long bone, but may extend distally into the adjacent metaphyseal region. It is mostly encountered in long bones such as femur, tibia, and humerus. Its presence may cause pain and often an enlargement of the affected part.

Radiographic examination reveals a well-defined area of bone destruction lying within the epiphyseal area of the bone. The lesion may be round or ovoid in shape and presents an appearance of a fuzzily mottled rarefied focus which tends to be limited by a well-defined narrow encircling line of sclerotic bone. The mottling of its shadow reflects spotty calcification within the lesional tissue.

Treatment of choice consists of opening into the cavity and thoroughly scraping out the cartilaginous contents. The resulting defect is then packed with bone chips taken from the iliac crest. Benign chondroblastoma is associated with a very minimal recurrence rate and exhibits no tendency to undergo malignant transformation.

CHONDROMYXOID FIBROMA

Chondromyxoid fibroma is a relatively rare benign tumor of bone believed to be derived from cartilage-forming connective tissue which exhibits certain chondroid and myxoid traits. The tumor is encountered most frequently in young adults and tends to involve the lower extremity, particularly the distal metaphysis of the femur, the proximal metaphysis of the tibia, the distal fibula, the metatarsals, and the calcaneus.

Radiographic examination reveals a radiolucent rounded or oval lesion which tends to be located eccentrically in the metaphysis of the involved bone. More often than not it is surrounded by a shell of cortical bone which may appear scalloped.

Treatment of choice consists of opening into the cavity and thoroughly scraping out the contents and packing the resulting defect with bone chips taken from the ilium. Depending on the size of the lesion and its location, the tumor could also be treated by local resection.

Chondromyxoid fibroma appears to exhibit a slight tendency to recur locally. A few instances of chondrosarcomatous transformation have been reported.

II. Bone Origin

OSTEOID OSTEOMA

Osteoid osteoma is a not uncommon benign tumor of osteoblastic derivation identified by a rather characteristic radiographic and pathologic appearance and causing nagging pain in the patient.

The tumor is encountered mostly in children and young adults and appears to be somewhat more common in males. Although the lesion may occur anywhere in any bone, it is found most frequently in the lower extremity. Osteoid osteoma causes pain in the bone, often of a severe degree. If located in an accessible region, there may be a local tenderness to palpation, although no mass can usual-

FIGURE 9–4. Osteoid osteoma in distal tibia. Note the small oval clear space (nidus) surrounded by an area of sclerotic reactive bone. (Courtesy Dr. Leonard Ellenbogen, Atlantic City, N.J.)

ly be felt. The pain caused by osteoid osteoma is characteristically worse at night and, curiously, is often relieved by aspirin.

Typically, radiographic examination discloses a small oval clear space in bone, surrounded by a large area of sclerotic reactive bone (Fig. 9–4). The small oval clear space is called a nidus and contains the neoplastic tissue. This lesion must be differentiated from a small intracortical bone abscess and chronic sclerosing osteomyelitis.

Histologically, the lesion consists of varying proportions of osteoid tissue and fine new bone trabeculae in a vascular fibrous matrix.

Osteoid osteoma should be treated by operative removal of a block of bone containing the nidus. It is a good idea to radiograph the removed specimen to verify the presence of the nidus. Recurrence of the tumor is unlikely if the nidus has been completely removed.

OSTEOBLASTOMA

Osteoblastoma is a relatively rare benign vascular bone- and osteoid-producing tumor encountered most often in children and teenagers. It often causes pain and a tender swelling and is usually found in a bone of the lower extremity, vertebral column, or skull.

Radiographic examination discloses a well-circumscribed lesion which may appear radiolucent or mottled depending on the degree of focal calcification of osteoid and its conversion to bone. The tumor appears surrounded by a margin of sclerotic bone. Even if the overlying cortex is expanded by the tumor mass, the lesion would still be contained by a shell of periosteal bone. An osteoblastoma must be differentiated from osteoid osteoma, fibrous dysplasia, and giant cell tumor.

Treatment of choice consists of opening into the cavity and thoroughly scraping out the contents and packing the resulting defect with bone chips taken from the ilium. Depending on the size of the lesion and its location, the tumor could also be treated by local resection.

III. Blood Vessel Origin

HEMANGIOMA

Hemangioma is an uncommon benign tumor of bone composed of blood vascular channels of varied patterns. Hemangioma is most often encountered in the skull, vertebrae, and long bones of patients in the middle decades of life.

Radiographic examination discloses a characteristic distinctive vertically striated appearance to the lesion. If the lesion occurs in the spine, it is not unusual for the roentgenogram to show involvement of two or more contiguous vertebral bodies.

Hemangiomata involving the spine may cause symptoms because of direct pressure on the spinal cord or spinal nerve roots. Hemangioma is not believed to undergo malignant transformation.

Radiation therapy is usually satisfactory treatment for a hemangioma.

IV. Fibrous and Connective Tissue Origin

SUBPERIOSTEAL CORTICAL DEFECT

Subperiosteal cortical defects are completely asymptomatic, small, eccentrically placed cortical bone craters filled with fibrous tissue. It has been estimated that these lesions can be detected in as many as 20 per cent of all children at some stage during skeletal growth. They are associated with no clinical findings, represent true incidental findings on a radiograph, and require no treatment. They are sometimes referred to as "bone islands."

NONOSSIFYING FIBROMA

Nonossifying fibroma is the name given to an extremely common bone defect found most frequently in the long bones of the lower extremity during the patient's first two decades of life. The lesion consists of a localized area of bone tissue destruction with replacement by collagenous fibrous tissue.

Radiographic examination reveals an irregularly circular area of radiolucency, frequently exhibiting a scalloped border of sclerotic bone (Fig. 9–5). The typical location of a nonossifying fibroma is an eccentric position in the distal end of a long bone of the lower extremity. This lesion must be differentiated from bone cyst and fibrous dysplasia.

The majority of these lesions cause no symptoms and are discovered only when a radiographic examination is made for another reason. Occasionally the lesion may cause pain, and rarely it will cause pathologic fracture.

FIGURE 9–5. Nonossifying fibroma of distal tibia. Note its characteristic eccentric location.

FIGURE 9-6. Aneurysmal bone cyst of fourth metacarpal. Note bubble-like appearance.

It is believed that the natural course of a nonossifying fibroma is to undergo spontaneous healing. For this reason, definitive treatment of the lesion is rarely necessary.

ANEURYSMAL BONE CYST

Aneurysmal bone cyst is a benign, usually solitary expansile lesion of bone most often occurring in the metaphysis of long bones, vertebrae, and flat bones. As it grows, it causes a rather characteristic bubble or ballooning of the overlying cortex. Growth of the lesion containing blood-filled spaces tends to destroy and expand the host bone and stretch the overlying periosteum. The periosteal layer, so stimulated, lays down reactive bone that forms a shell around the tumor and contributes to the bubble-like appearance seen on the radiograph (Fig. 9–6).

Aneurysmal bone cysts are encountered most commonly during the second and third decades of life. Pain is the presenting complaint and a mass may be palpated if the tumor arises in a superficial bone. Extensive bleeding may occur if the overlying cortical bone shell is broken. Pathologic fracture through an aneurysmal bone cyst is not uncommon.

The rate of growth of aneurysmal bone cysts is unpredictable and may be rapid or quite slow. The tumor may involve more than one bone owing to expansion and is the only benign bone tumor that may extend from one bone to another in the vertebral column.

If feasible, treatment of choice is surgical curettage followed by packing of the resulting defect with bone graft material. If the lesion is in a site not easily accessible to surgery, as for example a vertebral body, radiation should control the lesion by sclerosing the blood vessels.

UNICAMERAL BONE CYST

Unicameral bone cyst is a benign cystic lesion of bone encountered most frequently in the upper end of the humerus and femur in children between three and fourteen years of age. The word *unicameral* means single chamber. This single-chamber cyst is lined with a grayish-white membrane and usually contains a clear yellowish or serosanguineous fluid. Bone cysts typically form just distal to the growth line but tend to migrate toward the center of the shaft as the bone grows.

Almost invariably the unicameral bone cyst is an asymptomatic lesion for most of its existence. Frequently, vague complaints of ache or mild discomfort in the area are overlooked. In about half of the patients, a unicameral bone cyst is discovered on roentgenographic examination made because a fracture occurs through the involved area following some traumatic incident (Fig. 9–7). Healing of this pathologic fracture occurs readily following immobilization of the part. In a few instances fracture healing has been noted to bring about spontaneous obliteration of the cyst, but this does not usually occur.

Radiographic examination discloses a round or oval defect in the metaphyseal region of the involved bone, often juxtaposed to the growth line. The long axis in these lesions is parallel to the long axis of the host bone. There often is thinning of the cortex and expansion secondary to slow growth within the medullary cavity. A dense line of cortical bone surrounding the margins of the cystic area is usually present, and ridging of the inner surface of the cyst may give a false multiloculated appearance. Evidence of fresh fracture through the cyst wall may be noted. In lesions through which prior fractures have occurred, an increased periosteal reaction and loculation may be noted.

A typical unicameral bone cyst is a solitary lesion that needs to be differentiated from aneurysmal bone cyst, eosinophilic granuloma, enchondroma, giant cell tumors, and solitary foci of fibrous dysplasia. The presence of multiple bone cysts should suggest hyper-

FIGURE 9-7. Unicameral bone cyst in proximal humerus of a child.

parathyroidism (see p. 122). Unicameral bone cysts have demonstrated no tendency to undergo malignant transformation. Their natural pathologic course would appear to be toward spontaneous healing.

Treatment of a bone cyst is surgical, although sporadically reports appear detailing good results after injection of various medications into the cyst. For many years the surgical treatment of choice consisted of opening the cyst cavity at operation and thoroughly scraping the cyst walls down to bleeding bone. The resulting defect was then filled with bone chips removed from the iliac crest. Long-term follow-up studies of the results obtained by this form of surgical therapy have shown a disappointing 20 to 30 per cent recurrence rate, which has awakened interest in other forms of surgical therapy. One of the most promising is subperiosteal diaphysectomy with total removal of the cyst-bearing portion of the bone. In this technique the periosteal tube surrounding the segment of diaphysis containing the cyst is elevated and the entire cyst-bearing segment of diaphysis is removed. Length is maintained by packing the periosteal tube with bone graft material and using postoperative traction. No recurrences following subperiosteal diaphysectomy have been reported to date.

GIANT CELL TUMOR

Giant cell tumor is a benign but potentially aggressive locally destructive neoplasm that develops within bone and apparently arises from the mesenchymal cells of the connective tissue framework. Giant cell tumors range the whole gamut from those that respond satisfactorily to treatment, through those that are more aggressive and prone to recur locally, to those that may eventually become sarcomatous and metastasize. Typically the lesion develops in the region of the epiphysis of long bones after the growth plate has closed, and it extends by growth into the metaphyseal area. The majority of giant cell tumors develop in the lower end of the femur, the upper end of the tibia, and the lower end of the radius in young adults, with the highest incidence in the third decade. As the lesion grows, it destroys bone and expands the overlying cortex, even to the point of erosion. The tumor may extend to the joint cartilage but usually not beyond.

Radiographic examination discloses an area of rarefaction in the end of a bone with a thinned and expanded cortex and no evidence of periosteal new bone formation over the thinned expanded cortex. The tumor not infrequently may present as a multilocular appearing cyst resembling an accumulation of soap bubbles (Fig. 9–8).

Grossly, the tumor consists of soft hemorrhagic material that has been likened to currant jelly. Microscopically the tumor consists of a moderately vascularized network of stromal cells and multinucleated giant cells meagerly interspersed with collagenous fibrils.

Treatment for this tumor depends upon the bone involved. Follow-up studies have shown that the surgical technique of thoroughly curetting out the tumor material and packing the resulting defect with iliac bone chips is followed by tumor recurrence in 50 to 60 per cent of patients. If the tumor is well-defined and in a surgically accessible area, local resection of the segment of bone containing the tumor and using bone graft material to restore bone continuity is the preferred method of surgical treatment.

If the tumor is encountered in an area that is not surgically accessible, radiotherapy may be used. However, both local recurrence and malignant transformation have been reported after radiation treatment.

Approximately 10 per cent of benign giant cell tumors undergo malignant transformation. A majority of malignant giant cell tumors are fibrosarcomas; a few are osteosarcomas.

FIGURE 9–8. Recurrent giant cell tumor in proximal tibia.

MALIGNANT BONE TUMORS

I. Cartilage Origin

PRIMARY CHONDROSARCOMA

Primary chondrosarcoma is a malignant cartilaginous tumor whose cells produce hyaline cartilage that is usually lobulated. Chondrosarcoma is the second most common primary malignant tumor of bone, with osteogenic sarcoma being the most frequent. In total frequency, however, chondrosarcoma occurs only about half as often as osteosarcoma. These are predominantly tumors of adulthood and old age and are somewhat more common in males. The majority of chondrosarcomas involve the pelvic bones, but other sites may include rib, femur, humerus, spine, scapula, and tibia.

Chondrosarcomas tend to grow slowly, extending along pathways of least resistance, and becoming large bulky tumors. Patients with primary chondrosarcomas appear to have a better survival record than those with the other primary malignant bone tumors. Patients with a well-differentiated chondrosarcoma do considerably better than those with a poorly differentiated tumor. The usual chondrosarcoma is well differentiated, and metastases occur in less than one-half of the patients. When metastases do occur, it is usually hematogenous to the lungs. Spread to regional lymph nodes may occur, but it is much less frequent. Pathologic fracture is uncommon because the periosteum frequently lays down new bone that protects against fracture. The greatest clinical problem with chondrosarcoma is local recurrence of the tumor.

Radiographic examination discloses a large multi-chambered area of bone destruction containing scattered areas of calcification (Fig. 9–9). Periosteal new bone formation may be seen around the tumor and the outline of a large bulky mass may be noted beyond the confines of the bone.

Treatment is amputation of the part containing the tumor or a large block excision depending on the site and size of the tumor. Radiation therapy and chemotherapy appear to be ineffective treatment modalities at this time.

FIGURE 9–9. Chondrosarcoma of scapula, showing bone destruction and scattered areas of calcification.

Secondary Chondrosarcoma

Chondrosarcoma may arise superimposed upon a pre-existing benign cartilaginous neoplasm. In this situation, the tumor is spoken of as secondary chondrosarcoma. Some of the primary conditions that may precede the development of secondary chondrosarcoma include osteochondroma, enchondroma, and Paget's disease.

II. Bone Origin

Osteosarcoma (Osteogenic Sarcoma)

Osteosarcoma is a malignant primary bone tumor consisting of malignant stroma with evidence of malignant osteoid, bone, and/or cartilage formation. Except for the marrow tumors, osteosarcoma is the most frequent and most fatal of the primary malignant bone tumors. The peak age incidence for this tumor is between 10 and 20 years with a slight predilection for males. Until recently five-year survival rates for this tumor have ranged from 10 to 20 per cent, with the average patient surviving for only about 18 months after diagnosis before succumbing to pulmonary metastases. Recent advances in chemotherapy for the treatment of osteosarcoma have begun to alter the pessimism in this disease with some five-year survival rates as high as 55 per cent being reported.

The tumor usually begins in the metaphysis of a long bone, particularly about the knee and shoulder, but practically never involves the joint space. Less often, the tumor may involve flat bones such as ilium or ribs. Most, if not all, osteosarcomas penetrate the cortex and invade the surrounding soft tissue before treatment can be instituted. The tumor tends to creep insidiously proximally up the medullary canal of the involved bone. Not infrequently "skip metastases" occur in the canal or bypass joints with subtle microfoci that can defy early detection.

Because this tumor destroys, erodes, and expands bone, pain is a constant and significant complaint. With time the pain becomes progressively more severe and persistent. As the tumor grows beyond the confines of the bone, it produces an obvious swelling or enlargement of the part. Pathologic fracture is rare as a presenting sign but may occur later in the disease process. Approximately one-half of the patients will exhibit an elevated alkaline phosphatase. Metastatic spread to the lung may occur quickly and early in an otherwise healthy appearing patient.

Radiographic examination discloses an irregular and ill-defined

FIGURE 9–10. Osteosarcoma of distal femur, showing bone destruction with erosion of tumor into soft parts and the formation of periosteal reactive bone.

area, usually in the metaphysis of a long bone, showing evidence of both bone destruction and bone formation with destruction of the cortex (Fig. 9–10). The tumor destroys bone in irregular fashion and erodes through the overlying cortex to grow out into the soft tissue. The tumor cells may produce a type of tumor bone that gives a density and a mottling through the tumor area on the radiograph. Reactive and neoplastic bone may be deposited along the blood vessels running through the tumor, giving the so-called "sun burst" effect frequently seen on radiographs. In addition, as the tumor grows it raises the periosteum, which is stimulated to lay down reactive bone. This reactive bone may be reflected on the radiograph as Codman's triangle, "onion-skin" appearance, or both.

Treatment of choice is amputation or disarticulation of the part bearing the tumor as soon as the diagnosis is established. Osteosarcoma is not sensitive to radiotherapy and no beneficial results have been reported from its use. Chemotherapy has recently shown exciting promise in prophylactically suppressing pulmonary micrometastases after surgical removal of the primary lesion.

Osteosarcoma has been known to develop secondarily in a pre-existing lesion in bone, such as Paget's disease or fibrous dysplasia, or in a previously irradiated bone. Malignant sarcomatous degeneration may arise in a bone that has been subjected to heavy irradiation. The tumors are mainly osteosarcomas and fibrosarcomas with an occasional chondrosarcoma. Survival rates are low, and most patients succumb to widespread metastases.

III. Marrow Origin

EWING'S SARCOMA

Ewing's sarcoma is an uncommon primary malignant tumor of bone apparently arising from immature reticulum cells or the primitive mesenchyme of the medullary cavity. Characteristically, it affects children and adolescents and usually involves the flat bones such as ilium, ribs, and vertebrae and the shafts of long bones, but it has been seen in almost all bones of the body. Males predominate in incidence in a ratio of approximately two to one.

Ewing's tumor begins in the medullary region of the bone and destroys bone from within. It may gradually erode to the cortex to grow out into the surrounding soft tissues. Spread of the tumor within the marrow cavity frequently causes a great deal of bone necrosis, but pathologic fracture is uncommon.

Extensive bone necrosis produced by Ewing's tumor may cause pain, swelling of the part, and local heat. In addition, the patient may present fever, leukocytosis, anemia, and an elevated sedimentation rate. These features, suggestive of infection, in association with radiologic evidence of bone destruction, may lead to a mistaken diagnosis of osteomyelitis.

Radiographic examination reveals an irregular area of bone destruction, usually in the shaft of a long bone and involving both the marrow cavity and overlying cortex (Fig. 9-11). As the tumor bursts through the confines of the bone, it raises the periosteum and so stimulates it to lay down strips of reactive bone. This is reflected on the radiograph as lamellation of the cortical bone or "onion-skin" appearance.

The microscopic picture of Ewing's sarcoma is fairly characteristic, consisting of small rounded closely packed cells forming dense sheets or nests.

Treatment for Ewing's tumor involves a combination of irradiation and long-term chemotherapy. Irradiation is used for its local effect and drug therapy for its systemic effect. Other than for biop-

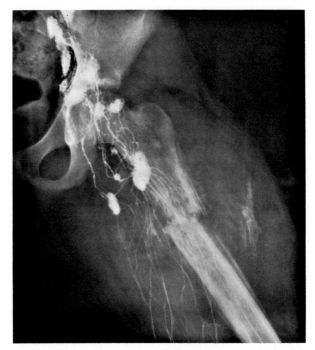

FIGURE 9-11. Ewing's tumor of femur. Note bone destruction involving marrow cavity and cortex, pathologic fracture, and "onion-skin appearance" along lateral cortex. Radiopaque material represents a lymphangiogram performed to detect regional lymph node metastasis. (Courtesy Dr. John Hope, The Children's Hospital, Philadelphia, Pa.)

sy, surgery plays a very limited role in the treatment of Ewing's sarcoma.

Until recently the mortality associated with Ewing's sarcoma was high because the tumor is aggressive and exhibits a propensity to spread to other bones as well as to the viscera and lungs. The average patient had a life expectancy of less than two years after onset of the tumor.

Aggressive chemotherapy is beginning to brighten the outlook for these patients. A combined modality therapy protocol consisting of Adriamycin, cyclophosphamide, vincristine, and brain irradiation has resulted in dramatic improvement in survival rates.

RETICULUM CELL SARCOMA

Reticulum cell sarcoma, a relatively uncommon tumor, is believed to represent an isolated focus of lymphoma apparently arising from the medullary cavity of bone. Reticulum cell sarcoma is the slowest growing and least malignant of the marrow tumors. Histologically its cellular picture is often quite difficult to distinguish from that of Ewing's sarcoma. Reticulum cell sarcoma, however, affects an older age group than Ewing's tumor, is less malignant, and may be associated with a 50 per cent 10-year survival rate.

The tumor is found in both long and flat bones. It may produce widespread bone destruction with expansion into the surrounding soft tissues. It frequently causes pain and may be associated with a palpable lump and pathologic fracture. Unlike Ewing's tumor, however, bone necrosis is not a feature of reticulum cell sarcoma, and consequently a systemic response suggesting infection is absent.

Radiographic examination reveals an irregular destructive process, usually in the shaft of long bones, involving medullary cavity and cortex. The presence of the tumor may cause an expansion of the affected shaft. Reactive bone formation within the tumor area gives the lesion a characteristic granular or mottled appearance on the radiograph (Fig. 9–12).

FIGURE 9–12.   Reticulum cell sarcoma of humerus with pathologic fracture.

Treatment for reticulum cell sarcoma consists of a combination of irradiation and long-term chemotherapy. Irradiation is used for its local effect and drug therapy for its systemic effect. Surgery is limited to biopsy and possibly to treatment of pathologic fractures of long bones.

Plasma Cell Myeloma (Multiple Myeloma)

Plasma cell myeloma is a neoplastic proliferation of the plasma cells of the bone marrow that may present as a clinically localized osseous lesion or as a systemic disease. It is generally accepted that plasma cell myeloma has its origin in the primitive reticulum cell.

It is only rarely encountered prior to 40 years of age but is the most commonly encountered primary malignant bone tumor beyond that age. The disease is seen more frequently in males than females in a ratio of approximately two to one.

The earliest lesions of myeloma are usually found in flat bones such as skull, pelvis, and vertebral bodies. The bone lesions cause erosion of the marrow cavity and overlying cortex, giving rise to bone pain and resulting quite frequently in pathologic fracture. Involvement of vertebral bodies may result in compression fractures and back pain. Other symptoms and signs that may be observed include weakness, neurologic involvement, kidney impairment, fever, anemia, and hypercalcemia. Amyloid deposits occur in approximately 10 per cent of patients with plasma cell myeloma.

Laboratory examination is of great help in establishing the diagnosis. Examination of marrow tissue taken by biopsy from the sternum or iliac crest frequently demonstrates myeloma cells. Hypercalcemia and hyperuricemia are frequently observed. The tumor produces large amounts of abnormal protein belonging to the globulin fraction. This abnormal protein, called *Bence Jones protein,* is excreted through the urine, and its presence may be detected in approximately 50 per cent of patients with multiple myeloma by examining a collected 24-hour urine sample. The production of abnormal protein results in an elevation of the value of total serum protein and a reversal of the normal albumin-globulin ratio. The electrophoretic pattern for total serum protein gives a characteristic tracing with abnormalities noted in the globulin fraction. Urine electrophoresis may also be a helpful study.

Radiographic examination characteristically reveals multiple discrete "punched out" areas, frequently affecting multiple bones, such as skull, vertebrae, pelvis, and shafts of long bones (Fig. 9–13). The lesions cause destruction of bone and appear as rounded, sharply demarcated "holes" in the bone. As a rule, no associated

FIGURE 9-13. Multiple myeloma involving humerus. Note pathologic fracture.

bone sclerosis or reactive bone formation around the lesions is seen on the radiograph.

Treatment consists of a combination of irradiation and long-term chemotherapy using Cytoxan (cyclophosphamide) and Alkeran (melphalan). Radiation is used for its local effect and drug therapy for its systemic effect. Surgery plays no definitive role in the treatment of plasma cell myeloma except for biopsy purposes or in the treatment of pathologic fractures.

Generally the disease has been noted to be fatal within one to three years after onset. The use of improved chemotherapeutic agents may improve the prognosis.

IV. Blood Vessel Origin

ANGIOSARCOMA

Angiosarcoma is a very rare malignant bone tumor apparently having its origin in the vasculature or precursor cells of bone blood vessels. It is a destructive and generally expansile lesion most frequently encountered in the femur of adults. It may involve multiple bones or several sites in a single bone.

The microscopic pattern is that of new blood vessel formation with endothelial proliferation.

Treatment consists of local tumor resection or amputation combined with radiotherapy. The prognosis for survival is poor.

V. Fibrous and Connective Tissue Origin

FIBROSARCOMA

Fibrosarcoma is a relatively rare malignant bone tumor believed to arise from the connective tissue of bone, either centrally (medullary) or peripherally (periosteal). It is a fibroblastic tumor which produces bundles of collagen fibers but no neoplastic bone, osteoid, or cartilage either in the primary tumor or in its metastases. The tumor may develop at any age but shows a predilection for patients in the adult and older age group. Fibrosarcoma usually involves long bones and many arise from femoral or tibial metaphyseal bone adjacent to the knee joint. The principal presenting symptom is pain. Pathologic fracture is infrequent.

Radiographic examination reveals an irregular, poorly defined area of bone destruction showing no evidence of bone formation either within the tumor proper or in the surrounding bone tissue.

Treatment of choice, depending on size and location of the tumor, is either local resection or amputation of the part. Irradiation and chemotherapy have been used in conjunction with surgery but no convincing beneficial effects of these additional modalities have been reported as yet. Prognosis for cure is poor with reported five-year survival rates ranging from 5 to 35 per cent.

In addition to primary tumors there are secondary fibrosarcomas of bone that may be associated with fibrous dysplasia, Paget's disease or giant cell tumor and fibrosarcomas seemingly induced by chronic osteomyelitis or irradiation.

Soft tissue fibrosarcoma may also occur and must be carefully distinguished from fibrosarcoma of bone. Treatment for soft tissue fibrosarcoma differs from that for bone involvement, and prognosis for cure is much better with soft tissue fibrosarcoma than with the bone tumor.

VI. Notochord Origin

CHORDOMA

Chordoma is one of the rarer primary tumors of bone and is encountered most frequently at either end of the axial skeleton, the basi-cranial area, or the sacrum and coccyx. It arises from primitive notochordal remnants in the intervertebral disc. The tumor is locally invasive and tends to destroy and replace the bone at its site of development. Chordoma grows slowly over a number of years and metastasizes rarely. It is encountered in males twice as frequently as females and rarely under 30 years of age.

Radiographic examination discloses an expanded rarefied destructive lesion in the affected bone.

Treatment is surgical excision if possible. This is frequently difficult to accomplish because of the extent of the growth. Thus local recurrence is a common problem. Occasionally high voltage irradiation is helpful.

VII. Metastatic Carcinoma

Primary carcinomas arising particularly in breast, prostate, kidney, thyroid, and lung may secondarily invade the bone tissue by direct extension or by way of blood stream or lymphatic transportation. Metastatic malignant tumor deposits in bone are more common than any of the primary malignant bone tumors. The tumor that most frequently metastasizes to bone is adenocarcinoma of the breast.

Some metastatic cancer deposits in the bone, such as breast cancer, may cause purely destructive lesions while others, such as prostatic carcinoma, may cause lesions characterized by reactive bone formation (Fig. 9–14). The bones most often affected are skull, spine, pelvis, femur, and humerus. It is believed that metastatic cancer deposits may be present in bone tissue for some time before causing enough destruction to be detected on standard radiographs. Usually, however, bone scan is positive if cancer deposits are present in bone even before their presence can be detected on radiographs.

Usually the first symptom to be noted is bone pain. This is particularly suggestive if the patient has had a prior diagnosis of a primary malignancy of a tissue such as breast or prostate. Pathologic fractures are rather common with metastatic carcinoma because

FIGURE 9–14. *A*, lytic lesions in femoral shaft due to metastatic adenocarcinoma of breast. *B*, same patient after "prophylactic" nailing using "stacked" intramedullary rods.

these lesions are frequently associated with marked bone destruction.

In some patients aspiration biopsy of the metastatic lesion can be carried out to establish the diagnosis and identify the primary site, while in other people open surgical biopsy may be required. Metastatic deposits in bone usually reproduce some of the cellular patterns characteristic of its tissue of origin.

Treatment depends to a great extent on the type and origin of the primary carcinoma that has metastasized to bone. Irradiation, hormones, chemotherapy, and surgery all play some role in the treatment program.

Surgery is most effective in the treatment of pathologic fractures, particularly of the major long bones. Whenever possible "prophylactic" internal fixation of major long bones should be considered if the presence of a large lesion presages an impending pathologic fracture. This spares the patient the excruciating pain of a long bone fracture.

The development of methyl methacrylate or "bone cement" has added another dimension to the palliative treatment of metastatic tumors of long bones with or without pathologic fracture. Large segments of diseased bone can be replaced by "bone cement" used in conjunction with sturdy internal fixation or prosthetic devices. Although not curative or even definitive, such surgical methods help to improve the quality of survival for patients with metastatic carcinoma and enable them to maintain a functional state for a longer period.

References

Aegerter, E. E., and Kirkpatrick, J. A., Jr.: Orthopedic Diseases: Physiology, Pathology, Radiology, 4th Edition. Philadelphia: W. B. Saunders Co., 1975.

Barnes, R., and Catto, M.: Chondrosarcoma of bone. J. Bone and Joint Surg., 48–B:729, 1966.

Enneking, W. F. (Ed.): Osteosarcoma. Clin. Ortho. and Rel. Res., No. 111, 1975.

Gartland, J. J., and Cole, F. L.: Modern concepts in the treatment of unicameral bone cysts of the proximal humerus. Ortho. Clin. of N.A. Vol. VI, No. 2, Philadelphia: W. B. Saunders Co., 1975.

Harrington, K. D., Sim, F. H., Enis, J. E., Johnston, J. O., Dick, H. M., and Gristina, A. G.: Methlymethacrylate as an adjunct in internal fixation of pathologic fractures. J. Bone and Joint Surg., 58–A:1047, 1976.

Larsson, S. E., Lorentzon, R., and Boquist, L.: Fibrosarcoma of bone. A demographic, clinical and histopathological study of all cases recorded in the Swedish Cancer Registry from 1958 to 1969. J. Bone and Joint Surg., 58–B:412, 1976.

Pomeroy, T. C., and Johnson, R. C.: Combined modality therapy of Ewing's sarcoma. Cancer, 35:36, 1975.

Price, C. H. G., Zhuber, K., Salzer-Kuntschik, M., Salzer, M., Willert, H. G., Immenkamp, M., Groh, P., Matejovsky, Z., and Kehl, W.: Osteosarcoma in children. A study of 125 cases. J. Bone and Joint Surg., 57–B:341, 1975.

Simon, M. A., and Enneking, W. F.: The management of soft-tissue sarcomas of the extremities. J. Bone and Joint Surg., 58–A:317, 1976.

Spjut, H. J., Dorfman, H. D., Fechner, R. E., and Ackerman, L. V.: Tumors of bone and cartilage. Armed Forces Institute of Pathology, Washington, D. C., 1971.

Sutow, W. W., Gehan, B. A., Vietti, T. J., Frias, A. E., and Dyment, P. G.: Multidrug chemotherapy and primary treatment of osteosarcoma. J. Bone and Joint Surg., 58–A:629, 1976.

CHAPTER 10

DISORDERS OF THE SHOULDER

INTRODUCTION

The term shoulder is used clinically to encompass the entire shoulder girdle. The shoulder girdle comprises the upper humerus, scapula, clavicle, and sternum, articulating through the glenohumeral, acromioclavicular, and sternoclavicular joints (Fig. 10–1). Although the glenohumeral joint, or shoulder joint proper, is the major and most important element of the shoulder girdle, all component parts play a role in successful arm trunk movements. Injury or disease affecting any part of the shoulder girdle may result in a painful shoulder or a disturbance of shoulder function.

As an element of the shoulder girdle, the clavicle acts as an outrigger to hold the arm and the scapula outward and backward. Full elevation of the arm in the direction of either forward flexion or abduction takes place chiefly through the glenohumeral joint, but must be accompanied by rotation of the scapula on the thorax to be completed. Rotation of the scapula is dependent upon movement through the acromioclavicular joint and rotation of the clavicle through the sternoclavicular joint. Thus it can be seen that an apparently simple maneuver, such as raising one's arm, depends upon a complicated interdependence of several joints working in rhythm and involves all the component parts of the shoulder girdle.

244

FIGURE 10–1. Functional components of the shoulder joint. *A*, sternoclavicular joint. *B*, acromioclavicular joint. *C*, glenohumeral joint. *D*, thoracocapsular joint. (From De-Palma, A. F.: Surgery of the Shoulder, 2nd ed. Philadelphia: J. B. Lippincott Co., 1973.)

GENERAL CONSIDERATIONS

The shoulder joint proper, or glenohumeral joint, is the pivotal joint of the upper extremity. Consider how difficult everyday motions such as reaching up to a shelf or scratching your back would be without an extremely movable shoulder joint. There is a price for this mobility, however, and that price is a sacrifice in stability. A glance at the anatomy of the joint shows that it is indeed constructed for mobility rather than stability.

The shoulder joint, like the hip, is a ball and socket joint. In contrast to the hip joint, however, the humeral head presents a small area of bony contact to the glenoid which, in turn, constitutes a very shallow socket. Both bony parts are enclosed in a loose capsule. The overhanging coracoacromial arch prevents upward displacement of the humerus at the shoulder joint, but the joint depends mainly upon muscles for its stability. Four short muscles, the teres minor, the infraspinatus, the supraspinatus, and the subscapularis, arise closely around the humeral head and support it. Their tendons blend with one another and with the joint capsule to form a conjoined tendon that inserts in and about the greater tuberosity of the humerus. This conjoined tendon is spoken of as the musculotendinous or rotator cuff of the shoulder, and its chief function is to stabilize the humeral head in the glenoid cavity. The long muscles that pass across the joint, such as the biceps, coracobrachialis, deltoid, latissimus dorsi, triceps, pectoralis major, and teres major, are the prime movers of the joint.

A joint that presents loose bony contact and depends upon muscles for stability will indeed be flexible, but it will also be structurally weak. For this reason, the majority of orthopaedic problems encountered about the shoulder joint involve the soft tissue components of the joint rather than the bony parts. Degenerative arthritis of the shoulder joint, for example, is most unusual. It should also be noted that the shoulder is the only joint in the body in which recurrent dislocation is common.

Contrast the function and behavior of the shoulder joint with that of the hip joint, which is the counterpart pivotal joint of the lower extremity (see p. 377). In the hip joint, mobility is sacrificed for stability.

INTERVIEWING AND EXAMINING THE PATIENT

The majority of patients presenting with a shoulder problem do so because of pain, ache, or some type of discomfort. Less commonly the presenting complaint is stiffness, weakness, or deformity. Pain in the shoulder area may arise from a problem primarily in the joint, or it may be referred to the part from a problem originating elsewhere in the body. Referred pain can usually be traced to cervical spine disorders, cardiac disorders, gall bladder disease, or diseases involving the mediastinum or diaphragm. Referred pain, however, is less likely to be accompanied by local tenderness and limitation of motion. A good searching history and complete physical examination should enable the examiner to distinguish between primary and referred causes of shoulder pain.

THE INTERVIEW

The patient should be asked to describe the complaint and to point to the area involved. Many times an important clue can be obtained immediately. If the complaint is pain, its type should be determined. Pain in some shoulder disorders is brought on only by movement, while in others the pain is present constantly. The type and location of any radiating pain should be ascertained.

A clear statement should be obtained about the duration of symptoms, beginning with the type of onset and the subsequent progress. It is important to determine if the patient has previously had similar episodes and, if so, how they were treated. The patient should be questioned concerning a history of trauma or possible occupational diseases.

Primary shoulder disorders present symptoms that are definitely related to shoulder and arm motion. This pain should be clearly delineated by the history. Many shoulder problems are characteristically aggravated by certain activities, such as combing the hair, putting on a coat, reaching into the back pocket, or finding a comfortable position for the arm in bed at night. It is also important to question the patient about activities that relieve the complaint.

THE EXAMINATION

It is necessary that the patient be sufficiently undressed for the examination. Males may be stripped to the waist. Females should be gowned in such a manner that both arms and shoulders and the upper chest are exposed. The local examination of a patient with shoulder complaint begins at the sternal notch and covers the entire shoulder girdle, utilizing the unaffected side as the control.

Inspection. The examiner should look for any evidence of deformity, atrophy, redness, or swelling or for any abnormality that might distinguish one shoulder from the other.

Palpation. The area is palpated for evidence of swelling, deformity, muscle spasm, or local painful areas with special reference to the sternoclavicular joint, clavicle, acromioclavicular joint, shoulder joint, rotator cuff, and bicipital groove.

Range of Motion. The range of joint motion is assessed both actively and passively. Both shoulders are put through a full active range of flexion, extension, abduction, adduction, and internal and external rotation, and any differences are noted. Observation is made of the shoulder rhythm in relation to glenohumeral motion and scapular rotation (Fig. 10–2). It must be remembered that shoulder girdle motion also occurs between the scapula and the posterior thoracic wall. When the arm is abducted to 180 degrees at the shoulder, there is approximately 1 degree of scapulothoracic

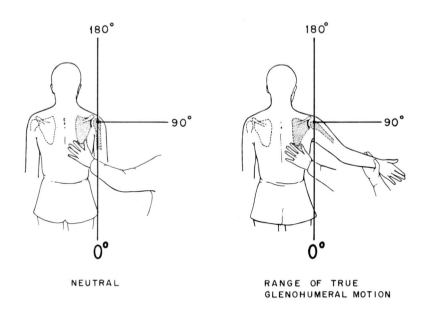

NEUTRAL

RANGE OF TRUE
GLENOHUMERAL MOTION

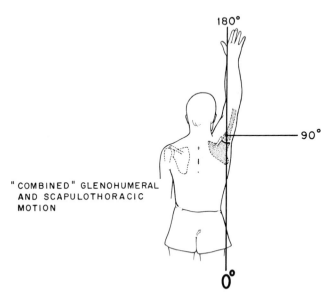

"COMBINED" GLENOHUMERAL
AND SCAPULOTHORACIC
MOTION

FIGURE 10–2. Elevation of the arm at the shoulder joint involves both the glenohumeral and scapulothoracic components. (Courtesy of American Academy of Orthopaedic Surgeons.)

motion for each 2 degrees of glenohumeral motion. The same motions are checked passively to uncover any joint tightness.

Special Maneuvers. Special maneuvers are required for specific diagnoses, such as evaluating the strength of the rotator cuff in case of suspected cuff tear or determining if forced supination of the forearm gives pain in the bicipital groove.

Neurologic Examination. The examiner should evaluate muscle power, not only in the shoulder girdle region, but in the entire upper extremity. The presence of muscle clonus or spasticity and evidence of sensory changes should be noted. The biceps, triceps, and brachioradialis reflexes should be compared.

Radiographic Examination. The most useful routine views are anteroposterior projections taken with the shoulder in internal and external rotation. The lateral view of the shoulder joint is difficult to interpret because of overlap of the thoracic contents. An axillary view of the shoulder joint is occasionally helpful, particularly if a posterior dislocation of the shoulder joint is suspected.

Arthrography is indicated for patients in whom the cause of the shoulder pain is in doubt. It provides information not available without exploratory surgery and demonstrates soft tissue injuries that are not seen on standard roentgenograms and may not be noted by physical examination. Arthrography of the shoulder joint can aid in the diagnosis of a variety of lesions including rotator cuff tear, subluxation and recurrent dislocation of the shoulder, subluxation and rupture of the biceps tendon, anterior capsular derangements, frozen shoulder deformity, and combinations of these abnormalities.

DISORDERS OF THE STERNOCLAVICULAR JOINT

DISLOCATION

A force applied to the arm, shoulder, or chest may cause a traumatic dislocation of the medial end of the clavicle at the sternoclavicular joint. The displaced clavicle rides upward causing a visible and palpable prominence of the joint. The prominence is apparent when the injured joint is compared with its counterpart joint on the opposite side. In rare instances, the dislocation may be posterior. Radiographic examination confirms the diagnosis.

In most instances, the dislocation can be reduced by closed manipulation. If closed reduction is unsuccessful, open reduction can be performed with the reduction maintained by the temporary use of metallic pin fixation.

OLD DISLOCATION

Occasionally, a patient presents with an unreduced sternoclavicular dislocation of long standing. No treatment is attempted if the dislocation is asymptomatic. If it is causing pain or distress because of its instability, reconstruction of the joint aided by temporary internal fixation may be carried out. Some orthopaedic surgeons prefer to excise the dislocated end of the clavicle as an alternative procedure to relieve pain.

DEGENERATIVE ARTHRITIS

Degenerative arthritis may affect the sternoclavicular joint and give rise to a painful thickening and swelling of the joint. A patient may seek attention because of a "lump" in the neck area.

In the acute stage, the joint may be warm, thickened, and tender. Later, all symptoms and signs may subside, but the thickness and enlargement usually remain. This condition may be related to Tietze's syndrome, which is characterized by pain, swelling, and tenderness of the second and third costochondral junction (see p. 328).

Pain may be relieved by warm applications and by the use of orally administered anti-inflammatory agents. Sometimes it is necessary to inject hydrocortisone into the sternoclavicular joint. Surgical treatment is usually not required.

DISORDERS OF THE ACROMIOCLAVICULAR JOINT

The acromioclavicular joint is not uncommonly injured by athletic and industrial accidents. A direct blow or fall upon the shoulder may tear the supporting ligaments and cause varying degrees of disruption of the joint. After this type of injury, the weight of the dependent arm pulls the acromion down and the lateral end of the clavicle may displace out of the joint and become prominent beneath the skin.

Degenerative arthritis may also affect the acromioclavicular joint to cause shoulder girdle pain.

SUBLUXATION

If the injury tears the joint capsule and overlying musculature, but spares the conoid and trapezoid ligaments linking the coracoid process to the clavicle, the degree of joint disruption is minimal and injury is described as a subluxation of the joint. To demonstrate incomplete displacement of the acromioclavicular joint radiographically, the film must be taken with the patient in the standing position while holding a weight in the hand of the affected side. The weight tends to pull the acromion downward and allows some upper migration of the lateral end of the clavicle.

Most subluxations can be treated by a combination of a pressure strapping centered over the joint and sling support for the arm. This holds the joint together until healing occurs. Occasionally the strapping will have to encircle both the shoulder and the elbow in order to elevate the acromion enough to bring about a reduction.

DISLOCATION

Complete dislocation of the acromioclavicular joint occurs when the injury ruptures the joint capsule and overlying musculature along with the conoid and trapezoid ligaments. This is the "shoulder separation" so often sustained by athletes. With the arm dependent, displacement of the clavicle is obvious both clinically and radiographically (Fig. 10–3).

FIGURE 10–3. Complete traumatic dislocation of acromioclavicular joint (shoulder separation). (Courtesy Dr. Phillip Marone, Methodist Hospital, Philadelphia, Pa.)

Treatment for this injury varies with the experience and judgment of the physician. Nonoperative treatment utilizes some type of encircling bandage designed to reduce the dislocation and hold the parts together until healing occurs. Easy-to-apply splints are now available from commercial manufacturers and appear to be quite efficient in maintaining reduction of the dislocation. Many surgical techniques are available for the operative treatment of acromioclavicular dislocations and most give satisfactory final results. A satisfactory operative treatment in older patients or those in sedentary occupations is excision of the distal pole of the clavicle.

ACQUIRED DEGENERATIVE ARTHRITIS

Acquired degenerative arthritis in the acromioclavicular joint may be a cause of shoulder area pain seen for the most part in the older patient. The condition is more frequent in males, particularly those who have subjected the joint to repeated trauma from either athletic or occupational demands. Movement through the acromioclavicular joint is limited to its role in the shoulder girdle mechanism, but the joint can be subjected to compression and shearing forces. For this reason, adduction of the arm across the chest and abduction above the horizontal are the motions that cause shoulder pain when the acromioclavicular joint is involved. For the same reason, these patients frequently experience pain in the affected shoulder when they sleep on that side.

In most patients, the joint margins will be felt to be enlarged and roughened, and visible enlargement of the joint is frequently observed. Direct pressure on the joint may elicit pain. Often surprisingly little actual damage to the joint is noted on radiographic examination even in patients presenting marked clinical findings. This is because the majority of the changes involve the soft tissue and cartilage components of the joint, which are not visible on the radiograph. Thus, there is usually no direct proportional relationship between the severity of the clinical findings and the degree of degenerative change noted on the radiograph. The pain due to acquired degenerative arthritis of the acromioclavicular joint can be relieved in the majority of patients by hydrocortisone injected into and around the involved joint. Local hydrocortisone may be combined with appropriate oral doses of an anti-inflammatory agent and with local heat applied to the joint. If the symptoms cannot be controlled by these measures, the distal end of the clavicle may be removed by operation. This widens the joint and relieves the pain.

FIGURE 10-4. Fracture of left clavicle in child.

FRACTURE OF THE CLAVICLE

The clavicle may be broken by a fall on the arm or shoulder. The injury is encountered much more frequently in children than in adults. Occasionally the clavicle of the newborn infant is fractured during a difficult delivery. The bone usually breaks cleanly through its midportion, but on rare occasions, a bone fragment may protrude through the skin or pierce the subclavian artery. As a consequence of the clavicular fracture, the shoulder loses its outrigger strut, and the shoulder tends to droop downward and forward, adding to the displacement of the fragments (Fig. 10-4).

TREATMENT IN CHILDREN

Fracture of the clavicle is a fairly common injury in children. Satisfactory reduction can be achieved in most children by applying a figure-of-eight bandage made either of elastic bandages or plaster, which will tend to hold the shoulders upward and backward. Open reduction is not necessary in children because of the capacity of growing bone to reshape and remodel its contours.

TREATMENT IN ADULTS

In adults it is important to obtain and maintain good apposition of the fracture fragments. It may be possible to reduce the fragment satisfactorily by moving the shoulders upward and backward. The reduced position, once obtained, may be maintained by a plaster of paris figure of eight bandage or shoulder spica.

Open reduction of clavicular fractures is rarely indicated in adults except for complicated fractures or possibly electively in the management of patients with multiple injuries.

FRACTURE OF THE SCAPULA

Fracture of a portion of the scapula is an unusual injury and is caused most frequently by a direct blow. It is usually seen in association with other injuries in patients sustaining severe trauma. Displacement of the fragments is rare because the scapula is encased in a heavy muscular envelope.

Most fractures of the scapula heal readily when treated with simple support to the arm and local measures to the scapular area to relieve pain and swelling.

DISORDERS OF THE SHOULDER JOINT (GLENOHUMERAL)
Trauma

SPRAIN

An injury caused by twisting the upper extremity or shoulder region can result in a stretching of the capsule or muscles about the shoulder joint that may produce a temporary painful disability. This may be associated with bleeding into the joint (hemarthrosis) that will give the shoulder region a swollen appearance. Radiographic examination will be negative except for possible capsular swelling. Simple sling support, combined with cold compresses, is helpful in relieving pain. Motion should be encouraged as soon as comfort permits. Moist heat to the area is beneficial as motion begins to return.

FRACTURE

In an elderly person, a fall on the hand or arm frequently causes a fracture of the humerus through the surgical neck region. Immediate pain and disability are noted by the patient. Although the radiograph may disclose varying degrees of impaction, comminution, or displacement of the fragments, the position is usually acceptable in the majority of these older patients and no actual reduction is necessary (Fig. 10–5). The arm and shoulder are immobilized in a Velpeau bandage for three weeks, after which activity may be resumed. A satisfactory range of shoulder motion is usually regained even if the fragments heal in a moderately deformed position.

FIGURE 10–5. Comminuted fracture through surgical neck region of humerus.

If the displacement of the fragments is too severe to expect return to a functional range of shoulder motion, open reduction can be carried out to replace the fragments in a more anatomic position. If comminution is so severe that open reduction is impractical, the fragments can be excised and replaced with a metallic humeral head prosthesis. Total shoulder prostheses are now being developed for use in those few patients in whom severe trauma or disease has resulted in destruction of the shoulder joint, including, in some patients, loss of the rotator cuff. The units of a total shoulder prosthesis are fixed to the humeral shaft and scapula with methyl methacrylate bone cement.

Occasionally, fractures through the greater tuberosity of the humerus require open reduction. In such instances, the attached musculotendinous cuff has retracted and pulled the tuberosity fragment up towards or under the acromion. The only treatment of value is to reattach the fragment in its proper position by suture or screw fixation (Fig. 10–6).

DISLOCATION

A force applied to an upper extremity may result in an abnormal degree of abduction and external rotation to the humerus and

FIGURE 10–6. Fracture through the surgical neck of the humerus with marked upward displacement of the greater tuberosity fragment. (Compare with Figure 10–5.)

force the humeral head to tear out of the joint and lodge beneath the coracoid process of the scapula (Fig. 10–7). This injury is called an anterior shoulder dislocation and may occur in any age group. In order for the joint to dislocate anteriorly, the subscapularis muscle must stretch or tear along with the anterior joint capsule. Rarely, the shoulder may dislocate posteriorly. A posterior dislocation may be difficult to appreciate on routine shoulder radiographs and an axillary view would be needed to demonstrate its presence.

A patient with an anterior dislocation of the shoulder joint seeks medical attention because of shoulder pain and severe disability. Inspection reveals a typical flattening of the normally rounded shoulder contour when compared to the uninvolved side. Palpation reveals displacement of the humeral head from its normal position beneath the acromion to the subcoracoid region. Both before and after reduction, the examiner must always check the integrity of the axillary, radial, median, and ulnar nerves and the arterial circulation.

As soon as the diagnosis is confirmed by radiographic examination, the dislocation is reduced by manipulation, and the arm and shoulder are immobilized in a Velpeau bandage for three or four weeks.

Associated fracture of the humeral head or greater tuberosity sometimes accompanies dislocation of the shoulder joint in middle-aged or elderly patients. In most of these patients, however, successful reduction of the dislocation also reduces the accompanying fracture.

Less frequently, a complete fracture through the upper shaft of the humerus may be seen in association with dislocation of the humeral head. This is a serious and complex injury, and open reduction with internal fixation is required to secure the fragments in position.

FIGURE 10-7. Anterior dislocation of the right shoulder with fracture through greater tuberosity.

RECURRENT DISLOCATION

Dislocation of the shoulder joint in a younger patient carries with it a high recurrence rate, estimated to be as great as 40 per cent. This predilection for redislocation is unique to the shoulder joint. Recurrence is not prominent in middle-aged or elderly patients because of the normal tendency of the subscapularis muscle to tighten with age, thereby effectively limiting the motion of external rotation. Authorities are not agreed upon the cause of recurrent dislocation. Undoubtedly some type of capsular or tendinous stretching occurs with the initial dislocation that does not completely heal, but there is not universal agreement about its exact nature. The tendency for redislocation is definitely related to the inherent anatomic instability of the shoulder joint. Although recurrent dislocation may occur posteriorly, the great majority of patients with this disorder sustain recurrent anterior dislocation.

Anterior dislocation may occur on abduction and external rotation of the arm. Some patients experience multiple shoulder dislocations following unguarded movements of the arm, and many patients become adept at reducing their own dislocations. Recurrence can become so frequent as to preclude rigorous physical activity in an otherwise healthy person.

No amount of immobilization will cure the tendency for the shoulder joint to dislocate repeatedly. Operative repair is necessary for a permanent correction of this condition. Many different successful surgical techniques are available to tighten the soft tissue components of the joint to prevent redislocation.

RUPTURE OF THE BICEPS TENDON

The tendon of the long head of the biceps brachii muscle lies in the bicipital groove of the humerus, where it may undergo degenerative changes with resulting loss of tensile strength. Shoulder pain may be noted by the patient as the degenerative tendon and tendon sheath changes occur. Some evidence has been presented that implicates the use of hydrocortisone injections into the tendon sheath of the biceps tendon in degenerative changes of the tendon tissue (see bicipital tenosynovitis, p. 265).

By lifting or lowering a heavy object, the patient may apply a sudden force to this weakened tendon and may cause it to fray apart in the bicipital groove, with resulting pain and weakness in the arm. The small proximal piece of tendon remains in position in the bicipital groove, but the distal fragment with the attached muscle belly retracts toward the elbow. The torn biceps muscle belly shortens, giving a ball-like appearance to the arm muscle. The lower shoulder and upper arm area is tender to palpation and a muscular gap can be felt. The tissues appear swollen and indurated, and the overlying skin becomes ecchymotic. Weakness in flexion of the elbow and supination of the forearm are noted by the patient.

Operative repair may be carried out. The distal tendon fragment with the attached muscle belly is located and fastened to the bicipital groove of the humerus with sutures or a metallic staple.

Less commonly, the rupture may occur at the elbow where the biceps tendon inserts distally on the bicipital tuberosity of the radius. In this instance, the muscle belly retracts towards the shoulder and must be reattached to the bicipital tuberosity by operation.

TEARS OF THE ROTATOR CUFF

The musculotendinous or rotator cuff of the shoulder, which acts to stabilize the humeral head in the glenoid cavity so that the motion of shoulder abduction can be initiated, normally undergoes some degenerative changes with advancing age. Asymptomatic "worn out" spots may appear in the cuff. If a sudden adduction force is applied to such a cuff while the arm is being held in abduction, particularly in a patient over 40 years of age, traumatic tears of the cuff tissue can occur that may make it impossible for the patient to initiate the movement of shoulder abduction.

The patient may be aware of immediate pain in the shoulder. Local tenderness may be noted over the cuff and the patient may be unable to initiate or maintain active abduction of the arm at the shoulder joint. If the examiner passively places the arm in abduction at the shoulder, the patient may be unable to sustain this position and the arm will drop to the side. Full passive mobility of the shoulder joint, however, is not lost.

Routine radiographic examination of the shoulder is negative unless there is an associated fracture. The diagnosis may be confirmed by injecting air or dye into the shoulder joint and observing its escape into the subdeltoid bursa on a radiograph. This study is called an *arthrogram*.

The initial treatment of a tear of the rotator cuff is conservative, because many patients sustain only incomplete ruptures and they gradually recover strength and motion spontaneously. The arm is supported in a sling, and hot applications may be used on the shoulder. Surgical exploration of the rotator cuff area is reserved for those patients who do not recover on a conservative program after a four to six week trial. These patients have usually sustained massive tears or complete ruptures of the rotator cuff that will necessitate operative repair.

Derangements of the Subacromial Mechanism

The painful shoulder is a complaint that is fairly common to all age groups in both sexes, and in order to treat these patients satisfactorily, a diagnosis of the exact cause must be determined in each patient. The use of "bursitis" as an all-inclusive term denoting the diagnosis and basis for therapy in the painful shoulder syndrome is irrational. Excluding the traumatic causes already discussed, shoulder pain may radiate from a lesion of the cervical spine or may represent irritation from some other organ, such as gall bladder or heart. Most frequently, however, it originates in the shoulder joint proper as some derangement of what is known as the subacromial mechanism.

The subacromial mechanism of the shoulder joint is bounded above by the acromion and the coracoacromial ligament and below by the humeral head. Its component structures include the subacromial and subdeltoid bursa, the musculotendinous or rotator cuff, the articular capsule of the shoulder joint, and the tendon-tendon sheath gliding mechanism of the tendon of the long head of the biceps brachii muscle (Fig. 10–8).

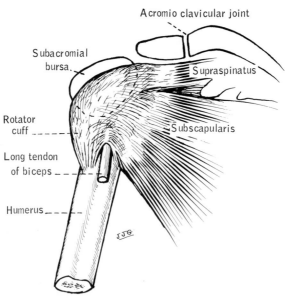

FIGURE 10–8.   Subacromial mechanism of shoulder.

The majority of patients with shoulder pain will be found to have some lesion involving a component of this mechanism. The use of the blanket term "bursitis" to explain all the derangements of the subacromial mechanism is overly simplistic in the face of all the possible causes of a painful or stiff shoulder. All lesions of the subacromial mechanism may secondarily involve the subdeltoid bursa, but only rarely is a true primary subdeltoid bursitis encountered. The most frequently seen derangements of the subacromial mechanism causing shoulder pain are calcific deposits in the musculotendinous cuff, bicipital tenosynovitis, lesions of the acromio-clavicular joint, and frozen shoulder deformity or adhesive capsulitis of the shoulder joint.

Calcium Deposits

Amorphous calcium deposits may occur in many soft tissue sites throughout the body, giving rise to pain and dysfunction. By far the most common site for the deposition of amorphous calcium is the musculotendinous or rotator cuff of the shoulder. Calcification usually occurs in the supraspinatus portion of the cuff. This is the condition most commonly referred to erroneously as "bursitis."

Calcium deposits in the shoulder are seen most frequently during the third, fourth, and fifth decades of life and are slightly more common in the male. There is a high incidence in "white collar" workers and housewives. The mechanism by which calcium is deposited in the area is unclear. Vascular profusion studies of the rotator cuff tendon reveal a "critical zone" or zone of poor blood supply near the area of attachment of the supraspinatus tendon to the greater tuberosity. Since this area also corresponds to the common site of calcium deposits in the shoulder, it has been postulated that both vascular and mechanical factors play a role in the deposition of calcium.

The physical characteristics of the calcium deposit will greatly influence the type of pain experienced by the patient. If the calcium is in a liquid or soft state, an acute process will ensue, characterized by severe throbbing shoulder pain and marked disability. If the deposit is dry, gritty and hard, a chronic picture is produced, characterized by less intense shoulder ache and a "catching" pain on certain motions associated with raising the arm above the horizontal plane.

Acute Stage. The acute stage is characterized by severe, disabling shoulder pain that has been known to reduce an adult to tears. It is often described as a constant throbbing or beating type of pain. Although markedly aggravated by motion of the shoulder, the pain is constantly present even when the shoulder is immobile. This point is useful in distinguishing the acute stage from the chronic stage or from a bicipital tenosynovitis. In the latter two conditions, shoulder pain is not present constantly, but rather is brought on by movements of the arm and shoulder.

The onset of shoulder pain may be sudden and surprising or may be preceded by a few days of shoulder ache. The pain originates in the shoulder cuff region, but it may radiate up into the neck or down into the forearm and hand. Exquisite tenderness may be produced by palpation over the area of the calcium deposit. The patient usually holds the arm splinted to the side.

Anteroposterior radiographs of the shoulder joint, taken with the arm in both external and internal rotation, reveal the amorphous calcium deposit in the rotator cuff area (Fig. 10–9).

FIGURE 10–9. Calcium deposit lying in the rotator cuff just above the greater tuberosity of the right humerus.

Chronic Stage. The chronic stage is characterized by ache or pain in the shoulder brought on by movement of the arm. The patient may be aware of a constant ache or an uncomfortable sensation in the shoulder, but it is never as severe or disabling as an acute process. Usually the patient can get along quite well if certain motions of the shoulder, such as raising the arm above the horizontal plane and throwing a ball, are avoided. This type of motion produces the so-called "painful arc syndrome" in which pain is caused by impingement of the hard calcified material underneath the coracoacromial ligament as the arm is raised in abduction. The patient with a chronic calcium deposit usually has had discomfort for many months and has learned to avoid painful movements. Those patients notice pain when they attempt to lie on the affected shoulder at night, or they complain of difficulty in finding a comfortable position for the arm in bed. Radiographic examination of the shoulder joint will reveal the presence of a calcium deposit.

Mixed Stage. Occasionally a patient with a dry, hard calcium deposit in the rotator cuff (chronic stage) will sustain fresh trauma to the affected shoulder and, in the space of a few hours, develop severe disabling shoulder pain. In this instance, the fresh trauma has caused the hard, dry calcified material to pass into the liquid or soft state. The clinical picture produced is identical to that described for the acute stage. Gardening, lifting heavy objects, shoveling, and carrying heavy suitcases are activities that frequently bring about this change in the physical characteristics of the calcium deposit.

Treatment. "Needling" of the calcium deposit is frequently very effective treatment. Once the site of the calcification has been localized by clinical and radiographic examination, the deposit is entered with an 18-gauge needle under local anesthesia. Multiple needle puncture of the calcium deposit is carried out by moving the point of the needle rapidly into and out of the deposit. This maneuver serves to break up the localized calcium deposit and lessen its tension, and it also tends to change the local tissue pH to the acid side by bringing fresh blood to the area. This is helpful because calcium tends to go into solution in an acid medium. Calcium can sometimes be aspirated into the syringe, although this is not necessary in order to effect a cure. Before the needle is withdrawn, hydrocortisone may be injected into the deposit area for its "anti-inflammatory" effect. Some physicians combine "needling" with the oral administration of anti-inflammatory drugs. If this treatment is successful, the patient will notice a rapid disappearance of the constant beating pain and a gradual return of normal shoulder motion and function.

Surgical excision of the calcium is advised when the deposit is too large to be needled effectively, when there are repeated recurrences, or when the radiograph shows the calcium deposit to be burrowing into the bone.

Under no circumstances should heat, in any of its forms, be applied to a shoulder during the acute stage of a calcium deposit. This usually results in increased shoulder pain. Ice packs to the shoulder are more soothing. After the acute stage has been treated, heat is helpful in restoring motion to the joint.

BICIPITAL TENOSYNOVITIS

Mechanical tenosynovitis involving the tendon-tendon sheath gliding mechanism of the long tendon of the biceps in the bicipital groove of the humerus is a common cause of shoulder pain. The long tendon of the biceps muscle arises from the supraglenoid fossa of the glenoid cavity, extends through the space between the superior part of the capsule of the shoulder joint and the humeral head, and passes into the fibrous tunnel formed by its theca covering the bicipital groove. The tendon is ensheathed in a synovial membrane and extends as an outpocketing from the joint into the bicipital groove and makes up the tendon part of the gliding mechanism. Actually, the tendon does very little gliding within the groove. It is the humerus that glides on the tendon and irritates the inflamed tendon sheath.

This gliding mechanism is readily disturbed by excessive activity of the arm, particularly when the arm is made to work at a disadvantage, or by direct trauma to the area of the bicipital groove. Once the process is precipitated, all activities that require much motion of the humerus on the tendon will produce pain. Abduction and external rotation, as well as internal rotation and extension, are the movements of the arm most likely to irritate the biceps tendon and cause pain. Such movements are required, for example, in combing the hair, putting on a shirt or coat, fastening a brassiere, or reaching for a telephone.

Clinical Picture. The onset of pain in this condition may be slow and gradual, or it may be more acute, following sudden vigorous activity of the arm such as in shoveling snow. Trauma to the arm may produce a strain or snap of the tendon in the bicipital groove, causing an irritation of the tendon sheath. The pain originates in the anterior and medial aspects of the shoulder, but it may radiate along the course of the biceps muscle to the elbow or even to the forearm and fingers. Occasionally pain may radiate to the posterior aspect of the shoulder joint and to the neck.

Bicipital tenosynovitis is more common in the female, and its greatest incidence is in 45 to 65 year old patients. The pain is always brought on by the motions previously described and is relieved by resting the arm.

Invariably, these patients describe great difficulty in finding a comfortable position for the affected arm in bed. Point tenderness may be found over the biceps tendon and in the bicipital groove, or along the anterior aspect of the humerus. A combination of abduction, external rotation, and extension of the arm at the shoulder may cause pain in the region of the bicipital groove. Forced flexion of the elbow against resistance and forced supination of the forearm against resistance with the elbow flexed will frequently cause pain in the area of the bicipital groove. If bicipital tenosynovitis is present for several weeks, it may cause a frozen shoulder deformity because of the patient's disinclination to move the shoulder and bring on pain. Since bicipital tenosynovitis involves the soft tissues of the shoulder joint, radiographic examination is negative.

Treatment. A period of rest to the arm and shoulder is helpful. This may be supplied by a sling. Too much immobilization must be avoided, however, to prevent the complication of a frozen shoulder or adhesive capsulitis. Moist heat applied to the area of the bicipital groove is quite soothing to the patient. Hydrocortisone injected directly into the tendon sheath within the bicipital groove is effective in relieving the tendon sheath irritation if it is not given too frequently. In some patients, injected hydrocortisone may cause degenerative lesions of the biceps tendon and may be associated with the eventual rupture of the biceps tendon. Injected hydrocortisone may be combined with orally administered anti-inflammatory drugs to relieve the pain of bicipital tenosynovitis. Diathermy and ultrasound treatment to the painful area have been used, but they do not seem to be as effective as the anti-inflammatory agents.

Rarely, operative intervention may be required for relief of pain if all other treatment methods have failed. At operation the biceps tendon is permanently anchored to the bicipital groove of the humerus by suture or by means of a metal staple. Anchoring the tendon firmly to the underlying bone obliterates the tendon-tendon sheath gliding mechanism and the stimulus for pain.

Disorders of the Acromioclavicular Joint

Disorders of the acromioclavicular joint may be classified under trauma or under derangements of the subacromial mechanism. They may occur frequently, and if not readily recognized and treated, may result in considerable shoulder pain and discomfort. These disorders have already been discussed earlier in this chapter.

Frozen Shoulder Deformity — Adhesive Capsulitis of the Shoulder

Any number of painful shoulder conditions may ultimately be associated with a tightening or stiffening of the soft tissue components of the joint, resulting in a painful restriction of motion. Such a condition, regardless of cause, is termed a "frozen shoulder" deformity. The primary causative factor for the development of a frozen shoulder is pain associated with elevating the arm in a person who tends to self-protect the extremity. The pain may arise from the shoulder joint itself and may follow dislocation, fracture, or other upper extremity trauma, bicipital tenosynovitis, calcium deposits in the rotator cuff, or painful lesions of the acromioclavicular joints. The pain may arise primarily away from the shoulder, but radiate to this region with enough intensity to result in a frozen shoulder. Such pain transference may be seen after myocardial infarction, radical mastectomy, and thoracic surgical procedures. Regardless of cause, the pain is of sufficient unpleasantness to discourage shoulder movements; the joint, self-protected from painful elevation, gradually and insidiously becomes stiff and more painful. Continued immobility of the shoulder joint allows the capsule to adhere to the proximal humerus, resulting in a stiffened or frozen shoulder deformity.

Clinical Picture. The patient with a frozen shoulder presents with a tight, stiff shoulder joint that developed following some primary cause of shoulder pain (Fig. 10–10). The original cause of pain, as noted, may be one of several possibilities and may already have been corrected. Passively the glenohumeral joint is tight and contracted in all planes of motion. Actively the patient may superficially appear to have a greater range of motion than passively, but this appearance is the result of compensatory scapulothoracic motion. The overlying shoulder muscles may appear atrophic. Many times these tense patients present with associated muscle spasm that produces pain running from the occiput to the wrist. Frequently, associated vasomotor effects in the hand and fingers are seen. The combination of neck, chest wall and arm pain sometimes mimics cervical radiculitis (see p. 320).

Treatment. The treatment of a frozen shoulder involves locating and treating the primary cause of pain if it is still present. The characteristics of the problem should be carefully explained to the patient, since it may take months to recover a normal range of

FIGURE 10–10. Patient with frozen shoulder deformity on right: glenohumeral rhythm is grossly disturbed on the right side. The scapula on the right side rotates outward with elevation of the right humerus, indicating loss of glenohumeral joint motion. (From DePalma, A. F.: Surgery of the Shoulder, 2nd ed. Philadelphia: J. B. Lippincott Co., 1973.)

shoulder motion and these patients will need reassurance and encouragement. Range of motion exercises must be initiated and maintained. Generally, the prognosis for recovery is good if the patient understands the problem and the need for a conscientious and vigorous exercise program.

Injections of hydrocortisone into the glenohumeral joint space frequently aids in relieving pain and makes the initiation of a vigorous exercise program more tolerable. Inflating the shoulder joint with a relatively large volume of normal saline solution, mixed with local anesthetic and a corticosteroid, frequently peels the adherent capsule from the humeral head. Combined with gentle manipulation of the shoulder this treatment, called *infiltration brisement*, is often quite beneficial. Manipulation of the tight shoulder joint under anesthesia is not favored, because it may cause fracture or rupture of an important tendon. In an occasional patient, the tightness may be sufficiently severe to require surgical release of the tight structures about the shoulder joint.

References

Abbott, L. C., and Lucas, D. B.: The function of the clavicle. Its surgical significance. Ann. Surg., *140*:583, 1954.

Bailey, R. W.: Acute and recurrent dislocation of the shoulder. J. Bone and Joint
Surg., *49-A*:767, 1967.

DePalma, A. F.: Surgery of the Shoulder, 2nd Edition. Philadelphia: J. B. Lippincott
Co., 1973.

Inman, V. T., Saunders, J. B. deC. M., and Abbott, L. C.: Observations on the function of the shoulder joint. J. Bone and Joint Surg., *26*:1, 1944.

Rothman, R. H. (Ed.): Symposium on surgery of the shoulder. Orthop. Clin. North
Am., Vol. 6, No. 2, April 1975.

Wolfgang, G. L.: Surgical repair of tears of the rotator cuff of the shoulder. J. Bone
and Joint Surg., *56-A*:14, 1974.

CHAPTER 11

THE UPPER EXTREMITY

In Chapter 10, the reader's attention was drawn to the great mobility possessed by the shoulder joint. This mobility characterizes the entire upper extremity. Our upper limbs are free and possess great range of movement. Our ability to survive and flourish depends, to a considerable extent, on this capability. Unfortunately, we are also prey to many diseases and disorders that may seriously impair this mobility through pain, deformity, or muscle weakness. This impairment may arise primarily in a segment of the upper extremity, or it may radiate secondarily to the part from a primary focus in the neck or shoulder area.

When a complaint is referable to the upper extremity, the examiner must be prepared to differentiate between the primary and secondary causes. It is well to remember that the examination of the upper extremity begins at the sternal notch and works out gradually to the fingertips. For this reason, the patient should be suitably draped so that the neck, shoulders, and both upper extremities are exposed for examination and comparison.

For descriptive purposes, the disorders of the upper extremity are presented under the headings of upper arm, elbow, forearm, wrist, and hand.

THE UPPER ARM

GENERAL CONSIDERATIONS

Pain localized to the upper arm area may arise from a local cause or may be radiating to the area from an origin in the neck or shoulder. Pain arising in the neck is discussed on page 315; that arising in the shoulder on page 249. Two conditions that affect the shoulder, bicipital tenosynovitis and rupture of the biceps tendon, overlap anatomically into the arm area and may cause symptoms predominantly localized to the upper arm area.

Bone tumors may involve the humerus. The more common benign tumors seen in this area include unicameral bone cysts, osteochondroma, giant cell tumor, and benign chondroblastoma. Primary malignant bone tumors, such as osteosarcoma, fibrosarcoma, and Ewing's tumor, occasionally arise in the humerus. Metastatic carcinoma from a primary site, such as the breast, kidney, prostate or lung, not infrequently involves the humerus. The presence of a tumor in the bone may be a cause of pathologic fracture (see p. 29).

Although more rare, benign and malignant soft tissue tumors may also be found in the upper arm area.

False aneurysms may be found in the upper extremity and have been reported following angiographic studies, surgical procedures, or penetrating wounds. They have been observed most frequently in the area of the antecubital fossa and at the wrist. Once their presence has been confirmed, they should be treated by evacuation of the clot and either repair or ligation of the vessel.

FRACTURE OF THE SHAFT OF THE HUMERUS

Injury to the humerus may result in a transverse or spiral fracture to the midshaft of the bone (Fig. 11–1). Whenever possible, closed reduction is the treatment of choice, using a sugar-tong splint with a Velpeau bandage, a hanging cast, or a shoulder spica as the immobilizing agent. If open reduction is deemed necessary, either intramedullary pin fixation or compression plate fixation is usually employed.

The two major complications of fractures of the shaft of the humerus are nonunion of the bone and radial nerve palsy. Nonunion occurs in 5 to 12 per cent of patients and requires bone graft operation for its cure.

Injury to the radial nerve adjacent to the musculospiral groove may accompany humeral shaft fractures and may result in the pa-

FIGURE 11–1. Displaced fracture through upper shaft of right humerus.

tient's losing the power to actively dorsiflex the wrist and elevate the thumb. The wrist hangs limply in a flexed position. The condition is called "wrist drop" and occurs in about 12 per cent of patients. However, because it is likely that the radial nerve is only bruised and not severed in association with the humeral shaft fracture, nerve function returns in the majority of patients within three to nine months, unless there is further trauma from the treatment itself. The wrist should be splinted in the dorsiflexed position (position of function) while awaiting nerve regeneration. Periodic electromyographic examination and nerve conduction tests are helpful in monitoring return of nerve function.

RADIAL NERVE PALSY

Radial nerve palsy, as previously noted, may complicate a humeral shaft fracture. A penetrating wound of the arm may damage or sever the radial nerve, resulting in a temporary or permanent wrist drop. Temporary radial nerve palsy may also result from direct pressure against the nerve trunk. This is occasionally caused by improper use of crutches or by a person's falling asleep with the arm draped over the back of a chair or bench. Complete return of nerve function can be expected in instances of temporary radial nerve palsy. Complete severance of the radial nerve requires surgical repair or, if this is impossible, wrist fusion and tendon transfers to restore both dorsiflexion ability to the paralyzed wrist and elevation for the thumb.

THE ELBOW

From an anatomical standpoint, the elbow is the most complicated joint of the upper extremity. This consideration accounts for many of the complications that follow involvement of the elbow by trauma or disease. The distal end of the humerus and the proximal ends of the radius and ulna are specially constructed together to form the elbow articulation (Fig. 11–2). Normal appearance and normal range of motion of the elbow require that this structural relationship be maintained.

Basically, the elbow is a hinge joint and allows only flexion and extension through an arc of 150 degrees (see Fig. 1–4). Mechanically, this motion occurs through the humeroulnar component of the joint, with the radius playing only a passive role. The radius is more directly concerned with the motions of pronation and supination of the forearm. Like the knee joint, the elbow depends upon strong collateral ligaments for lateral stability. The muscles are massed in front and behind in order to flex and extend the joint.

When the elbows are flexed to a right angle and held firmly at the sides, the forearms can be rotated into almost 90 degrees of pronation and supination. A normal range of pronation and supination requires smooth rotation of the radial head on the capitellum of the humerus in addition to mobility through the superior radioulnar joint at the elbow and the inferior radioulnar joint at the wrist. A bone block at any of these levels will obliterate the motion of pronation and supination.

When the forearm is viewed from the front with the elbow joint completely extended, it is seen that the forearm projects outward from the arm at an angle of 10 to 15 degrees. This is known as the *carrying angle* and depends for its existence on a proper relationship between the various bones making up the elbow joint. The carrying angle can best be appreciated when the subject is standing erect, both arms stiffly at the side with palms facing forward. It can then be seen that the forearms project away from the sides of the body. This allows one to carry an object without bumping it against

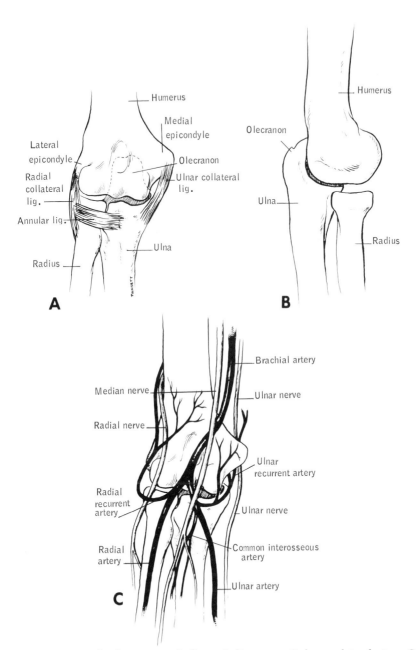

FIGURE 11-2. Skeletal anatomy of elbow. *A*, ligaments. *B*, bones, lateral view. *C*, nerves and arteries.

the legs. If the carrying angle is abnormally increased by trauma or disease, the deformity is called *cubitus valgus*. Decrease in the carrying angle is known as *cubitus varus* (see Fig. 4–8).

The relationship of the ulnar nerve, median nerve, and brachial artery to the elbow must be continually borne in mind in considering problems involving this joint. The ulnar nerve lies in a vulnerable position as it passes beneath the medial epicondyle. At the level of the elbow joint, the brachial artery and median nerve overlie the anterior aspect of the humerus and the brachialis muscle.

GENERAL CONSIDERATIONS

The elbow joint may fall victim to the same general problems that beset all joints.

Arthritis. Rheumatoid arthritis may destroy the joint, causing deformity and stiffness. If both elbow joints should undergo ankylosis as a result of rheumatoid arthritis, the functional disability to the patient would be enormous. Attempts are being made to develop total elbow joint implants in an effort to restore a useful range of motion to these destroyed and stiff joints. Degenerative arthritis is not a common problem at the elbow since this disorder primarily involves weight bearing joints. Bleeding into the elbow joint is a frequent occurrence in hemophilia and may result in permanent joint damage.

Infection. Pyogenic infection and tuberculosis may involve the elbow joint and must be quickly recognized and vigorously treated if permanent joint damage is to be avoided.

Tumors. Benign and malignant bone and soft tissue tumors may appear in the elbow joint area, although none has a particular affinity for the site.

Traumatic Myositis Ossificans. On occasion, hemorrhage into a muscle may produce irregular masses of bone complete with cortex and medullary cavity. This condition, known as traumatic myositis ossificans (Fig. 11–3), is most commonly seen over the anterior surface of the femur following hemorrhage into the quadriceps muscle and over the flexor surface of the elbow following hemorrhage into the brachialis anticus muscle. In almost all instances, the hemorrhage is produced by injury and the resulting bone mass lies alongside the normal bone or may be attached in part to the underlying normal bone.

The process is thought to represent metaplasia of fibroblasts and is characterized by heterotopic calcification and ossification. It may result from the seeding of a muscle with endosteum or periosteum following injury to an adjacent bone. As time passes, the bone

FIGURE 11–3. Lateral radiograph of elbow, showing an area of mature myositis ossificans overlying the flexor aspect of the joint.

becomes more mature and dense. It can complicate fractures and dislocations at the elbow and can become a major functional problem by acting as a block to flexion.

Traumatic myositis ossificans must be differentiated from osteosarcoma and *myositis ossificans progressiva*, a rare congenital disease characterized by the formation of sheets of bone in muscles, ligaments, and fascia. Careful study of the characteristics of the bone mass, its radiographic appearance, and the histologic sections should permit this essential distinction.

Treatment depends on the stage of activity of the process. During the active phase, rest and immobilization are essential. Misguided attempts at forceful exercise or early surgical removal will be rewarded with further bone formation. If there is functional impairment, surgical excision of the bone mass should be carried out, but only after the ectopic bone has become dense and mature, a state usually not reached until six months to one year after the bone first appears.

Trauma

Subluxation of the Radial Head. This condition, known as "nursemaid's elbow," is seen exclusively in infants and young children. Forceful pulling on a child's hand or forearm may cause the cartilaginous radial head to slip partially out of the encircling orbicular ligament. As a result, the child refuses to use the arm because of pain and holds it in a semiflexed and slightly pronated position. Radiographic examination is of no help because the radial head at this age is cartilage and will not show on the film.

Reduction is quite easy, requires no anesthesia, and is achieved by first rapidly turning the forearm into full supination and then following with sudden flexion of the elbow. As the maneuver is carried out, the radial head can be felt to "click" back into place. The reduction is usually stable, and no immobilization is required. The child can be encouraged to use the arm normally.

Dislocation of the Elbow Joint. A fall on the outstretched hand in a child or adult not infrequently causes a traumatic dislocation of the elbow joint. The joint gives way under the force and most commonly the lower end of the humerus is driven over the coronoid process of the ulna and out through the torn anterior capsule. The ulna and radius are forced backward, and the ulna finally lodges behind the lower end of the displaced humerus. This is described as a posterior dislocation of the elbow. Anterior dislocation of the elbow is quite rare.

The injury results in a painful deformity of the elbow soon accompanied by marked swelling. Normally, the point of the olecranon lies ahead of the line connecting the medial and lateral humeral epicondyles. In the presence of a posterior dislocation of the elbow, the point of the olecranon typically lies behind this line. Radiographic examination will confirm the diagnosis of dislocation (Fig. 11–4). The possibility of associated nerve or circulatory damage must always be considered.

Closed manipulative reduction under adequate anesthesia should be carried out as soon as possible. The elbow is immobilized in a posterior plaster splint in a safe degree of flexion for three weeks. The elbow joint has poor tolerance for injury and immobilization, and it may be months before full motion returns.

Unlike the shoulder joint, however, the elbow joint rarely suffers recurrent dislocation. Occasionally dislocation is accompanied by circulatory or nerve damage. Traumatic myositis ossificans may be seen as a complication of dislocation.

Supracondylar Fracture of the Humerus. The supracondylar area of the humerus is the lower flared end of the bone just above the elbow joint. Fractures through this area occur commonly in children and uncommonly in adults. They are occasionally accompanied by frightening complications and distressing physical deformity. Immediate deformity may superficially resemble that caused by a posterior dislocation of the elbow, except that the relationship between the olecranon and the epicondyles is not disturbed. Radiographic examination serves to differentiate the two conditions.

FIGURE 11–4. Lateral view of elbow, showing traumatic posterior dislocation of the joint.

On the lateral radiographic view it can be recognized that normally the lower end of the humerus, containing the condyles, tilts forward at an angle of approximately 30 degrees with the shaft. A fracture through the supracondylar area results in a broken bone of two fragments (Fig. 11–5). The small distal fragment consists of the lower flared condylar portion of the humerus to which are attached the elbow joint and forearm. The larger proximal fragment is the remainder of the humeral shaft. Most often following fracture, the small distal fragment is displaced backward, but rarely it may be displaced forward depending on the direction of the fracturing force. This displacement results in a loss of the normal forward angulation of the lower end of the humerus. In addition to being displaced backward, the small distal fragment usually rotates on the larger proximal fragment. If the backward displacement of the distal fragment is not corrected and the forward angulation not restored, permanent alteration in the range of flexion and extension at the elbow joint will occur. If the rotatory displacement is not corrected,

FIGURE 11–5. AP and lateral views of supracondylar fracture of the humerus. (Compare with Fig. 11–6.)

it will result in permanent abnormality of the carrying angle with the appearance of a cubitus varus or cubitus valgus deformity.

Every child with a suspected elbow fracture should have a radiographic examination of both elbows for comparison. The normally present growth lines at the lower end of the humerus sometimes make the detection of a fracture line difficult. If a radiograph of the child's uninjured elbow is made for comparison, detection can be facilitated (Fig. 11–6). Such comparison is usually not necessary in an adult, however, because growth lines are no longer present to cause confusion.

Immediate check should be made to determine the existence of any circulatory embarrassment or nerve damage. Treatment of the fracture should be undertaken as soon as the radiographs are reviewed and the diagnosis is established. This is one injury that brooks no delay. Swelling about the elbow enlarges rapidly and increases the danger of bony and vascular complications.

Reduction of a displaced supracondylar fracture involves restoring the normal forward angulation of the distal end of the humerus in addition to correcting the rotational spin of the distal fragment. If these objectives are not accomplished, permanent limitation of motion or deformity will result. The choice of a method of reduction depends on the severity of the individual fracture and the training and experience of the physician. Many of these fractures can be successfully reduced by closed manipulative methods, but others may require skin or skeletal traction. Post-reduction fixation of the fragments by percutaneous pinning is favored by some orthopaedic surgeons. Open reduction of this fracture is not usually considered necessary. Immobilization in plaster for a total of six weeks is normally sufficient to insure adequate bone healing. The prognosis for return of normal function is excellent in a well-reduced fracture that heals without complication.

Complications may arise following a supracondylar fracture of the humerus because of: (1) inadequate or incomplete reduction of the fracture, (2) damage to nerves passing over the fracture site, or (3) circulatory impairment heralded by a weak or absent radial pulse.

Inadequate reduction will result in permanent limitation of motion or an obvious physical deformity such as cubitus valgus or cubitus varus (see Fig. 4–8).

Stretching or contusion injuries to the median, ulnar, or deep muscular branch of the radial nerve have been noted in approximately 6 per cent of patients sustaining a supracondylar fracture of

FIGURE 11–6. AP and lateral views of normal child's elbow. Note open growth lines.

the humerus. The nerve damage in almost all patients proves to be temporary and disappears in time without any specific treatment. It is important, however, to recognize evidence of nerve damage, if present, before fracture treatment is started.

The most dreaded complication of a supracondylar fracture of the humerus is circulatory embarrassment, which is expressed as an extremely weak or absent radial pulse. If present before reduction, such embarrassment is usually due to antecubital edema, impingement of a bone fragment against the brachial artery, or rarely a torn or lacerated brachial artery. If the embarrassment appears after reduction, it is probably due to vascular obstruction secondary to tight bandages or to a position of acute or extreme flexion. An absent radial pulse in the presence of a supracondylar fracture of the humerus demands maximum effort to determine its cause and bring about correction. If it is ignored or not corrected within a four- to eight-hour period, the severe deforming and crippling condition of the hand and arm known as Volkmann's ischemic contracture may result.

Volkmann's Ischemic Contracture. This tragic condition begins as a forearm compartment syndrome in which increased pressure within a limited space compromises the arterial and venous circulation and function of tissue within that space. If allowed to continue unchecked, the resulting ischemia leads to massive muscle infarction with gradual replacement of muscle by fibrous tissue and a binding down of tendons and nerves with scar. In the upper extremity, the final result may be a hard atrophic forearm with a stiff clawhand deformity which is frequently anesthetic and paralyzed. It is this final state that is called Volkmann's ischemic contracture.

Compartment syndrome in the forearm is seen most commonly after supracondylar fractures of the humerus, but it may also follow other fractures about the elbow joint and forearm bones, crush injuries to the forearm, excessive use of the forearm muscles, and tight dressings. Compartment syndrome may also involve the lower extremity, particularly in association with fractures of the femur or tibia. It has been described as occurring in the lower extremity subsequent to the use of Bryant's traction in small children.

Compartment syndrome in either the upper or lower extremity must be recognized and treated promptly, certainly within a four- to eight-hour period, in order to avoid irreversible ischemia to muscles and nerves. The first rule is to think of the possibility when dealing with any condition of the extremities that might be complicated by impaired peripheral circulation. Avoid tight casts and bandages or severely flexed positions that could cause acute venous obstruction. Check the peripheral circulation frequently, with special reference

FIGURE 11-7.   Displaced fracture of olecranon and dislocation of radial head.

to the arterial pulses and the color, temperature, and presence of swelling of the fingers or toes.

Certain cardinal signs warn the observer of an impending or an actual compartment syndrome: (1) pain in the part usually out of proportion to the anticipated clinical situation; (2) muscle weakness or paralysis of the compartment musculature; (3) pallor of the part; (4) pulselessness; (5) pain elicited on passive stretching of the compartment muscles; (6) hypesthesia in the distribution of the nerves in the compartment; and (7) tenseness of the fascial boundaries of the compartment.

Diagnostic aids available to support a clinical diagnosis of a compartment syndrome include the use of compartment tissue pressure monitoring devices, such as a large bore needle, tubing, and a manometer or a wick catheter or an infusion technique for continuous monitoring over several days and the use of a portable nerve stimulator to monitor neuromuscular function.

If the diagnosis of a compartment syndrome is made and an impending ischemia is suspected, all constricting bandages should be released immediately and the extremity elevated. If the condition shows no sign of correcting itself within a one- to two-hour period of close observation, the fascial planes of the deep and superficial compartments should be promptly opened surgically in order to insure adequate decompression of the compartment.

Fractures of the Olecranon.   Fracture of the olecranon is more common in adults than in children and is caused by a direct fall on the elbow or by forceful contraction of the triceps muscle following a fall on the hand with the elbow flexed (Fig. 11–7). Many times associated laceration of the lateral aponeurosis of the triceps tendon allows marked separation of the fragments. Since this fracture involves the humeroulnar component of the joint, an inadequate reduction may result in limitation of extension at the elbow.

Although many olecranon fractures can be reduced satisfactorily by immobilizing the extremity in a cast with the elbow in complete extension, it may take two or three months for the fracture to heal and several more months for the patient to regain elbow joint motion. This has led to a general tendency towards operative treatment because it offers the advantage of earlier motion. In general, two surgical methods are in use: (1) open reduction of the fracture may be performed with the fractures held in position by means of internal metallic fixation devices, such as screws or wire loops; (2) if the proximal fragment is not too large, it may be excised and discarded and the triceps muscle resutured to the ulnar shaft.

Fracture of the Radial Head. Fracture of the radial head is common in adults and is caused usually by a fall on the outstretched hand. Because this fracture tends to cause joint stiffness if immobilized, the key to its successful treatment is early motion. The choice of treatment depends on the degree of displacement of the fragments, but all methods have in common the use of early motion.

If displacement of the fragments is minimal or absent, the fracture may be safely ignored and early motion stressed. Pain can be controlled by aspirating blood from the distended radiohumeral joint and keeping the elbow at rest in a posterior plaster splint for 48 hours. After this period, the immobilization is eliminated and motion started.

If the fracture is comminuted or if the displacement is such that interference with pronation and supination can be anticipated, operative excision of the radial head is carried out, preferably within 24 hours of injury, and early motion of the joint is encouraged in the immediate postoperative period.

Although not as common, similar injuries may be seen in children. In this instance, trauma causes a fracture of the radial neck or a separation of the upper radial epiphysis. In either case, reduction must be carried out if there is displacement of the fragments. If closed reduction is unsuccessful, open reduction is used. The radial head should not be removed in a child, because a growth deformity might develop. Subsequent overgrowth of the ulna at the wrist might produce a clubhand deformity.

SPECIFIC CONDITIONS

Osteochondritis Dissecans. Osteochondritis dissecans is a joint condition in which a fragment of articular cartilage, with or without subchondral bone, becomes partially or completely separated from the parent bone. It occurs most commonly in the knee joint, but it may also be seen in the elbow, ankle, and hip joints. The area of involvement in the elbow joint is usually the capitellum of the humerus. The condition is described in more detail in the discussion of the knee joint (see p. 419).

The presence of osteochondritis dissecans in an elbow joint may cause pain, joint swelling, and restriction of motion. If the separated piece becomes a loose body, it may wedge between the bones of the joint and cause locking or a block to extension. The lesion is visible on clear radiographs.

If the diagnosis is made before the fragment completely separates, healing by "creeping substitution" may take place if the joint is put at rest. If this does not occur or the fragment becomes a loose body, surgical excision is indicated.

Loose Bodies. Joints, on occasion, may be found to contain loose fragments of bone or calcified tissue that, by their presence and mobility, cause pain, joint irritation, and locking. These fragments are known as loose bodies or "joint mice" and arise as a result of trauma or disease.

Loose bodies are most commonly found in the knee joint, but the elbow, shoulder, hip, and ankle joints may also contain them. As stated earlier, osteochondritis dissecans may be a cause of loose bodies. Other causes may be fracture of the articular surface, fracture of an osteoarthritic spur, fracture of articular hyaline cartilage, and osteochondromatosis (see p. 420). Treatment is operative removal in order to relieve the symptoms caused by the presence of these fragments and to save the joint from further damage.

Tennis Elbow. The term "tennis elbow" refers to a common condition that is characterized by pain in the region of the lateral epicondyle of the humerus with radiation down the extensor surface of the forearm. This predicament is brought on by activity that combines excessive pronation and supination of the forearm with an extended wrist, particularly in a person not accustomed to it. Thus, tennis, badminton, sculling, or using a screwdriver may be inciting causes.

Although the mechanism producing "tennis elbow" is understood, the actual cause of the pain has never been clearly established. Several causes probably exist: among them radiohumeral bursitis, tendonitis at the common extensor origin, and traumatic epicondylitis or periostitis at the lateral epicondyle. The patient exhibits an area of palpable tenderness over the lateral epicondyle of the humerus or the radiohumeral joint. Pain can be characteristically aggravated by forced dorsiflexion of the wrist against resistance, which puts tension on the common extensor origin and reproduces pain.

Radiographic examination of the elbow is usually negative, but calcium deposits have been noted on rare occasion.

Most patients respond to moist heat, analgesics, and local injections of corticosteroids at the site of maximum tenderness. Occasionally it is necessary to rest the extensor tendons in a plaster splint with the wrist fixed in dorsiflexion. In a few patients, operative release of the common extensor origin from the lateral epicondyle of the humerus may be required.

Medial Epicondylitis. On rare occasions, the region of the medial epicondyle of the humerus may become painful as a result of activity that puts excessive strain on the common flexor origin. Local palpable tenderness will exist in the region of the medial epicondyle. Pain is aggravated by forced palmar flexion of the wrist against resistance. Wrist motion places tension on the common flexor origin and reproduces pain. The same modalities used in treating lateral epicondylitis or tennis elbow can be used in a patient suffering from medial epicondylitis.

Olecranon Bursitis. Trauma to the point of the elbow often results in marked swelling of the olecranon bursa, giving rise to a large knob in this area. Following trauma, the fluid contained in the bursal sac frequently is bloody and the bursa walls become permanently thickened. Tender swelling of the bursa may also be seen with gout and rheumatoid arthritis.

Treatment consists of aspiration of the fluid and local instillation of corticosteroid, followed by application of a pressure dressing. If the problem cannot be controlled locally, operative excision of the thickened bursa may be carried out.

Traumatic Ulnar Neuritis. Because of its vulnerable position in the ulnar groove behind the medial epicondyle of the humerus, the ulnar nerve may be impinged upon by deformities of the elbow, giving rise to a traumatic ulnar neuritis.

It is known that the ulnar nerve is unusually mobile in some people and will, as a consequence, dislocate across the tip of the medial epicondyle on flexion and return to its normal location on extension of the elbow. A certain percentage of these patients ultimately develop a traumatic ulnar neuritis from friction alone. Other causes of traumatic ulnar neuritis include osteoarthritic spur formation growing into the ulnar groove, scarring following laceration or contusion of the soft tissues near the medial epicondyle, and any congenital deformity of the elbow that increases the carrying angle.

The most common cause of traumatic ulnar neuritis, however, is residual deformity of the elbow from a previous fracture, specifically a cubitus valgus deformity following a supracondylar fracture of the humerus or displaced fracture of the medial epicondyle of the humerus. In these instances it may be years before the ulnar neuritis develops. In one reported case, neuritis developed fifty years after the elbow fracture. For this reason the condition is known as tardy ulnar neuritis.

The patient with ulnar neuritis may complain of numbness, tingling, and pain over the ulnar distribution, particularly the fourth and fifth fingers. A feeling of clumsiness in the affected hand is often noted by the patient. This can progress from the stage of interossei weakness with muscle wasting to complete interossei paralysis.

Traumatic ulnar neuritis is treated by displacement of the ulnar nerve from the area of irritation, preferably before motor changes occur and while sensory complaints are still reversible. This is accomplished by surgically transposing the nerve anteriorly to the front of the medial epicondyle and burying it beneath the mass of soft flexor muscle tissue.

THE FOREARM

The forearm is the lever for the hand and as such is an important segment of the upper extremity. Trauma or disease affecting the forearm may therefore seriously impair the function and efficiency of the entire part. The motions of flexion and extension of the forearm are, for the most part, controlled by the elbow joint. The motions most often limited by forearm problems are pronation and supination. This range of motion is usually limited in the direction of pronation.

GENERAL CONSIDERATIONS

The motion of pronation and supination requires a rolling of the radius and the ulna on each other along their longitudinal axes. Equal amounts of motion take place at the superior and inferior radioulnar joints, which requires that the radial head not impinge on the capitellum of the humerus. Fracture or dislocation of the radial head or trauma involving the superior or inferior radioulnar joints may seriously impair this forearm motion.

TRAUMA

Fracture of the Forearm Bones. Because of the intimate relationship between the radius and the ulna, a force strong enough to break either forearm bone commonly breaks both bones simultaneously. Fracture of a single forearm bone usually results from a direct blow applied to the bone. Fractures of both bones of the forearm are often the consequence of a fall on the outstretched arm and are more common in children than in adults. Their management, however, poses a more difficult problem in the adult.

In children, closed reduction with immobilization in a long arm plaster cast is usually sufficient for a good result, with correction of the forearm bowing deformity. Frequently in children, the bones will be broken on the convex side of the deformity, but the cortex will appear intact on the concave side. Such fractures are spoken of as "greenstick" fractures. To obtain complete reduction and stabilization of a "greenstick" fracture, it is necessary to complete the fracture of both cortical surfaces manually during reduction. If this is not done, the bowing deformity of the forearm bones may recur within the cast.

The management of a fracture of both forearm bones is a much more difficult problem in the adult patient. Strong muscle pull results in marked positional deformity of the fragments, and interposition of muscle tissue between the fragments frequently makes adequate closed reduction difficult or even impossible to achieve. Malunion and nonunion are relatively common following closed reduction treatment of fractures of both bones of the forearm. As a result, more than half of all adult patients with forearm fractures will require open reduction of the fractures. At the time of surgery some form of internal fixation, such as compression plate fixation, is used. Frequently, the use of internal fixation is combined with the addition of bone graft material around the fracture site. For better functional results, the decision to employ open reduction should be made within a few days of injury.

An occasional complication of fracture of both bones of the forearm is *synostosis* or *cross union* between the two bones. This bony growth connecting the two forearm bones may occur at either radioulnar joint or anywhere along the shafts, usually opposite the site of fracture. It arises along injured periosteum or interosseous membranes or within a hematoma. Its presence may effectively limit the motion of pronation and supination by preventing one bone from rolling on the other. Surgical release at the point of obstruction may successfully restore a functional range of pronation and supination.

Mechanical Tenosynovitis. Acute post-traumatic tenosynovitis of the flexor tendon sheaths in the forearm is a form of compartment syndrome and is usually caused by strenuous and unaccustomed use of the hand and wrist. As a result of the overactivity, serous fluid accumulates in the flexor sheaths and the distention results in severe temporary discomfort and disability of the part.

Clinically, the flexor compartment of the forearm may appear swollen and may be tender. Motions of the wrist and hand may be markedly limited by pain. There is usually no vascular or nerve complication.

The condition usually responds to local heat and rest. The rest may have to be afforded by plaster immobilization.

THE WRIST

The wrist is a movable bridge that connects the hand to the forearm. It comprises the distal end of the radius and ulna plus eight carpal bones arranged in a proximal and distal row. The stability of the wrist joint is maintained by strong ligaments that lash the bones together.

The lower end of the radius is broad and thick and articulates with the proximal row of carpal bones (Fig. 11–8). This is the radiocarpal joint, which is responsible for the major portion of the motions of dorsiflexion or extension, palmar flexion, radial deviation, and ulnar deviation of the wrist joint. As previously described, pronation and supination of the wrist joint is dependent upon a movable forearm. The distal ulna does not articulate with any of the carpal bones and can be surgically removed if necessary without causing any particular disturbance to wrist joint mechanics.

It is important to note that normally the tip of the radial styloid lies ahead of the tip of the ulnar styloid at the wrist. Fractures in this region are frequently accompanied by an alteration in the relationship of these landmarks.

The carpal bones on the volar aspect of the wrist are bridged by the volar carpal ligament. The deep passage beneath this wide transverse band is called *carpal canal* or *carpal tunnel*. The structures that pass through this canal are the median nerve and all the flexor tendons of the wrist (Fig. 11–9). The radial artery, ulnar artery, and the ulnar nerve lie outside the carpal tunnel.

On the dorsal or extensor surface of the wrist, the dorsal carpal ligament contributes to the formation of the osteofibrous tunnels that house the extensor tendons as they pass over the dorsal surface of the radius.

GENERAL CONSIDERATIONS

Because malposition of the wrist can seriously impair the use of the hand, every effort must be made to keep this joint in the position

Distal phalanx
Middle phalanx
Proximal phalanx

Metacarpal
Lesser multangular
Greater multangular
Hamate
Pisiform
Capitate
Triquetrum
Navicular
Ulnar styloid
Lunate
Radial styloid

Radius

Ulna

Radial neck
Radial head
Lateral condyle of humerus
Olecranon

FIGURE 11–8. Bones of the forearm and hand. (Redrawn from Marble, H. C.: The Hand.)

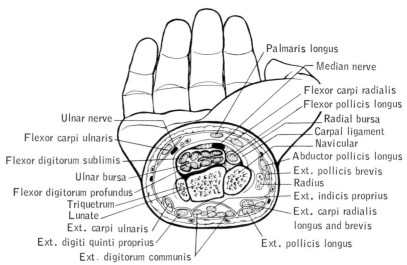

Palmaris longus
Median nerve
Flexor carpi radialis
Flexor pollicis longus
Ulnar nerve
Radial bursa
Flexor carpi ulnaris
Carpal ligament
Navicular
Flexor digitorum sublimis
Abductor pollicis longus
Ulnar bursa
Ext. pollicis brevis
Flexor digitorum profundus
Radius
Triquetrum
Ext. indicis proprius
Lunate
Ext. carpi radialis
Ext. carpi ulnaris
longus and brevis
Ext. digiti quinti proprius
Ext. pollicis longus
Ext. digitorum communis

FIGURE 11–9. Cross-sectional anatomy of the hand through the proximal row of carpal bones. (Redrawn from Marble, H. C.: The Hand.)

of function during the treatment period of an injury or a disease. Position of function of the wrist is 30 degrees of dorsiflexion or extension and 10 degrees of ulnar deviation.

Arthritis. Rheumatoid arthritis may involve the wrist, resulting in joint destruction with pain and progressive loss of motion. A severely involved wrist joint may progress to ankylosis. Disability is greatly lessened if the wrist stiffens in the position of function. Osteoarthritis, unless induced by trauma, is not a frequent problem here since the wrist is not a weight bearing joint.

Infection. Pyogenic infection may affect the wrist proper or the tendon sheaths lying in relation to it. Acute suppurative tenosynovitis may involve the wrist area by extension from the hand. Pyogenic arthritis and acute suppurative tenosynovitis are serious problems that require immediate treatment including surgical drainage when necessary.

Tuberculous tenosynovitis is occasionally seen as a diffuse granulomatous thickening of the tendon sheaths around the wrist, particularly on the extensor surface. Excision of the tuberculous tissue, combined with adequate chemotherapy, frequently arrests the process and preserves joint mobility.

Tumors. Benign and malignant bone and soft tissue tumors may appear in the wrist joint area, but none are particular to the location.

Ganglion. Ganglion is a term used to describe a smooth cystic swelling that may appear in relation to any of the extremity joints, but is seen most frequently about the wrist. Ganglia are thought to arise from degeneration in connective tissue close to joints and tendon sheaths. They subsequently become unilocular or multilocular encysted swellings containing thick, colorless, viscous fluid. Although they may cause symptoms of pain and weakness secondary to the pressure of the local swelling, they have never been known to become malignant.

About the wrist, ganglia most commonly arise from the joint capsule and present on the dorsal surface as visible and palpable cystic tumors. They may also appear on the volar wrist surface. The patient may be aware of a gradual onset, or the swelling may arise suddenly. Trauma seems to be a factor in about half the cases.

Ganglia can be treated by aspiration or by excision. A treatment combining aspiration of the fluid contents through a large bore needle with the instillation of hydrocortisone and the use of a pressure dressing is successful in decompressing the cystic swelling in a high percentage of patients. However, it may be necessary to repeat the treatment several times before a clinical cure is obtained.

If surgical excision is elected, it is well to remember that a ganglion is like an iceberg, with the greatest amount of its mass submerged.

Surgery is thus carried out in a field made bloodless by use of a tourniquet. The surgeon must be prepared to expose the joint capsule in order to excise the entire ganglion and its capsular base.

TRAUMA

Because of its exposed position and its role as a defensive shield for the rest of the body, the wrist is frequently subjected to trauma, including lacerating injuries, dislocation, and fractures.

Laceration. The wrist is the narrowest segment of the upper extremity. The tendons that flex and extend the fingers and the nerves that motivate these tendons, plus the arterial and venous circulation, must pass through this narrow neck on the way to the hand. Lacerating injuries at this level, therefore, possess the capability of severing tendons, arteries, and nerves and of inflicting grievous damage to the hand. The hand is well supplied with blood by arterial arches formed by the radial and ulnar arches. A lacerated or severed artery can usually be ligated without danger of compromising the circulation.

Severed tendons and nerves must be repaired in order to restore function to the hand. This is often a task of the greatest magnitude and is certainly no job for the surgical novice. Successful restoration of hand function following such an injury requires detailed knowledge of the anatomy of the area, sound surgical judgment, and, frequently, the use of microsurgical techniques.

Dislocation of the Wrist. A fall on the palm may displace the hand dorsally and cause a dislocation of the wrist joint. The actual dislocation may occur at the radiocarpal joint or through the bones of the carpus. Careful radiographic examination, with films of the normal wrist for comparison, should reveal the type of dislocation present.

Usually, dislocations of the wrist joint can be readily reduced by closed manipulation followed by immobilization for three or four weeks. If closed reduction is unsuccessful, open reduction of the dislocation is carried out.

Dislocation of the Lunate Bone. A fall on the palm of the hand that forces the wrist into sudden extension may dislocate the lunate bone out of its position in the proximal row without causing any other damage to the wrist. The lunate dislocates forward, tearing the capsule, and comes to rest in the carpal tunnel. In this position, the bone presses against the flexor tendons and causes the hand to be held with the wrist and fingers in semiflexion. Motion of the wrist and fingers is painful.

The dislocated bone also presses against the median nerve, causing a median neuritis characterized by pain, paresthesia, atrophy, and weakness or paralysis of the muscles of opposition.

This injury occasionally goes unnoticed on the radiograph and must be considered in evaluating trauma to the wrist.

If diagnosis is made early, closed reduction may be successful. If it is not, operation will be necessary to reduce the dislocated lunate bone and repair the capsular tear.

Some authorities favor excising a lunate bone that has been dislocated for a period longer than three weeks, because of the likelihood of the development of avascular necrosis of the bone.

Colles' Fracture. The most common bone injury produced by a fall on the outstretched hand is Colles' fracture, defined as a fracture through the distal end of the radius with or without a fracture of the ulnar styloid. An associated fracture of the elbow or shoulder may accompany a Colles' fracture. As a rule, there are no accompanying nerve or circulatory complications with Colles' fracture.

Clinically, the wrist appears puffy and deformed. The distal radial fragment is displaced and tilted dorsally, giving rise to the characteristic hump or "silver fork" deformity seen when the wrist is viewed from the side. Backward displacement of the distal radial fragment causes shortening of the radius and an alteration in the normal position of the radial styloid in relation to the ulnar styloid. The normal volar concavity of the radius is lost and the area feels distended to the touch.

Radiographic examination will confirm the diagnosis and will also show if impaction or comminution of the fragments is present (Fig. 11–10).

Many Colles' fractures can be adequately reduced by closed manipulative reduction, provided effective muscular relaxation can be supplied by anesthesia. The goal of the reduction is to restore radial length and to replace the distal radial fragment in its normal anatomic position. Immobilization should include the elbow to prevent pronation and supination and can be achieved by the use of a sugar-tong splint or a long arm plaster cast. Every effort should be made during the healing period to maintain mobility and flexibility in the fingers and knuckles.

In some patients, the Colles' fracture may be quite comminuted and unstable. It may be impossible to maintain satisfactory reduction with plaster cast fixation. In this instance, a treatment technique such as pins and plaster fixation can be utilized. This technique is described in Chapter 2. Open reduction of Colles' fracture is almost never required.

Fracture of the Navicular. Fracture of the navicular is the injury most frequently sustained by the carpal bones and is found mainly in young adult males. Pain and disability are not great and many of these injuries are erroneously diagnosed and treated as "wrist sprains." For

FIGURE 11–10. *A* and *B*, AP and lateral views of wrist, illustrating the typical deformity of a Colles' fracture. *C*, lateral view of same wrist after closed manipulative reduction and plaster fixation.

FIGURE 11–11. AP view of the wrist, illustrating an established nonunion of the navicular bone.

this reason, nonunion of the fracture occurs in a high percentage of
patients. In one series, 76 per cent of the patients presented radiographic evidence of an established nonunion of the navicular at the
time of initial examination by an orthopaedic surgeon. The fracture
can be missed in routine anteroposterior and lateral radiographs, but
can be seen on the oblique view of the wrist (Fig. 11–11).

   If the diagnosis of a fracture of the navicular is made early, plaster
immobilization for three to six months is usually followed by healing.
If the patient is seen after nonunion has become established, some
type of surgical treatment such as bone grafting is required.

SPECIFIC CONDITIONS

   Madelung's Deformity. Madelung's deformity is a relatively
rare malformation of the wrist that gives the joint the cosmetic appearance of having sustained a forward dislocation. It is believed to arise

from an epiphyseal growth defect at the lower end of the radius that causes the radius to shorten and grow in a volar and ulnar direction. Comparative overgrowth of the ulna results in marked dorsal prominence of the lower end of this bone and instability of the distal radioulnar joint. The patient may present because the deformity causes a feeling of weakness and insecurity in the wrist.

The deformity can be greatly lessened by excising the distal end of the ulna and straightening the radius by surgical osteotomy.

Osteochondrosis of the Carpal Bones. As previously described, the osteochondroses are characterized by avascular necrosis of bone, with involvement limited to pressure epiphyses and the tarsal and carpal bones (see p. 96). Avascular necrosis of the lunate bone is known as *Keinböck's disease*; involvement of the navicular bone is known as *Preiser's disease*.

The process probably starts during the growth period, but symptoms at this age may be minimal or absent. Symptoms usually arise secondarily to mechanical disturbance or induced degenerative arthritic changes in the wrist joint. For this reason, a majority of patients presenting with this problem are adults. The chief complaint is aching pain or discomfort in the wrist with use. There may or may not be restriction of joint motion. A history of trauma is frequently obtained.

Occasionally the bone may become revascularized following prolonged immobilization. In certain selected patients, it may be beneficial to excise the flattened dense bone and fill the resulting defect with a silicone rubber prosthesis. If there is much secondary degenerative arthritis in the wrist joint, arthrodesis or fusion of the wrist may be required for pain relief.

Carpal Tunnel Syndrome. As mentioned previously, the carpal bones on the volar aspect of the wrist are bridged by the transverse carpal ligament forming the carpal tunnel for the passage of the finger flexor tendons and the median nerve. Normally, the carpal tunnel becomes tight and narrow when the fingers and wrist are held in forced flexion. If any soft tissue or extrusion of bone is insinuated into this tight canal, symptoms of median nerve compression may be experienced. Abnormal pressure on the median nerve in the tunnel gives rise to the clinical condition known as the carpal tunnel syndrome.

Causes of the abnormal pressure include dislocation of the lunate bone, malunited Colles' fracture, certain fractures of the navicular bone, arthritic deformities and spurs, hypertrophy of the volar ligament, soft tissue masses such as lipomas and ganglia, and thickening of the flexor tendon sheath secondary to rheumatoid arthritis or chronic tenosynovitis. In occasional patients, no definite cause can be determined.

Symptoms are produced by motions that tend to constrict the carpal canal, such as forced flexion and extension of the wrist. The patient may complain of pain with median nerve radiation associated with numbness and paresthesia of median nerve distribution. Manual compression of the carpal tunnel may accentuate the symptoms. Thenar atrophy and weakness of opposition of the thumb may develop. The diagnosis can usually be confirmed by electromyographic and nerve conduction studies.

Symptoms may subside following a period of immobilization of the wrist and avoidance of work that requires flexion of the joint. If this is not successful, the transverse carpal ligament may be divided surgically in order to decompress the median nerve.

THE HAND

The hand is man's universal tool, functioning at the end of a long jointed lever known as the upper extremity. Anatomic study of the hand reveals it to be a mechanism of extreme delicacy, refinement, and specialization. For this reason, trauma or disease affecting the hand is capable of causing severe functional impairment.

Considering the clearly evident importance of the hand, it is surprising to note that hand problems received little special attention for many years. During this period, treatment was often haphazard and results were uncertain. The past three decades, however, have seen the emergence of a new surgical specialist, the hand surgeon.

Trauma or disease affecting the hand may implicate skin, bones, joints, tendons, and nerves. The problems may overlap the fields of orthopaedic surgery, plastic surgery, and neurosurgery. The hand surgeon brings knowledge of all three specialties to bear on the problem for the maximum benefit of the patient.

GENERAL CONDITIONS

Pyogenic Infection. Pyogenic infections in the hand are serious problems because of their potential for causing severe tendon damage. Infection may destroy tendon sheath gliding mechanisms or cause actual tendon slough with resulting finger stiffness.

PARONYCHIA. Paronychia is a pyogenic infection of the tissues just lateral to the fingernail. Pus accumulates and forms a small abscess. Infection may spread around the base of the nail to the other side, or it may burrow beneath the nail to involve the nail bed.

Treatment entails hot soaks, antibiotics, and adequate surgical drainage, including removal of part or all of the nail if necessary.

FELON.   Felon is a pyogenic abscess in the distal pulp space of a finger, characterized by exquisite pain. The connective tissue of the distal phalanx forms a closed sac that includes part of the bone of the distal phalanx. An abscess in this area is, therefore, a closed space infection and pus may accumulate under considerable pressure. The pressure may cause an avascular necrosis of the bone, or infection may invade the bone tissue and result in osteomyelitis of the distal phalanx.

Treatment involves early recognition and adequate surgical drainage of the abscess.

TENDON SHEATH INFECTIONS.   Puncture wounds of the fingers may introduce pyogenic organisms, particularly staphylococcus, into the flexor tendon sheaths. Infection here is called *acute suppurative tenosynovitis* and may result in permanent loss of finger function through tendon necrosis and slough.

Tendon sheath infection causes a rapid uniform swelling of the finger, which is held stiffly in a semiflexed position. There is marked tenderness to palpation over the length of the tendon sheath and attempts to extend the finger passively cause severe pain.

If unchecked, tendon sheath infection may spread into the palm and forearm. Infection in the index, middle, and ring fingers spreads to the midpalmar space. Infection in the thumb and index finger may rupture into the thenar space. The forearm may be invaded by infection spreading through the tendon sheaths of the thumb and little fingers.

Tendon sheath infections are serious problems and true surgical emergencies. Incision and drainage should be carried out immediately in a bloodless field. Adequate antibiotic coverage is essential. Inadequate or delayed treatment may result in tendon slough and a stiff finger.

Rheumatoid Arthritis.   Rheumatoid arthritis may involve the metacarpophalangeal and finger joints, causing severe deformity from bone destruction and subluxation of the joints. A classic hand deformity caused by rheumatoid arthritis is "ulnar drift" of the fingers at the metacarpophalangeal joints.

This deformity can frequently be corrected and hand function greatly improved by surgically inserting silicone rubber implants (Swanson prosthesis) into the metacarpophalangeal joints. This usually results in a functional arc of stable motion at these joints.

Tumors.   Benign tumors of soft tissue and bone are relatively common in the hand. Fortunately, malignant tumors are rare.

GIANT CELL TUMOR (XANTHOMA).   The most common benign soft tissue tumor seen in the hand is the giant cell tumor, or xanthoma, which originates from tendon sheaths and other fibrous structures. It

FIGURE 11-12. A soft tissue giant cell tumor, arising from flexor tendon sheath, exposed at operation.

arises most frequently on the flexor or extensor surface of a finger and appears beneath the skin as a firm nodular, painless swelling. It may produce a pressure erosion of the underlying bone. On cross-section it presents a characteristic yellow-brown color when examined grossly. Treatment is complete surgical excision (Fig. 11–12).

GLOMUS TUMOR. This is a benign tumor involving the neuro-myoarterial glomus, which is a heat regulatory mechanism located in the skin. The tumor frequently, but not always, appears beneath a fingernail as a purplish dot. It causes exquisite pain on pressure and is extremely sensitive to temperature changes. Treatment is surgical excision.

GANGLION. The wrist joint area is the most common site for ganglia, with the fingers ranking second (see p. 289). Ganglia are often discovered accidentally as painless, firm cystic masses arising from flexor tendon sheaths. Occasionally the patient will notice pressure pain when an object is grasped firmly in the hand. Treatment is complete surgical excision.

Other benign soft tissue tumors and masses that may be seen about the hand include lipomas, hemangiomas, solitary fibromas, and foreign body granulomas.

ENCHONDROMA. Enchondroma is a benign tumor of cartilaginous origin that is the commonest bone tumor seen in the hand (see p. 221). The radiographic appearance in a phalanx is of a circular area of radiolucency with a bulging and thinned cortical border (see Fig. 9–3). Often this tumor is asymptomatic until minimal trauma causes a pathologic fracture through the weakened shell of bone. Once the tumor is diagnosed, treatment consists of complete curettage of the bone cavity, which is then filled in with chip bone grafts.

Primary malignant bone tumors are quite rare in the hand. Very infrequently, an osteosarcoma, chondrosarcoma, or Ewing's tumor may be seen. Metastatic carcinoma may occasionally involve the bones of the hand.

TRAUMA

Because the hand plays a role in almost every human endeavor, it is not surprising that it is often injured. It has been stated that more than 75 per cent of all injuries resulting in permanent partial disability occur in the hand and fingers. Joint dislocations and fractures are not uncommon. Lacerating and crushing injuries to the hand may sever tendons and nerves. Industrial accidents may result in traumatic amputation of fingers or even the entire hand. Treatment of hand trauma frequently poses perplexing problems that require specialized knowledge for their solution.

Dislocations. Dislocation of finger joints can occur at the interphalangeal or metacarpophalangeal level. As a rule, these dislocations reduce quite readily with manipulation. The affected finger is immobilized for one week (Fig. 11–13).

Occasionally, the end of a dislocating bone will "button-hole" through the capsule of the joint. When this occurs, the torn capsule may fold around the bone end, thus making closed manipulative reduction impossible. This situation is seen most commonly with dislocations of the metacarpophalangeal joint of the thumb and requires an open reduction with repair of the capsule for its treatment.

Fractures. Fractures of the phalanges and metacarpals may be spiral or transverse. Often there is no displacement of the fracture fragments and simple immobilization will suffice to insure healing. Finger fractures are immobilized for a 10- to 14-day period in gentle flexion. The positions of extension and acute flexion are unphysiologic and prolonged immobilization will lead to finger joint stiffness. Nondisplaced metacarpal fractures are immobilized for a three- to four-week period with the hand and wrist in a position of function.

Displacement of the fracture fragments leads to shortening and rotation of the involved finger. If the displacement cannot be reduced and held by closed methods, a more vigorous form of treatment must be sought. Some treating physicians elect skeletal traction, while

FIGURE 11–13. Dislocation of proximal interphalangeal joint, fourth finger.

others might favor percutaneous pinning of the fracture fragment or open reduction with pin fixation. Regardless of the type of treatment used, the deformity caused by the fracture must be overcome and every effort must be directed to early motion to minimize residual joint stiffness.

Occasionally a patient presents with a severely traumatized hand with extensive skin damage, lacerated tendons and nerves, and multiple fractures. In this instance, the fractures are best treated by intramedullary pin fixation. This provides a stable skeletal framework for the rest of the reconstructive procedures.

BOXER'S FRACTURE. The term boxer's fracture applies to a frequently seen fracture through the neck of the fifth metacarpal, most often obtained by striking an object with a clenched fist. The head of the fifth metacarpal is displaced into the palm and the patient presents with a flattening or loss of the knuckle prominence (Fig. 11–14).

It may be possible to reduce the depressed metacarpal head into normal alignment by pushing upward on the flexed proximal phalanx of the finger and pushing downward on the metacarpal shaft simultaneously. If it proves impossible to reduce the fracture, open reduction and pin fixation can be carried out. If it proves possible to reduce the

FIGURE 11–14. Displaced fracture through the neck of the fifth metacarpal bone (boxer's fracture).

fracture, but impossible to maintain position, percutaneous pinning of the fracture fragments may be carried out in order to maintain the reduction until the fracture heals.

BENNETT'S FRACTURE. Bennett's fracture is a fracture through the base of the thumb metacarpal, with a proximal displacement of the first metacarpal shaft away from the greater multangular bone. It is caused by a force applied to the end of the thumb and if not accurately reduced, can result in permanent disability to the thumb.

If the displacement is minimal, reduction may be obtained by immobilizing the hand and wrist with the thumb in wide abduction, but in most instances, the fragments are displaced and unstable and the fracture will require skeletal traction, percutaneous pinning, or open reduction with pin fixation for its correction.

Tendon Lacerations. Industrial and household accidents can result in lacerating injuries to the hand and fingers that sever flexor tendons (Fig. 11–15). Although these are potentially crippling injuries requiring specialized skill and knowledge for their repair, a few general principles concerning their management should be known to all physicians.

Each finger contains two flexor tendons: The flexor sublimus inserts on the middle phalanx and the flexor profundus inserts on the distal phalanx. The thumb has only one long flexor tendon inserting on the distal phalanx. These flexor tendons are contained in dense

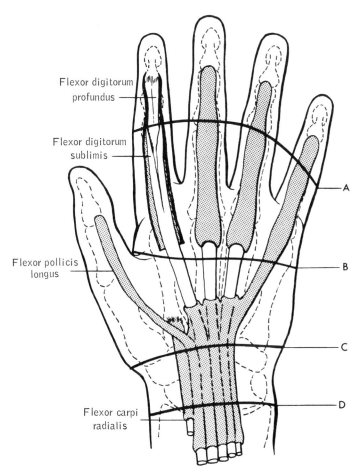

FIGURE 11-15. Flexor tendons and tendon sheaths on palmar surface of hand. Zones indicate common areas of tendon laceration: Zone A, flexor tendons may be repaired primarily distal to line A. Zone A-B, no man's land. No primary tendon repairs here. Delayed management requires a tendon graft. Zone B-C, repair one tendon only. If both are cut, repair flexor digitorum profundus. Zone C-D, may repair more than one tendon. Open carpal ligament. Zone D, more than one tendon may be repaired proximal to line D in forearm. Repair of median nerve takes precedence. Flexor pollicis longus may be repaired throughout its length, but leave tendon sheath open at repair site.

fibrous tunnels or sheaths in the area from the distal flexion crease of the palm to the distal finger joints. This is the area known to the hand surgeon as "no man's land," because primary repair of lacerated flexor tendons in this location frequently results in poor functional results owing to scar adherence between the tendons and the sheath.

Experienced hand surgeons are now reporting successful results following primary and secondary repair of lacerated flexor tendons in "no man's land," but they utilize careful selection of patients and an atraumatic surgical technique. For those surgeons less experienced in hand trauma, it is considered better initial treatment for tendon lacerations in this region to simply cleanse and close the wound, leaving the tendon unrepaired. Later, after complete wound healing has occurred, secondary repair or tendon grafting can be performed. Following this delayed type of repair, a tendon may not become adherent to the fibrous sheath by scar formation.

A laceration may sever both the flexor sublimus and flexor profundus tendons at the same level in the hand. If both tendons are repaired at the same level, they frequently will become adherent to each other with resulting finger stiffness. The proper treatment is repair of the profundus with excision of the sublimus tendon. This is feasible because the profundus runs to the distal phalanx and has sufficient strength to flex the entire finger even in the absence of the sublimus.

If a tendon does become adherent to the fibrous sheath by scar formation, resulting in a finger that has no motion, treatment includes complete excision of the tendon and replacement with a Silastic rod or a Silastic tendon prosthesis around which a new sheath can form. Months later the Silastic rod or Silastic tendon prosthesis can be removed and a flexor tendon graft inserted through the newly formed tendon sheath.

In some areas of the hand and fingers, primary tendon repair is the treatment of choice. However, timing is important. In cleanly incised wounds or in wounds with only minimal tissue damage or contamination, tendons may be repaired safely up to six or eight hours following injury. If the wound is contaminated or contused, or if the surgeon is in doubt about proper treatment, the best course of action is to cleanse and close the wound without tendon repair. Later after complete wound healing has occurred, secondary repair or tendon grafting can be performed.

Occasionally a patient will present with a severely mangled hand including loss of skin covering, multiple fractures, and severed tendons and nerves. The initial treatment of severe trauma to the hand involves meticulous surgical debridement, intramedullary pin fixation of fractures, and skin closure using skin grafts if necessary. The major nerves and the digital nerves should be sutured primarily if possible. If this is not feasible, they can be repaired at a second stage. In the severely mangled hand, severed flexor tendons are never repaired at the time of initial treatment. They are allowed to go unrepaired until complete wound healing has occurred and then are treated by tendon graft replacement.

Until quite recently, the success rate following surgical reimplantation of severed digits and extremities was poor. The adoption of microsurgical techniques to this type of surgery has dramatically increased the chance of success. Provided rapid access to a trained microsurgical team is available, it is presently possible to surgically reimplant severed digits and extremities with a high degree of success.

SPECIFIC CONDITIONS

Mallet Finger (Baseball Finger, Dropped Finger). Mallet finger is the term applied to the deformity that results when a direct blow on the tip of an extended finger forces the distal phalanx into sudden flexion and avulses the extensor tendon from its insertion. The extensor tendon may pull away cleanly or it may tear away along with a chip of bone from the distal phalanx.

The end of the finger exhibits a characteristic "droop" and the patient loses the ability to actively extend the fingertip. Initially the distal interphalangeal joint is swollen and painful. Later, the deformity may be annoying only because of the propensity of the dropped finger to get in the way or catch in clothing or pockets.

If the deformity is treated soon after onset, the distal phalanx may be splinted in the position of hyperextension with the proximal interphalangeal joint flexed for a period of six weeks. In an occasional patient, the deformity may be severe enough to warrant being treated by pin fixation. In either instance, the tendon usually reattaches to bone and a return to adequate function is usually obtained. In patients with the deformity of long duration, surgical repair is often unsatisfactory. However, fusion of the distal interphalangeal joint in the position of function gives good results in the occasional patient who is seen late and whose symptoms are sufficient to warrant surgery.

Trigger Finger. A trigger finger or snapping finger is one that locks in a flexed position and can be extended only with some difficulty associated with a "snap" or "pop." This curious behavior involving fingers and thumb is due to a narrowing or constriction of the flexor sheath at the level of the metacarpal neck. There is an accompanying nodular enlargement of the tendon that is probably secondary to the constriction. This "trigger mechanism," which is almost always located at the level of the metacarpal head, blocks free passage of the tendon, and if the tendon passes the point of obstruction, a click or snap is produced.

Occasionally the condition is relatively painless, but most often is accompanied by an aching pain as a mechanical tenosynovitis develops. Pressure on the trigger mechanism is painful.

In children involvement of the thumb is seen, but rarely involvement of the fingers. Because trigger thumb has been seen in newborns, it is suspected that the condition may be congenital in many instances. In the adult, the condition may involve fingers or thumbs, with the thumb being involved more frequently.

In many instances, hydrocortisone injected into the sheath at the level of the trigger mechanism may reduce local edema sufficiently to allow free tendon gliding to resume. If this does not succeed, surgical excision of the constricted portion of the sheath will effect a cure.

De Quervain's Disease. This is a term applied to a commonly seen, painful, mechanical tenosynovitis that affects the abductor pollicis longus and extensor pollicis brevis in their common sheath passing over the radial styloid to the thumb. The cause may be either trauma or repeated mechanical irritation. If the condition becomes chronic, the sheath may thicken and become stenotic.

De Quervain's disease is more common in women. Patients may complain of pain in the region of the radial styloid and thumb with use of the hand. Motions such as wringing out wet clothes and removing lids from jars may aggravate the pain. The patient may frequently drop lifted objects because of the pain. There may be tenderness to pressure over the affected tendon sheath and the radial styloid. The radial styloid may frequently appear sharply prominent because of the thickness of the overlying tissue which results from the inflammatory lesion. A confirmatory maneuver to elicit pain in this condition is to fold the thumb into the palm and then forcibly snap the wrist into ulnar deviation (*Finkelstein test*).

If the condition is of only a few weeks' duration, it may rapidly respond to local heat and plaster splint immobilization of the thumb and wrist or to local instillation of hydrocortisone into the tendon sheath. Chronic cases, or those not responding to local hydrocortisone, may need surgical release of the tendon sheath at the wrist.

Dupuytren's Contracture. This term is applied to a chronic hyperplasia of the palmar fascia that leads to progressive fibrosis and contracture of the hand. As the contracture matures, the pretendinous bands of the palmar aponeurosis to the fingers shorten and pull the fingers into positions of fixed flexion. The fingers most frequently affected are the ring finger and little finger (Fig. 11–16). The fibroblastic proliferation of the palmar fascia involves the skin and draws it

FIGURE 11-16. Bilateral Dupuytren's contracture. (Courtesy Dr. James Hunter and Dr. Lawrence Schneider, Thomas Jefferson University Hospital, Philadelphia, Pa.)

down into tight puckers and nodules. Firm nodules may be palpated in the palm or the base of the fingers.

Dupuytren's contracture is most common in men past middle age and is usually bilateral. The exact cause is unknown, but a hereditary pattern has been noted. Trauma is not thought to play a significant role since the condition occurs frequently in those who do not do heavy manual labor. A higher incidence in those with gout and diabetes has been observed. The condition, as a rule, is relatively painless, but it may be associated with disabling functional impairment of the hand.

There is no known effective conservative therapy except stretching exercises to the fingers. The treatment of choice is usually operative resection of all the involved palmar fascia. Some surgeons favor a limited or conservative resection, while others favor a radical resection of the palmar fascia with skin grafting if necessary.

Rupture of Extensor Pollicis Longus Tendon. A tendon may rupture as a result of excessive tension or secondary to degenerative or attritional changes in the tendon tissue. Examples already discussed are rupture of the biceps tendon and the mallet finger deformity. Another area that is sometimes affected is the thumb, with rupture of the extensor pollicis longus tendon.

Rupture of this tendon may follow a Colles' fracture and is secondary to attritional or degenerative changes in the tendon substance induced when the tendon rubs against an irregular bony surface. It sometimes occurs in certain occupations, such as those of drummer, polisher, and carpenter. It results in loss of extension of the distal thumb joints and partial loss of extension in the proximal joints with consequent impairment of grasp. Direct suture of the tendon through the ruptured area is frequently not feasible because of loss of tendon length. If this should occur, it is considered better treatment to repair the deformity by use of a free tendon graft or to substitute for its function by means of a tendon transference operation.

References

American Academy of Orthopaedic Surgeons: Symposium on Tendon Surgery in the Hand. St. Louis: C.V. Mosby Co., 1975.

Boyes, J.H.: Bunnell's Surgery of the Hand, 5th Edition. Philadelphia: J.B. Lippincott Co., 1970.

Eyler, D.L., and Markee, J.E.: Anatomy and function of the intrinsic musculature of the fingers. J. Bone and Joint Surg., 36-A:1, 1954.

Flatt, A.E.: The Care of the Rheumatoid Hand. St. Louis: C.V. Mosby Co., 1968.

Flynn, J.E.: Hand Surgery, 2nd Edition. Baltimore: Williams and Wilkins Co., 1975.

Kaplan, E.B.: Functional and Surgical Anatomy of the Hand, 2nd Edition. Philadelphia: J.B. Lippincott Co., 1965.

Landsmeer, J.M.F.: The coordination of finger-joint motions. J. Bone and Joint Surg., 45-A:1654, 1963.

Markee, J.E.: Anatomy of the Hand. Am. Academy of Orthopaedic Surgeons Instructional Course Lectures, Vol. XIV:149. Ann Arbor: J.W. Edwards, 1957.

Swanson, A. B.: Flexible Implant Resection Arthroplasty in the Hand and Extremities. St. Louis: C. V. Mosby Co., 1973.

CHAPTER 12

DISORDERS OF THE JAW, THE NECK, AND THE THORAX

THE JAW

The orthopaedist is rarely confronted with problems involving the jaw. Consultation may be requested regarding fractures, tumors, or infections of the mandible, but in most instances these conditions are treated by oral surgeons. It is more likely that consultation may be requested by patients complaining of pain, snapping, locking, or stiffness involving the temporomandibular joints.

TEMPOROMANDIBULAR JOINT

A patient may be seen with a complaint of pain accompanied by a snapping or "popping" sound in the region of one or both temporomandibular joints. Medical attention is sought when it becomes difficult for the patient to eat because of pain and the accompanying loud noise. Examination may disclose local tenderness over one or both temporomandibular joints, and a palpable click or snap may be felt in the area when the mouth is opened and closed. On a few occasions, a patient may present with locking of the jaw.

It is believed that the most common cause of pain in the temporomandibular joint is chronic joint subluxation resulting from dental malocclusion. This is not difficult to understand when it is

307

realized that, unlike other paired joints in the body, the two temporomandibular joints must move simultaneously and in harmony, being at the complete mercy of the teeth. Two situations may develop, either in association with the dental malocclusion or independently of it, to cause the pain, snapping, and occasional locking. (1) The articular disc of the temporomandibular joint may develop a mechanical derangement — similar to a semilunar cartilage in the knee — to cause pain, snapping, or locking of the joint. (2) Recurrent dislocation of the temporomandibular joint may develop with the condyles of the mandible slipping forward when the mouth is opened. Repeated joint subluxation over a long period of time gradually leads to joint degeneration.

Radiographs of the temporomandibular joint taken with the mouth in the opened and closed positions are necessary for proper investigation of the complaint.

Replacement of missing teeth and correction of malocclusion may be curative if treatment is started before joint degeneration begins. Acute pain in the joint may be effectively treated by local heat and by rest to the jaw and occasionally by the use of intra-articular corticosteroids. Chronic symptoms, particularly if associated with locking, may require surgery. If an internal derangement of the articular disc is found, the disc is removed. Chronic subluxation or dislocation can be treated by condylectomy or a bone block operation.

A sensation of stiffness in the temporomandibular joint may accompany subluxation. True stiffness with actual loss of joint motion may be seen with rheumatoid arthritis, as a late result of trauma, or occasionally as a result of osteomyelitis of the temporal bone secondary to middle ear infection. As a consequence of these disease states, bony ankylosis of one or both of the temporomandibular joints may occur. This results in a serious deformity with profound nutritional implications.

Some motion may be restored to the jaw by resecting the condyles or by performing a surgical arthroplasty of the temporomandibular joint.

THE NECK

The neck, or cervical spine, is an extremely flexible segment of the vertebral column, bridging the space between the head and the relatively rigid thorax. Anatomically, the neck consists of seven cervical vertebrae with their intervertebral discs and articulations, anterior and posterior ligaments, and the anterior and posterior cervical musculature. These structures are compactly associated with the spinal cord, the nerve roots, and the two vertebral arteries with their associated sympathetic nerves. The cervical vertebrae are shaped primarily to give flexibility to this segment of the spine. The upper two cervical vertebrae, the atlas and the axis, are structurally different from the rest of the vertebrae, to allow free mobility of the head. The cervical spine is not only a flexible support between two rigid elements, the head and the thoracic spine, but when normal and intact also acts as a protective bony encasement for the spinal cord, nerve roots, and vertebral arteries with their associated sympathetic nerves.

GENERAL CONSIDERATIONS

Most complaints about the neck develop as a result of congenital deformities or acquired problems such as degenerative joint conditions and trauma. Infection and tumor may involve the cervical spine, but this is less common.

Problems arising in the neck mainly produce pain and restriction of neck motion. Radiation of the pain from the cervical area may involve the head, the anterior chest, the interscapular area, the shoulders, and the upper extremities. Sensations of numbness and tingling in the hands and fingers may be associated complaints. Pain of neck origin is frequently aggravated by the use of a pillow while lying in the recumbent position. For this reason, patients often describe great difficulty in achieving comfort in bed. It is also a common observation that patients suffering from neck problems declare that the period immediately following arising from bed is the time of their worst pain and stiffness. Unguarded movements of the head during sleep and the propped-up position of the head in relation to the shoulders produced by the pillow are believed to irritate the neck.

EXAMINATION OF THE NECK

The position of the head and neck in relation to the whole body and to the shoulder girdle and trunk in particular should be observed and any deviation from normal posture noted. As a result of pain or deformity, the head may be held rigidly in a neutral posture or may be carried in a tilted or rotated position. The presence or absence of spasm or tenderness in the anterior or posterior cervical musculature should be ascertained.

The range of motion allowed by the neck is determined next (Fig. 12–1). Motions of the cervical spine are flexion, extension, ro-

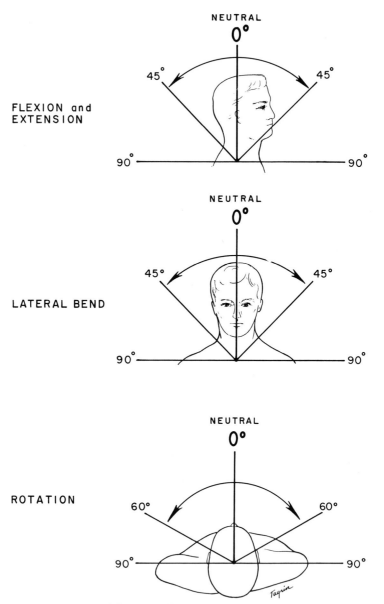

FIGURE 12–1. Motions of the cervical spine. (Courtesy American Academy of Ortho-paedic Surgeons.)

tation to the right and left, and lateral tilt or bend to the right and left. It is important to note whether the neck motions are unrestricted and whether movements of the head on the neck aggravate or reproduce pain.

Any areas of local tenderness along the anterior or posterior column of the neck are noted. It is not uncommon to find areas of local tenderness to palpation in the region of the scalene muscles anteriorly or the trapezius muscles posteriorly or along the spinous process and interspinous area of the cervical spine.

The pattern of any radiating pain must be carefully analyzed and the motion causing it accurately noted. Arm pain does not necessarily originate in the arm itself, but rather may radiate to the arm from the neck or shoulder region. It is important for the examiner to make this distinction carefully. In addition, neck pain may radiate to the head, anterior thorax, interscapular area, and shoulder. Almost always any radiating pain originating in the cervical spine area will be reproduced or aggravated by motions of the head or by a compressive force on the head.

If the symptoms suggest spinal cord or nerve root involvement, neurologic examination of both upper extremities is routinely carried out. This should include evaluation of the biceps, triceps, and brachioradialis reflexes, as well as detection of any abnormalities in motor or sensory pattern.

Examination of the cervical spine is not considered complete without radiographic study of the area. Anteroposterior, oblique, and lateral views with the neck in neutral position are the most useful. Special views are obtained when indicated.

Congenital Deformities

TORTICOLLIS (CONGENITAL WRY NECK)

Torticollis is a congenital abnormality of the sternocleidomastoid muscle that results in a typical positional deformity of the head. In almost all patients, there is an obstetrical history of some type of abnormal delivery such as breech presentation. The most widely held theory of etiology postulates intrauterine malposition of the fetus causing a pressure ischemia of the sternocleidomastoid muscle. This frequently results in fibrosis and ultimate contracture of the muscle. It may also involve the platysma and the scalene muscles. Not infrequently, a firm lump representing a hyperplastic fibrous mass can be palpated in the substance of the sternocleidomastoid muscle.

FIGURE 12–2. Residual torticollis, right, in older boy.

Clinical Picture. The infant lies with the head in a characteristic position. The head is tilted to the side of the deformity and the chin points toward the opposite shoulder (Fig. 12–2). The mother usually notices some restriction of the infant's neck motions. A firm lump may be palpated in the substance of the sternocleidomastoid muscle, but the lump usually regresses in size and ultimately disappears in a few months. Regression may be complete with ultimate resolution of the deformity. In many instances, however, regression is apparently incomplete and a fibrous contracture ensues, resulting, finally, in secondary contracture of most of the soft tissues of the neck.

After several months of deformity, in the more severe cases, a flattening and asymmetry of the face may develop on the side of the contracture. This facial asymmetry usually corrects itself if treatment is completed by about the third year of life. If untreated, the deformity of the head tends to increase with age because of the inability of the fibrotic sternocleidomastoid muscle to grow at relatively the same rate as the cervical spine. If allowed to persist, torticollis will eventually be accompanied by a compensatory curvature of the cervical and upper thoracic spine, elevation of one shoulder, and ocular imbalance.

A significant number of infants with congenital torticollis have an associated congenital dislocation or congenital subluxation of the hip.

Radiographic examination usually reveals a normal appearing cervical spine. Occasionally a torticollis deformity is seen in association with a congenital skeletal abnormality of the cervical or upper thoracic vertebrae such as hemivertebrae or Klippel-Feil syndrome.

Acquired torticollis may appear later in life as a result of trauma or infection in the throat, neck, or cervical spine. It may also be caused by disease of the central nervous system or by psychogenic factors.

Treatment. When the deformity is relatively mild and noted shortly after birth, it can frequently be corrected by gently stretching the head and neck into the overcorrected position. This is done several times daily by the parents.

Surgical treatment is advised for all patients in whom contracture has not been corrected by the age of two years or earlier if the deformity is severe. Usually, surgical division of the sternal and clavicular insertions plus all tight fascial structures is sufficient to obtain correction. In late or very tight cases, the insertion of the muscle into the mastoid process may also have to be cut. A collar, brace, or traction device is used in the immediate postoperative period followed by the continuation of stretching exercises. Recurrence of the deformity may occur because of reattachment of the tight fibrotic muscle ends, necessitating further surgical correction.

CERVICAL RIB

A cervical rib is a congenital overdevelopment of the transverse process of the seventh cervical vertebra and may vary in size from simple enlargement of the process to a complete supernumerary rib. The process attaches to the first rib either by a fibrous band or by bone. This anomaly occurs more often on the right side than on the left but is frequently bilateral.

This abnormality may be significant because the subclavian artery and lowest branch of the brachial plexus arch over the rib. If local pressure occurs, neurologic and vascular symptoms may develop in the arm. However, a cervical rib may be completely asymptomatic.

Clinical Picture. The patient may complain of pain and paresthesia in the forearm and hand, particularly on the ulnar side. An area of sensory loss or anesthesia may be detected in the forearm or hand. Weakness of the hand may be associated with wasting of the thenar interosseous or hypothenar muscles. Vascular manifestations may range from dusky cyanosis of the forearm and hand to gangrene of the fingertips associated with a diminution of the radial pulse. The patient characteristically notices aggravation or relief of symptoms in relation to the position of the arm.

Treatment. No treatment is indicated in the asymptomatic patient. Symptoms can frequently be relieved by the use of a Thomas collar or by various physical therapy devices, such as cervical traction. If symptoms persist, surgical excision of the rib is indicated.

KLIPPEL-FEIL SYNDROME

Klippel-Feil syndrome is a rare congenital malformation of the cervical spine that combines elements of many skeletal deformities. All or part of the cervical vertebrae are fused together. Frequently, many of the laminar arches are open and spina bifida is present. In addition, other developmental deformities of the cervical vertebrae, such as hemivertebrae, may be present and there may be an associated cervical rib.

The clinical result is extreme shortening of the neck, with the head appearing to rise from between the shoulders. Cervical spine motion is markedly restricted and torticollis may be present.

There is no effective treatment.

Acquired Conditions

RHEUMATOID ARTHRITIS

Approximately 30 per cent of patients with chronic rheumatoid arthritis and severe peripheral joint disease will show radiologic evidence of cervical spine subluxation. Often this cervical spine abnormality is not associated with neurologic symptoms, but in approximately 5 per cent of patients with significant cervical subluxation, signs of neurologic involvement or spinal cord compression can be detected on careful examination. These abnormal neurologic findings may vary from frank quadriplegia to minimal proprioceptive loss in either the upper or lower extremities.

Most often, rheumatoid arthritis affects the upper levels of the cervical spine usually producing fusion of the cervical spine elements in children and cervical spinal subluxation in adults. The commonest form of subluxation encountered in rheumatoid arthritis is an anterior subluxation of C1 on C2. Patients with significant C1 on C2 subluxation are at potential risk from falls, from "whiplash" injuries, and from excessive head movements during anesthesia or operations. Long-term studies of rheumatoid patients with cervical spine subluxation indicate that approximately one quarter will worsen, one quarter will improve, and one half remain stable.

Treatment of a rheumatoid patient with cervical spine subluxation associated with neurologic involvement or spinal cord compression includes the use of firm cervical support, a halo cast apparatus, or, eventually, surgical fusion of the involved cervical spine segment.

DEGENERATIVE DISEASE OF THE CERVICAL SPINE

Degenerative disease of the cervical spine is an extremely common clinical problem. Three more or less separate clinical states can be recognized under the general heading of degenerative disease of the cervical spine. These three clinical states are *cervical disc degeneration, degenerative arthritis of the cervical spine,* and *herniated cervical disc.* Although the basic etiologic cause for these conditions has not yet been defined, it is quite likely that it will be similar for all three. The pathologic changes seen in these conditions are quite similar, differing only in degree.

Cervical disc degeneration and degenerative arthritis of the cervical spine basically cause symptoms of pain and stiffness in the neck. In addition, degenerative arthritis of the cervical spine and herniated cervical disc may cause compression of the adjacent spinal nerve roots. If this complication occurs, the patient may complain of pain radiating into the shoulder, arm, or hand and may exhibit signs and symptoms of cervical nerve root compression.

Cervical Disc Degeneration. Degeneration of the cervical intervertebral disc represents premature aging of this particular tissue. The pathophysiology of disc degeneration has been described (see p. 367), but the reason one patient has it and another does not is still unclear.

Rapid depolymerization of the acid mucopolysaccharide and dehydration of the nucleus pulposus of the disc converts this normally gel-like substance into a thinned fibrous scar tissue that can no longer function as an adequate shock absorber. This change most frequently involves the C5–C6 intervertebral disc. Characteristically, disc degeneration results in narrowing of the involved interspace that can best be appreciated on the lateral radiographic view of the cervical spine.

CLINICAL PICTURE. The patient with symptoms related to cervical disc degeneration is generally younger than the patient with symptoms caused by degenerative arthritis in the cervical spine. Females appear to be affected more frequently than males.

The patient will present with acute onset of neck pain usually localized to one side of the neck with extension of the pain into the interscapular area. Symptoms may come on spontaneously or may be induced by some traumatic episode. The neck pain is reproduced or aggravated by motions of the head. Typically, the neck pain is worse in the morning upon arising from bed. The neck pain is commonly associated with occipital headache. Frequently, there is a diffuse radiation of pain into the area of the trapezius muscle and into the general area of the shoulder.

On examination, neck motion is usually restricted because of pain. Palpation along the paracervical muscle masses and over the trapezius muscle generally elicits tenderness. Tenderness over the spinous processes and the interspinous ligaments of both the cervical and upper thoracic spine is a common finding. The neurologic examination is negative.

Radiographic examination typically reveals a normal appearing

FIGURE 12–3. Lateral view of cervical spine, showing changes indicative of disc degeneration at C5-C6 and C6-C7 levels.

cervical spine except for narrowing of the involved interspace (Fig. 12–3).

TREATMENT. The neck is put to rest and pressure is removed from the involved interspace by the use of a soft collar. It is especially important for these patients to wear a collar during sleeping periods. Moist heat to the neck in the form of hot applications or hot showers is most beneficial.

The salicylates and the anti-inflammatory drugs in adequate doses are useful in alleviating pain and stiffness. Cervical traction is not indicated in these patients since they do not have cervical radiculitis.

The vast majority of patients with symptoms caused by cervical disc degeneration obtain relief with conservative measures. Interbody fusion of the affected interspace can be carried out through the anterior cervical approach in those few patients who do not satisfactorily respond to a conservative program.

Degenerative Arthritis of Cervical Spine. Degenerative arthritis of the cervical spine is a diffuse degenerative process that appears simultaneously to involve the intervertebral disc, vertebral bodies, ligamentous structures, and apophyseal joints. With multiple disc degeneration and narrowing of multiple disc spaces, hypertrophic bone changes appear in the form of osteophytes or spurs. These osteophytes form circumferentially about the marginal attachments of the anulus fibrosus to the vertebral bodies, but they are usually more prominent anteriorly than posteriorly. As the narrowing process continues, the apophyseal joints sublux, resulting in additional degeneration of these synovial joints with osteophyte formation at their margins.

CLINICAL PICTURE. The typical patient with symptoms related to degenerative arthritis of the cervical spine is past middle life and complains of stiffness and neck pain. The stiffness is characteristically worse following periods of immobility of the head and is relieved to a certain extent by motion. Pain, on the other hand, is characteristically aggravated by movement of the head and by certain sleeping positions. The pain may localize in the neck, but may radiate to the head, anterior chest, thoracic spine region, or the shoulders.

Motions of the cervical spine are restricted by both pain and stiffness. There is usually diffuse tenderness to palpation over the posterior neck structures and the trapezius muscles.

Radiation of pain to the arm or hand may signal the complication of cervical nerve root compression by bony encroachment on the adjacent spinal nerve roots.

Radiographic examination reveals involvement of multiple cer-

FIGURE 12–4. Lateral radiograph of cervical spine, showing changes indicative of degenerative arthritis.

vical interspaces (Fig. 12–4). The involved intervertebral disc spaces are narrowed, and spur formation may be present along the anterior and posterior aspects of the vertebral bodies. The subjacent bone shows hypertrophic changes with involvement including the apophyseal joints. The C4–C5, C5–C6, and C6–C7 interspaces are the most frequently involved. Narrowing of the intervertebral foramina, reactive bone changes about the apophyseal joints, and bone spurs projecting posteriorly into the nerve root foramina may be present to account for the signs and symptoms of cervical nerve root compression if this is disclosed by examination of the patient.

It is interesting to note that many patients demonstrate these typical radiographic changes indicative of degenerative arthritis of the cervical spine, yet are completely asymptomatic. The fact that almost all persons in the seventh and eighth decades of life show radiographic signs of degenerative change in the cervical spine indicates the correlation between such degeneration and the aging process.

Not infrequently, patients may be seen for the first time with complaints of pain and stiffness in the neck dating from a recent injury.

Radiographic examination reveals the changes typical of degenerative arthritis, which are thought to take years to develop. Is there any connection in this instance between radiographic evidence of previously existing degenerative arthritis and recent trauma to the neck that can bring about a clinical state characterized by stiffness and pain?

As mentioned previously, a patient may show radiographic evidence of degenerative arthritis in the cervical spine segment, yet be completely asymptomatic as far as normal activities are concerned. Flexibility of the involved spinal segment, however, is decreased by the joint narrowing and spur formation. The addition of trauma, particularly of the "whiplash" variety, to this less resilient cervical segment may upset the functional balance of the neck. The neck may be unable to adjust to the additional insult, and the symptoms of neck pain and stiffness may present. In this instance, then, previously existing asymptomatic degenerative changes in the cervical spine may be sufficiently aggravated by trauma to produce the typical symptoms of stiffness and pain. The same may be true for a patient with a prior asymptomatic degenerative disc disease who sustains neck trauma.

TREATMENT. In the vast majority of instances, the symptoms caused by degenerative arthritis of the cervical spine can be alleviated by a nonoperative treatment program. Support to the head with a Thomas collar, particularly during sleeping periods, is especially beneficial. Moist heat applied to the neck musculature is most helpful. Orally administered anti-inflammatory drugs used in adequate doses are effective in the relief of pain and stiffness due to degenerative arthritis if no medical contraindication to their use exists. The blood count should be checked periodically if long-term use of these drugs is contemplated. The use of cervical traction is not indicated unless the complication of cervical radiculitis is present.

Surgery is rarely required in the treatment of degenerative arthritis in the cervical spine unless the problem is complicated by an intractable cervical radiculitis. If spinal fusion is believed to be necessary to control chronic neck pain, the procedure can be carried out through an anterior or posterior approach, depending upon the requirements of the individual case.

Herniated Cervical Disc. Herniation of an intervertebral disc or disc fragment may occur in the cervical spine, but this is much less common than lumbar disc herniation. If frank herniation does occur, however, it is usually secondary to rather severe trauma to the cervical spine and is seen most commonly in younger individuals. The reason for the rarity of this lesion in the cervical spine is that the spinal canal and foramina have relatively strong anatomic barriers to posterior and posterolateral herniation. Posteriorly, the posterior longitudinal ligament is much heavier than that found in the lumbar region. Posterolaterally, the uncus, which contributes to the so-called *joints of Luschka*, provides a bony barrier to nuclear herniation. Thus, in contradistinction to disc herniation in the lumbar spine, frank herniation of the nuclear material in the cervical spine through a defect in the annulus fibrosus and through the posterior longitudinal ligament is quite rare.

Occasionally, however, a piece of disc material escapes the protective anatomic barrier and protrudes laterally to compress an adjacent cervical nerve root. Symptoms of neck pain with radiation into the shoulder, arm, and hand are produced as a result of cervical nerve root compression. In other instances, the herniation may be blocked by anatomic barriers and cannot protrude posterolaterally to press on cervical nerve roots. Instead, it may protrude posteriorly in the midline through a bulging or rupture of the posterior longitudinal ligament to produce cord tract pressure symptoms with manifestations in the low back and legs.

When present, disc protrusions are found most commonly at the C5–C6 and C6–C7 interspaces because that is where maximal motion occurs. Routine films of the cervical spine may be negative. Myelography is helpful in confirming the diagnosis and in localizing the level of involvement. Electromyography is useful in confirming the presence or absence of nerve root irritation.

TREATMENT. Effective conservative treatment is based on decompressing a nerve root by the use of cervical traction and a head halter, preferably with the patient recumbent in bed. The neck is supported with a collar during periods when the patient is out of the traction. Local moist heat to the neck, muscle relaxant drugs, and appropriate analgesic drugs are beneficial.

Surgical treatment, consisting of disc excision and fusion of the interspace, is reserved for those patients who fail to respond to an adequate conservative program and for those showing a neurologic deficit significant in degree or progressive in nature.

CERVICAL NERVE ROOT COMPRESSION SYNDROME (CERVICAL RADICULITIS, CERVICAL ROOT SYNDROME)

Any condition of the neck that causes impingement or entrapment of a cervical nerve root or encroachment on its intervertebral

FIGURE 12–5. Relationship of cervical nerve roots to cervical vertebrae.

foramen may be accompanied by signs and symptoms of a cervical nerve root compression syndrome (Fig. 12–5). The most frequent causes of this condition are degenerative arthritis and herniated vertebral disc. In the cervical spine, degenerative change with posterior spur formation is a more common cause of nerve root irritation than is protrusion of an intervertebral disc. The opposite is true in the lumbar spine. Less frequent causes include cervical subluxation and dislocations, cervical fractures with backward displacement of the fragments, congenital anomalies of the cervical spine, and tumors.

Clinical Picture. The characteristic complaint of the patient with cervical nerve root compression or cervical radiculitis is shoulder and arm pain associated with numbness and tingling in the hand and fingers. The pain is described as severe and sharp and usually follows a radiating pattern from the shoulder to the arm and frequently into the forearm to the fingers. The pain may also radiate to the anterior chest or subscapular area.

Pain is characteristically aggravated by certain motions of the head, particularly turning towards the side of the pain. It is also intensified by coughing, sneezing, straining, or by jarring the neck, as in coming down heavily on the heels, or in the application of pressure to the top of the head. In general, the pain is related to movements of the head and the neck; it is not produced by movements of the shoulder and arm.

The objective signs presented by the patient are determined by the level of involvement. The most common areas of involvement are C5–C6 and C6–C7, with entrapment of the sixth and seventh cervical nerve roots.

If the compression involves the sixth cervical nerve root, the sensation of numbness and tingling will predominate over the lateral aspect of the forearm and hand and into the base of the thumb and index finger. Sensory loss may be noted over the dorsal and radial aspects of the thumb and hand. Weakness of the biceps muscle may be found with a diminished or absent biceps reflex.

If the seventh cervical nerve root is involved, the sensation of numbness and tingling will predominate over the dorsal surface of the wrist and hand and into the base of the index and middle fingers. Sensory loss may be noted over the dorsal surface of the hand and index and middle fingers. Weakness of the triceps muscle may be found with diminished or absent triceps reflex.

Diagnosis is established by an attentive history, a thorough physical examination, and a careful study of the radiographs. Electromyography or myelography may be indicated to aid in localizing the level of involvement.

Treatment. Treatment of cervical nerve root compression syndrome is determined to a certain extent by the cause of the nerve root compression. Surgical treatment is frequently required if the cause is tumor, cervical dislocation, or displaced cervical fractures.

If the cause is arthritic spur impingement or herniated intervertebral disc, the patient is put to bed in head halter cervical traction. A period of several weeks in traction may be required to relieve the nerve compression. Local heat, muscle relaxant drugs, and appropriate analgesics may be added to the program. A Thomas collar is used when the patient is allowed out of bed. Surgical treatment is reserved for those patients who fail to respond to an adequate conservative program and for those patients showing a neurologic deficit of significant degree.

Traumatic Deformities

Flexibility of the cervical spine is gained at the expense of stability, making the intricate soft tissue structures and the slender vertebral column extremely prone to injury. The cervical vertebrae are mechanically vulnerable to trauma, not only because of their shape, but also because of their function. Automobile accidents, falls from high places, diving accidents, and trauma incurred in body contact sports frequently produce injury to the neck.

Trauma to the neck may result in cervical sprain, subluxation or dislocation of one vertebra upon another, fracture of the bony parts, or fracture-dislocation of a vertebra. Some of these conditions result in damage only to muscles, ligaments, and bones. Others may be associated with the grave complication of spinal cord damage.

In the cervical region, the proximity of the spinal cord and nerve roots to the vertebral elements makes neurologic damage an ever present possibility with many of these injuries. Severe cord involvement is more common following cervical spine trauma than after trauma to the thoracic or lumbar regions. Any injury to the cervical spine that results in a decreased anteroposterior diameter of the vertebral canal may be accompanied by spinal cord or nerve root damage. Thus, dislocation of one vertebra upon another, fracture-dislocations of vertebrae, and vertebral fractures in which bone fragments are displaced backward into the vertebral canal are serious injuries associated with varying degrees of temporary or permanent paralysis.

A patient who sustains an apparent clinical spinal cord injury as a result of trauma to the neck should have an immediate thorough neurologic examination to determine if the spinal injury is complete or incomplete. A lesion is classified as complete if there is no perianal sensation and no voluntary control over the sacral innervated muscles, toe flexors, or rectal sphincter. Virtually no patient in whom this situation persists for 24 hours will have functional recovery.

The presence of any evidence of sacral sparing on initial examination as manifested by perianal skin sensation, sensitivity to sharp and dull pin prick, toe flexion, or sphincter control indicates a partial lesion. These patients may have marked functional return, including bowel and bladder control and ambulation. In general, the more sparing found beyond the level of the injury, the better the prognosis for neurologic improvement.

A high percentage of patients who have suffered injury to the neck present with bizarre complaints including dizziness, nausea, headache, transitory deafness, blurred vision, and loss of balance. There is reason to suspect that irritation of the cervical sympathetic nervous system and of the vertebral artery gives rise to a somatoautonomic reflex that accounts for these accompanying symptoms. This is known as the *posterior cervical sympathetic syndrome* or *Barré-Lieou syndrome*.

CERVICAL SPRAIN

The joints of the cervical spine, like other joints in the body, may be subjected to sprain injuries. Force applied to the head or neck may cause a stretching injury to the anterior and posterior cervical ligaments and muscles, with production of the clinical state known as cervical sprain.

The majority of cervical sprains occur as a result of "rear-end" automobile collisions, the impact from which causes hyperextension then hyperflexion of the neck. This is the injury frequently designated "whiplash" — a confusing and misleading term that should not be used by physicians, since it does not accurately describe either the injury itself or the clinical state produced.

The symptoms and signs of acute cervical sprain are those resulting from ligamentous and muscular damage. The initial symptoms may be slight and may go unnoticed in the excitement of the accident. However, after a lag period of hours or days, the patient becomes aware of increasing pain and stiffness in the neck.

The mechanism seems similar to the production of the muscle spasms seen in low back disorders (see p. 349). The anterior and posterior cervical ligaments and muscles are stretched at the moment of injury. These sprained tissues are then required to support the weight of the head while the patient remains ambulatory. This added demand upsets the muscular balance and, after a time (lag period), the paracervical muscles go into spasm, with an accompanying increase in pain and stiffness. The pain may radiate to the shoulders, chest, and upper extremities. It is aggravated by movement or jarring of the head. Injury to the neck muscles may cause pain upon swallowing. Many patients have associated complaints of headache, dizziness, blurred vision, nausea, and loss of balance.

On examination, the patient may be seen to splint the neck and voluntarily restrict motion of the head. When asked to turn the head, the patient may turn the trunk, shoulders, and head together as a unit. The neck muscles usually feel tense and tight and may be tender to palpation.

The neurologic examination usually fails to reveal any alteration in sensory, motor, or reflex pattern.

Radiographic examination is negative for evidence of bone or joint damage. The usual finding is loss of the normal lordotic curve regularly seen on the lateral radiographic view. This extension of the cervical spine is usually seen in association with spasm of the long neck muscles.

Effective treatment is dependent upon adequate and prolonged rest of the neck. This can often be obtained by the use of a Thomas collar. If this is not sufficient, collar support should be combined with bedrest. These measures may be supplemented with local heat, analgesics, and muscle relaxant drugs. Cervical traction is not indicated in the presence of acute post-traumatic muscle spasm.

SUBLUXATION OF A VERTEBRA

Subluxation is an incomplete forward or lateral dislocation of one vertebra upon the one below. Trauma to the head and neck may result in a stretching or tearing of the supporting ligaments, allowing one cervical vertebra to drift partially away from another.

Because the dislocation is incomplete, there is usually no spinal cord involvement. However, pressure or traction on cervical nerve roots typically occurs, and the signs and symptoms of a cervical nerve root compression syndrome are often produced.

Subluxation or partial dislocation of one vertebra upon another can be demonstrated on lateral radiographs of the neck taken in flexion and extension.

Reduction of the subluxation can often be achieved by allowing the patient's head to hang free over the edge of a bed or an examining table. The weight of the head may be sufficient traction to pull the vertebra back into normal alignment. If this procedure is not successful, mechanical traction or manipulative reduction is carried out. After reduction of the subluxation has been achieved, the neck is immobilized in a brace to allow the soft tissues to heal.

As noted previously, a significant number of patients with chronic rheumatoid arthritis will develop subluxation of one vertebra upon another, usually in the upper cervical segment. Mongoloid children also have a high incidence of acquired dislocation of the atlas (C1) on the axis (C2). Although the majority of these retarded children are asymptomatic in regard to the cervical dislocation, spinal cord compression can follow apparently trivial injury.

DISLOCATION OF A VERTEBRA

Anterior dislocation of one vertebral body upon another is a relatively common injury of the cervical spine and is frequently complicated by spinal cord damage with temporary or permanent paralysis below the level of the lesion. This injury results from a fall on the back of the head that causes rupture of the normally weak posterior ligaments, allowing one vertebra to displace forward upon another.

Routine anteroposterior and lateral radiographs will disclose the dislocation (Fig. 12–6).

Skeletal traction applied to the skull is needed to reduce the dislocation. If this is not successful, open surgical reduction is carried out, and the part is immobilized in a plaster cast or a halo cast apparatus. In some patients the reduction will prove to be unstable, allowing the dislocation to recur. Spinal fusion of the involved seg-

FIGURE 12–6. Lateral radiograph of cervical spine, illustrating fracture through posterior elements of C2, with forward and downward displacement of body of C2 and C3.

ment must then be carried out in order to regain stability of the segment.

FRACTURE OF A VERTEBRA

Fracture of a cervical vertebra, the so-called "broken neck," may or may not be a critical injury, depending upon whether there is spinal cord or cervical nerve root involvement.

Simple wedge compression fractures of the vertebral bodies without dislocation, fractures of the transverse and spinous processes, and fracture of the laminae and pedicles without displacement are almost never complicated by spinal cord or nerve root damage. The injury can be readily diagnosed by adequate radiographic examination and usually heals uneventfully following immobilization in plaster or brace.

On the other hand, displaced fractures of the cervical vertebrae with bone fragments encroaching upon the spinal canal and fracture-dislocations of the cervical vertebrae are grave injuries that may be associated with varying degrees of temporary or permanent paralysis or even death. Patients so afflicted require specialized experienced care in regard to first aid measures, transportation, and definitive treatment. Casual, inexpert care at any stage carries the grave implication of increasing the degree of paralysis or even causing death of the patient.

THE THORAX

The thoracic cage is conical in shape and exhibits elements of both rigidity and mobility. Rigidity is supplied by the sternum, ribs, and thoracic vertebrae. Mobility is supplied by the muscles of respiration. In addition to housing and protecting the cardiopulmonary apparatus, the thorax acts as a point of fixation for the upper extremities. The thorax may be affected or deformed directly or it may be involved secondarily by malformations or curvatures of the spine.

The orthopaedic surgeon's interest in the thorax centers about certain developmental and acquired lesions, fractures of the ribs and sternum, and occasionally tumors involving the ribs.

FUNNEL CHEST (PECTUS EXCAVATUM)

This is a developmental deformity of the chest wall characterized by a funnel-shaped depression of the lower end of the sternum and is associated with shortening of the central tendon of the diaphragm, posterior angulation of the costal cartilage, and an outward flare of the lower ribs. As a rule, there is little to no alteration of cardiopulmonary function. The condition is mainly a cosmetic liability and is best treated by a thoracic surgeon.

PIGEON BREAST (PECTUS CARINATUM)

This is a developmental or acquired deformity in which overgrowth of the costal cartilages buckles the sternum forward, causing it to project outward as a cosmetically objectionable ridge. Corrective surgery is best managed by a thoracic surgeon.

KYPHOSCOLIOSIS

The term kyphoscoliosis refers to a severe cosmetic deformity of the spine consisting of two components, *kyphosis* and *scoliosis*. It is most serious when it involves the thoracic spine because it frequently causes pulmonary and cardiac disability. It is encountered most frequently in association with congenital scoliosis and myelomeningocele, but may also be produced by tuberculosis of the spine and poliomyelitis resulting in paralysis of trunk and chest musculature.

Treatment involves management of the cause in addition to the obtaining of cosmetic correction. Mechanical treatment of the deformity is similar to that described for scoliosis (see p. 341).

TIETZE'S SYNDROME

This is an ill-defined painful condition of unknown cause involving the anterior chest wall, and is of importance mainly because it may be confused with a tumor. It is thought to represent inflammatory, traumatic, or degenerative changes involving the costochondral and costosternal junctions and occasionally the sternoclavicular joint. The condition causes pain, tenderness, and some enlargement of the affected part. It is most frequently seen affecting the second and third costochondral junctions. The condition usually subsides with supportive treatment and requires no definitive measures.

FRACTURE OF RIBS AND STERNUM

Trauma to the chest wall may cause fracture of one or more ribs or the sternum. All fractures in this area cause pain with movement of the thoracic cage and are associated with some degree of respiratory embarrassment. With no displacement of fragments, these fractures usually heal uneventfully if the chest is strapped or a rib belt is used for immobilization. Intercostal nerve block may be a helpful adjunct to treatment by relieving pain.

With displacement, bone fragments may penetrate the pleural cavity to pierce the lung or an intercostal artery. If this occurs, the fracture will be complicated by pneumothorax or hemothorax.

Severe trauma to the chest wall may cause multiple fractures of the ribs and sternum with the subsequent development of a flail chest. Unsatisfactory expansion of the lungs due to the flail chest causes distressing dyspnea. Skeletal traction to the chest wall gives stability to the thorax until sufficient bone healing has occurred.

FIGURE 12–7.   Eosinophilic granuloma of sixth rib.

BONE TUMORS

A variety of bone tumors may affect the bony thorax, particularly the ribs. In some cases, the tumor may cause pain and occasionally a pathologic fracture of the rib. In other cases, the tumor may come to light when the patient first notices a lump on the rib cage (Fig. 12–7). The diagnosis rests upon the radiographic findings and histologic interpretation of tissue obtained at biopsy.

Among the benign tumors most commonly affecting the ribs are enchondroma and fibrous dysplasia.

Primary malignant bone tumors affecting the ribs include chondrosarcoma, osteosarcoma, and Ewing's tumor. Involvement of ribs with metastatic carcinoma is relatively frequent. The primary site of these metastatic cancer deposits is usually the breast, lung, kidney, thyroid, or prostate.

References

Bateman, J.E.: The Shoulder and Neck, 2nd Edition. Philadelphia: W. B. Saunders Co., 1978.

D'Abreau, A.L.: Thoracic injuries. J. Bone and Joint Surg., *46-B*:581, 1964.

Fielding, J.W.: Normal and selected abnormal motions of the cervical spine from the second cervical vertebra to the seventh cervical vertebra based on cineroentgenography. J. Bone and Joint Surg., *46-A*:1779, 1964.

Fietti, V.G., and Fielding, J.W.: The Klippel-Feil syndrome: Early roentgenographic appearance and progression of the deformity. J. Bone and Joint Surg., *58-A*:891, 1976.

Friedenberg, Z.B., and Miller, W.T.: Degenerative disc disease of the cervical spine: A comparative study of asymptomatic and symptomatic patients. J. Bone and Joint Surg., *45-A*:1171, 1963.

Hohl, M., and Baker, H.R.: The atlanto-axial joint. Roentgenographic and anatomical study of normal and abnormal motion. J. Bone and Joint Surg., *46-A*:1739, 1964.

Jacobs, B.: Cervical fractures and dislocations. Clin. Ortho. and Rel. Res., *109*:18, 1975.

Johnson, R.M.: Some new observations on the functional anatomy of the lower cervical spine. Clin. Ortho. and Rel. Res., *111*:192, 1975.

Macnab, I.: Cervical spondylosis. Clin. Ortho. and Rel. Res., *109*:69, 1975.

Stauffer, E.S. (Guest Ed.): Spinal cord injuries. Clin. Ortho. and Rel. Res., *112*, 1975.

Southwick, W.O., and Kekki, K.: The normal cervical spine. J. Bone and Joint Surg., *46-A*:1767, 1964.

White, A.A.: Biomechanical analysis of clinical stability of the cervical spine. Clin. Ortho. and Rel. Res., *109*:85, 1975.

CHAPTER 13

THE SPINE,
THE LOW BACK,
AND THE PELVIS

THE SPINE

For our purposes, the spine may be defined as a series of articulated vertebrae that are assembled to form the vertebral column or back. The function of the vertebral column is to support the weight of the trunk, transmit the weight of the body to the lower extremities, and protect the spinal cord and spinal nerve roots from damage. It may be subjected to congenital, acquired, or traumatic deformities.

The thoracic segment of the spine usually consists of twelve vertebrae and the lumbar segment of five vertebrae. The sacral and coccygeal vertebrae are fused together in the adult and are considered clinically as single bones. Except for the sacrum and coccyx, the articulated vertebrae are separated by intervertebral discs that act as shock absorbers and greatly enhance the flexibility of the back. The spine is held erect by the paravertebral muscle masses, which act as lateral supports or guy wires. Their normal stimulus for postural tone is the upright position. These muscles are completely flaccid in the prone or supine position.

The back is an extremely important segment of the body from an orthopaedic point of view. Clinical problems referable to the back, particularly to the low back area, are common in orthopaedic

331

HEMIVERTEBRA

1. *ALL BONES APPEAR HEALTHY.*
2. *ANTERIOR HALF OF VERTEBRA IS <u>ABSENT, NOT COMPRESSED.</u>*
3. *ADJACENT VERTEBRAE ARE EXPANDED TO FIT DEFORMITY.*
4. *NO BULGING ANTERIORLY.*
5. *OTHER DEVELOPMENTAL ABNORMALITIES (RIB) MAY BE PRESENT.*
6. *INTERSPACES ARE WELL PRESERVED.*

SENILE AND JUVENILE OSTEOPOROSIS

END PLATES OF VERTEBRAE ARE BICONCAVE AND BODIES ARE NARROWED IN MIDSECTION; BONY TEXTURE RADIOLUCENT WITH OCCASIONAL RELATIVE SCLEROSIS OF PERIPHERY.

SCHEUERMANN'S DISEASE
(JUVENILE KYPHOSIS; KYPHOSIS DORSALIS JUVENILIS; OSTEOCHONDROSIS.)

VERTEBRAE WEDGED WITH UNDULATING END PLATES AND NUMEROUS SCHMORL'S NODES; SECONDARY LIPPING AND DEGEN-ERATIVE CHANGES LATER SUPERVENE

PATCHY AREAS OF BONE DESTRUCTION

IN FRESH COMPRESSION FRACTURES, A DISCONTINUITY EXISTS ANTERIORLY, AND A SCLEROTIC IRREGULAR FRACTURE LINE IS SEEN; THIS DISAPPEARS AFTER HEALING.

"MOTH-EATEN" AND COMPLETE COLLAPSE

COMPRESSION FRACTURE

METASTATIC NEOPLASM

FIGURE 13–1. Vertebral contour changes seen in various spinal conditions. (From Meschan, I.: Analysis of Roentgen Signs, Vol. 1. Philadelphia: W. B. Saunders Co., 1973.)

practice. Congenital and mechanical deformities may cause symptoms at any period of life. Trauma to the back takes on added significance because of the proximity of the spinal cord. Infections, metabolic diseases, and tumors not infrequently implicate the spine (Fig. 13–1).

EXAMINATION OF THE SPINE

When a patient's back is examined in the anteroposterior view, the spine should appear straight with the head balanced over the sacrum (Fig. 13–2). A plumb line dropped from the posterior occipi-

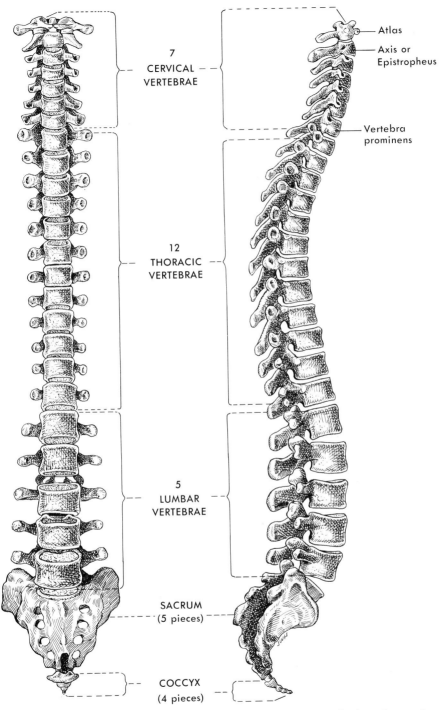

7
CERVICAL
VERTEBRAE

Atlas

Axis or
Epistropheus

Vertebra
prominens

12
THORACIC
VERTEBRAE

5
LUMBAR
VERTEBRAE

SACRUM
(5 pieces)

COCCYX
(4 pieces)

FIGURE 13-2. In the AP view the spine should be straight. In the lateral view the spine assumes four gentle physiologic curves.

tal tuberosity should fall directly over the intergluteal fold. Any lateral curvature or deviation is considered abnormal and has either a structural or a nonstructural cause. Nonstructural causes include not only poor posture, but also leg length inequality, pelvic tilt, contracture about the hip joint, paravertebral muscle spasm, and the "sciatic scoliosis" seen with herniated intervertebral disc. The principal structural cause is true spinal scoliosis.

When the back is examined in the lateral view, it is seen that the spine is not straight but rather consists of four gentle curves. Curvature exists with the convexity forward in the cervical and lumbar regions and the concavity forward in the thoracic and sacral regions. These are normal physiologic curves varying in magnitude from one person to another. In normal health or in normal mechanical alignment, however, the amplitude of the concave curves should just about balance the amplitude of the convex ones. In certain abnormal conditions, these curves may be either greatly accentuated or almost entirely obliterated.

The term "round back" refers to accentuation of the thoracic curvature — the deformity brought on by an increase beyond the normal physiologic curve of the thoracic segment of the spine. This may be the result of poor posture, particularly in tall, thin individuals. It may also be caused by the effects of Scheuermann's disease (p. 101), or it may be secondary to anterior wedging of the vertebral bodies as a result of osteoporosis of the thoracic spine in elderly people (p. 118).

When the thoracic spinal curvature passes beyond the "round back" stage and becomes a sharp angular deformity, it is referred to as a *kyphosis*, meaning knuckle. This is always a serious deformity because the sharp, bony curvature may produce an angular kinking of the spinal cord with resultant neurologic damage. This type of deformity may be caused by a compression fracture of the vertebral body or by tuberculosis of the spine.

The term *lordosis* refers to accentuation of the cervical or lumbar curvature beyond physiologic levels. In the lumbar region, the forward curve can be accentuated by lumbar vertebral deformities, such as spondylolisthesis, forward tilt of the pelvis, obesity, paralysis of the abdominal muscles, congenital dislocation of the hips, or hip flexion contractures. In both the cervical and lumbar regions, spasm of the paravertebral muscles may be associated with loss or flattening of the normal forward curve.

In general, the spine makes every effort to keep the head and trunk in balance. Deformity of one part of the spine is usually balanced by deformity in the opposite direction in another region of the spine in order to maintain the trunk erect and head centered over the pelvis. For example, a thoracic round back deformity would be accompanied by relative cervical and lumbar lordosis, while flattening of the lumbar spine would be associated with flattening of the thoracic spine. Lateral scoliotic curves are similarly associated with compensatory curves above and below the primary or main curve.

In some disease states, the portion of the spine that should compensate for a deformity may be too damaged or rigid to respond. In these instances, the trunk and head are forced out of line and out of balance, resulting in a severe disabling deformity for the patient.

Congenital Deformities

Congenital deformities of the spine are very common. It has been estimated that not more than one of five persons has a completely normal vertebral column by radiographic examination. The majority of congenital vertebral deformities occur in the lumbar spine, but fortunately, only a small number of these deformities cause symptoms.

The congenital anomalies most frequently seen on radiographic examination are variations in the structure of the lumbosacral joint, including spina bifida, variations in the number of lumbar vertebrae, and abnormalities of the lateral articulations. Some of these are occasionally associated with lumbosacral instability (Fig. 13–3).

HEMIVERTEBRA

Hemivertebra results from failure of development of the lateral half of a vertebral body due to a developmental error. This produces a wedge-shaped vertebra or one-half of a vertebra, which could occur in any area of the spine. The clinical effect of a hemivertebra is usually to produce a lateral curvature of the vertebral column that, with growth of the spine, may progress to a clinically significant structural scoliosis.

SPONDYLOLISTHESIS

The entity of one vertebra slipping forward on the one below is known as spondylolisthesis. The term "spondylo" means vertebra and "olisthesis" means to slip or slide down a slippery path. The

A

B

FIGURE 13-3. A, normal-appearing lumbosacral joint. B, congenital anomaly involving the lumbosacral joint, including sacral spina bifida occulta and sacralization of the fifth lumbar body.

term describes a deformity of the spine in which a vertebral body with the vertebral column above it subluxes or glides forward on the vertebral body below. The body and pedicles of the affected vertebra tend to slip forward, while the laminae and spinous process remain behind with the vertebra below (Fig. 13–4).

This state of affairs comes about because of the development of a defect or break in the pars interarticularis, giving rise to a bony

APOPHYSEAL JOINT, BEING FIXED, ACTS AS PIVOT. NO ANCHORAGE BECAUSE OF DEFECT.

POINT C MOVES LITTLE. POINT D MOVES THROUGH ARC D-D.

A

B

FIGURE 13–4. *A*, diagram illustrating the usual mechanism of spondylolisthesis. (Diagram from Meschan, I.: Analysis of Roentgen Signs, Vol. 1. Philadelphia: W. B. Saunders Co., 1973.) *B*, lateral view of spine showing moderate forward slipping of body of fifth lumbar vertebra on sacrum.

discontinuity between the anterior and posterior halves of the neural arch. It is now generally believed that the most frequent cause of spondylolisthesis is an undetected fatigue fracture occurring in a pars that is elongated and mechanically weak. A second type, seen most frequently in the lumbosacral joint, is believed due to a congenital developmental error. A third type, degenerative spondylolisthesis, occurs most frequently at the fourth lumbar vertebra in females in the fifth decade or over. This type is not associated with a neural arch defect, but frequently produces spinal stenosis (see p. 363) at the level of the vertebral slipping.

Spondylolisthesis commonly affects young adults; its incidence is believed to be 6 or 7 per cent in the western hemisphere. The defect is found most frequently at the lower end of the spine, with the fourth lumbar vertebra displaced forward on the fifth, or the fifth lumbar vertebra displaced forward on the sacrum. In addition to regular anteroposterior and lateral radiographs of the spine, it is necessary to obtain oblique views taken at a 45-degree angle to adequately visualize the pars interarticularis in order to be certain whether a bony defect is or is not present.

Patients are sometimes seen in whom the defect is visible on oblique radiographic views but in whom little to no displacement of the vertebral body has occurred. If there is no displacement of the vertebral body, the condition is called *spondylolysis*. However, before one can be certain no displacement exists, lateral radiographs of the lower spine made in the recumbent and the standing positions should be compared.

The major complaint of the patient with spondylolisthesis is chronic low back pain. In the majority of patients, no further vertebral slippage occurs and no neurologic involvement develops. In an occasional patient, fibrocartilage may pile up along the bone defect, causing pressure on the adjacent lumbosacral nerve root. If this occurs, the patient will develop the signs and symptoms of sciatica in addition to the back pain. Sciatica may also complicate spondylolisthesis when an intervertebral disc is herniated at a vertebral level just above the level of the spondylolisthesis.

Frequently, back pain in this condition can be controlled by the use of a back support, such as corset or brace, combined with back strengthening exercises and the avoidance of bending and lifting. Spinal fusion of the involved area is indicated in those patients who fail to respond to nonoperative treatment methods or those patients in whom further slippage can be demonstrated. If the condition has been complicated by neurologic compression, the loose bony elements should be removed to relieve the compression and the spine fused around the laminar defect.

Acquired Deformities

SCOLIOSIS

There are three basic types of spinal deformity, kyphosis, lordosis, and scoliosis, which may occur singly or in combination. The term scoliosis, derived from the Greek word meaning *curvature*, refers to a lateral curvature of a segment of the spine from the normally straight midline position. The term actually describes only a physical deformity, not a diagnosis. The known causes of scoliosis are many and include intrinsic deformity of the vertebrae, involvement of the muscle and nerve elements that support the spine and, occasionally, causes arising outside the spine itself. In general, two types of scoliosis are recognized: nonstructural scoliosis and structural scoliosis.

Nonstructural scoliosis is caused by postural influences on the spine and is not associated with any structural spinal changes. Nonstructural curves exhibit normal flexibility and tend to disappear when the patient is recumbent. The cause may be poor posture, leg length inequality, pelvic tilt, hip joint contractures, or paravertebral muscle spasm. As a rule, functional scoliosis poses no real orthopaedic problem.

Structural scoliosis is a lateral curvature of a segment of the spine that exhibits lack of normal flexibility and, unlike a nonstructural curve, tends not to disappear when the patient is recumbent. This ultimately results in a fixed lateral spinal curvature of varying severity and rigidity, associated with deformed wedge-shaped vertebral bodies and rotation of the vertebral bodies to the convex side of the curve. Structural scoliosis may have a congenital origin (hemivertebrae), or it may be associated with some neuromuscular disorders, such as cerebral palsy, poliomyelitis, or myelomeningocele. It may be found in association with neurofibromatosis and, occasionally, accompanies mesenchymal disorders, such as Marfan's syndrome. In the greatest majority of patients with structural scoliosis, however, the cause remains unknown. This form is called idiopathic scoliosis and is the type for which the orthopaedist is most frequently consulted.

IDIOPATHIC SCOLIOSIS

Idiopathic scoliosis is the most common of all forms of lateral curvature of the spine. It appears during the growing years in a previously normal straight spine. It is thought to begin insidiously and, because of the concealing effect of clothing, may reach considerable proportions before being noticed. The deformity caused by the curvature may worsen appreciably during the child's periods of rapid growth. It seems probable that idiopathic scoliosis is an inherited disease with the mode of inheritance being multifactorial. It occurs most frequently in the female, in an incidence reported to range from 2 per cent to 5 per cent of the adolescent population. Generally, the younger the patient at the time the curve is discovered, the worse the prognosis.

Clinical Picture. Several types of curvatures are recognized clinically and are classified by location. The most common is a primary or major curve that arises in the thoracic segment with the convexity to the right associated with a compensatory curve above in the cervical segment and one below in the lumbar segment, both with the convexity to the left. A compensatory curve is a curve above or below a major curve that tends to maintain normal body alignment. It may be structural or nonstructural. The parent's or patient's attention is usually first drawn to the deformity by the postural asymmetry caused by this combination of curves or by poorly fitting clothing.

The postural asymmetry resulting from a typical right thoracic, left lumbar scoliosis forces the child to stand with the right shoulder elevated and the left iliac crest prominently tilted upward. Rotation of the vertebral bodies to the right in the thoracic segment causes an increase in the posterior angulation of the rib cage on the same side and also prominence of the right scapula. The opposite side of the posterior thorax appears flattened. The asymmetry of the posterior thorax is accentuated when the spine is flexed (Fig. 13–5).

As a rule, a child with scoliosis does not have back pain despite the appearance of the deformity. When older, children may complain of back fatigue and pain, these being on a muscular basis secondary to the longstanding imbalance. Constant back pain usually signals the complication of degenerative arthritis within the affected vertebral segment. This complication is seen most frequently in adults in whom degenerative arthritis develops in the curve segment secondary to the bony malalignment of uncorrected scoliosis.

In patients with severe curvature, the organs of the chest and abdomen may be compressed by the resulting skeletal deformity. Marked thoracic scoliosis may result in cardiorespiratory distress. Almost all patients with thoracic deformity show some decrease in pulmonary vital capacity. Severe scoliosis may produce a restrictive ventilation abnormality. Chronically inadequate ventilation of the alveolar capillary bed may lead to pulmonary hypertension and kyphoscoliotic heart disease.

It was formerly believed that these curvatures did not increase

FIGURE 13-5. *A*, postural deformity caused by idiopathic thoracolumbar scoliosis. *B*, asymmetry of posterior thorax accentuated with patient flexed.

much in magnitude once spinal growth was completed. Studies have now shown that it cannot be assumed that curvature of the spine in the adult will not progress. Curves of the magnitude of 60 degrees or more in the adult are likely to progress, with increasing loss of pulmonary function. Most curves of less than 40 degrees in the adult do not progress or progress only minimally.

A complete radiographic study of the spine is needed to establish the diagnosis and to identify the characteristics of curvature in regard to flexibility and correctability.

Treatment. Spinal curves up to the magnitude of 25 degrees are considered mild deformities, and if the spine is flexible, a heel lift of sufficient thickness to level the pelvis might be prescribed. This should be combined with spinal stretching exercises designed to increase the flexibility of the vertebral column. The child must be observed carefully, and the status of the spinal deformity checked by radiographic examination every several months.

Patients with spinal curves in the magnitude of 30 to 50 degrees are treated with a Milwaukee brace and spinal exercises. This is a specially designed scoliosis brace with occiput and chin pieces, a molded pelvic girdle, lateral pads, and upright spinal bars. The brace affords comfortable passive support by distraction and the holding force of lateral pads. Use of the Milwaukee brace is indicated in most adolescent patients with idiopathic curves of moderate severity and in all young children, no matter what the etiology or magnitude of the deformity. In many patients, prolonged use of the brace results in permanent correction of the scoliosis. In others it may diminish the severity of the curve sufficiently to make subsequent surgery less extensive and formidable.

Surgical correction is generally recommended for curves of the magnitude of 60 degrees or greater. The definitive operation for scoliosis is spinal fusion of the involved segment. However, before fusion is performed, the spine should be straightened as much as possible. The use of preoperative stretching casts allows correction of some deformity before surgery. At the time the surgery is performed, metallic Harrington rods are hooked into the spine across

FIGURE 13–6. *A,* idiopathic thoracolumbar scoliosis of moderate severity. *B,* same patient after Harrington rod correction and spinal fusion.

the section of the curvature in order to maintain and hold the straightened spinal position until the spinal fusion has solidly healed (Fig. 13–6).

ARTHRITIS

The spine is a common site for the development of arthritic changes of various types.

The degenerative arthritis or osteoarthritis generally seen in older age groups frequently involves the spine, particularly the lumbar spine segment. In young individuals, degenerative arthritis may involve the thoracic or lumbar spine, particularly as a complication of some primary problem that causes malalignment of the vertebrae, such as Scheuermann's disease or scoliosis.

Ankylosing spondylitis is a systemic collagen disease that tends to begin in the sacroiliac joints, but often progresses from the lumbar area to involve the entire vertebral column (p. 146). It is seen most frequently in men between the ages of 20 and 40 years. The pathologic changes occurring in the joints are similar to the changes seen with rheumatoid arthritis. As the disease progresses, there tends to be involvement of the ligaments of the spine, with calcification and eventual rigidity of the spine.

INFECTION

Pyogenic infection of the spine is called *vertebral osteomyelitis* or *pyogenic spondylitis*. The infecting organism is usually bloodborne to the spine from some primary focus of infection elsewhere in the body. Rarely, infection may develop following spinal surgery or spinal puncture. Not infrequently, it may appear to commence as a disc space infection. Over the past few years, a startling increase in disc space and sacroiliac joint infections has been observed in drug addicts, with a high incidence of gram-negative organisms as the infecting agents.

The patient notices back pain that may or not be associated with systemic signs of infection. In spite of a paucity of local objective physical findings, the back pain is frequently quite severe and is often associated with functional disability. Radiographic examination eventually discloses evidence of bone destruction involving one or more vertebral bodies, accompanied by characteristic narrowing or loss of the intervertebral disc space (Fig. 13–7). Bone tissue exhibits a positive host response to invading pyogenic organisms and eventually the radiograph will show the presence of

FIGURE 13–7. *A*, pyogenic infection of the T12-L1 interspace. *B*, fifteen months later solid bony fusion existed.

reactive bone formation around the destructive lesion, illustrating a walling-off process.

Treatment is rest to the spine and adequate antibiotic therapy. In some instances, it may be possible to obtain material for culture from needle biopsy of the involved area. Rest to the spine may be obtained in bed or by the use of a plaster body cast or brace.

As healing occurs, serial radiographic examinations will show filling in or healing of the destructive lesions in the vertebrae. Frequently, the involved vertebrae may progress to spontaneous bony fusion. On rare occasions, it may be necessary to operate in order to drain the abscess, particularly if neurologic complications appear.

In years past, tuberculous infection of the spine, known as *Pott's disease,* was one of the commonest causes of vertebral kyphosis or "hunchback" deformity. The spine, particularly the dorsolumbar junction, is the skeletal area most frequently involved with tuberculosis (p. 187).

Radioisotope bone scanning techniques may be useful when the diagnosis of vertebral infection is not clear. There will be increased uptake in bone tissue in most inflammatory processes involving bone. In local skeletal lesions, such as infection, fractures, or tumor, the rate of mineral metabolism in the area of the lesion is increased. Appropriately selected radioisotopes given intravenously will accumulate at the site of the lesion, with resultant increased radioactivity over the area involved. The method is useful in the early diagnosis of dubious primary lesions and recurrences, but it cannot differentiate between various spinal infections, such as pyogenic spondylitis and tuberculosis.

TUMORS OF THE VERTEBRAL COLUMN

Benign tumors involving the vertebrae are unusual.

Hemangioma, a benign blood vessel tumor, may appear in the substance of a vertebral body giving rise to characteristic vertically striped trabeculation within the vertebral body as seen on radiographic examination. The tumor may weaken the structure of the bone, leading to pathologic fracture with collapse of the vertebral body (see p. 225).

Aneurysmal bone cyst is an expanded balloon of bone protruding from the cortical surface of a bone and containing a mass of vascular tissue. It is a benign bone tumor that may arise in the vertebrae (see p. 227).

Except for plasma cell myeloma, primary malignant bone tumors arising in the vertebral column are quite rare. Much more frequently, the spine is the site of metastatic cancer deposits from primary tumors in the breast, prostate, thyroid, kidney, and lungs. Secondary involvement of the vertebral column may also accompany leukemia, Hodgkin's disease, and malignant lymphoma.

Chordoma. Chordoma is an uncommon tumor that occurs in bone primarily at either end of the vertebral column. It develops from remnants of the embryonic notochord, such as nucleus pulposus or abnormal "rests" of notochordal tissue. More than half of the tumors occur in the bone of the sacrococcygeal region. The tumor is slow growing, affects mostly patients in the middle years of life, and is considered malignant because it is locally invasive.

Treatment is surgical excision, which is frequently incomplete because of the tumor's capacity for extensive growth (see p. 241).

Intraspinal Tumors. Although their treatment is not within the scope of orthopaedic surgery, intraspinal tumors may give rise to back and leg pain and should thus be considered in differential diagnosis of back pain, particularly of radiculitis. Approximately 1 per cent of patients operated upon for herniated lumbar disc are found to have an intraspinal tumor.

In general, two types of intraspinal tumors are described: extradural and intradural. A careful history and physical examination coupled with a close review of the radiographic findings and myelographic pattern help one to differentiate tumor from other causes of nerve root compression.

Usually, extradural tumors are secondary and represent metastatic carcinoma or spreading from lymphatic system tumors, such as Hodgkin's disease, lymphosarcoma, and reticulum cell sarcoma.

Intradural tumors are most often primary and include meningioma, neurofibroma, glioma, medulloblastoma, and ependymoma.

Traumatic Deformities

Fracture or dislocation involving the thoracic or lumbar segment of the spine is not accompanied by severe cord involvement as frequently as are similar injuries occurring in the cervical segment. Severe spinal cord involvement is the exception in the thoracic and lumbar regions, and consequently most patients who "break their backs" suffer no cord or spinal nerve root injury. Spinal injury statistics indicate that approximately 95 per cent of patients sustaining spinal fractures suffer simple skeletal injuries usually associated with relatively brief periods of disability and excellent prognosis. The remaining 5 per cent of patients sustaining spinal fractures will have neurologic deficit.

The cervical and lumbar segments of the spine are mobile, while the thoracic and sacral segments are relatively rigid. The thoracolumbar junction, therefore, marks an abrupt transition between rigid and mobile segments of the spine. If a force is applied to the body sufficient to produce motion of the spine beyond the physiologic range, the lumbar spine, because of its location between two relatively rigid segments, is highly susceptible to fracture or dislocation. For this reason, the great majority of spinal fractures occur in the lumbar and distal thoracic regions of the spine, usually as the result of hyperflexion injuries. The region from T12 to L2 accounts for more than 50 per cent of all vertebral body fractures, and approximately 40 per cent of all spinal cord injuries are at the T12 to L1 level. Neurologic deficit due to skeletal disruption at or above T10 is due almost entirely to cord damage. Between T10 and L1, neurologic deficit is usually due to both cord and spinal nerve root damage. Below L1, neurologic deficit is due entirely to spinal nerve root damage.

The most common fracture in the thoracic and lumbar spine is an anterior compression fracture of the vertebral body (Fig. 13–8). The next in frequency are fractures of the transverse and spinous processes. These fractures are almost never complicated by spinal cord or spinal nerve root involvement. These fractures can be expected to heal uneventfully following a period of bed rest and support to the spine.

Severely displaced fractures or fracture-dislocations in the tho-

FIGURE 13–8. Traumatic compression fracture of the body of L5.

racic and lumbar regions may encroach upon the spinal cord and cause neurologic damage. A person may recover from traumatic loss of spinal cord function if the injury is a reversible anatomic lesion or a physiologic disturbance without an anatomic lesion. However, loss of spinal cord function due to a major anatomic disruption of the cord has little to no chance for reversal.

The spinal cord ends, as a rule, at the level of the first or second lumbar vertebra as the conus medullaris. Fractures at the thoracolumbar junction causing injury to the conus are associated with saddle anesthesia, loss of sphincter control, and usually loss of ankle reflexes. Injuries to the lumbar spine below the first lumbar vertebra have a better prognosis from a neurologic standpoint because the cauda equina, having mobility, is less vulnerable to trauma. In addition, the abundant space available within the lumbar spinal canal contributes greatly to the generally more favorable neurologic prognosis for injuries in the lumbar spine as compared to the thoracic spine.

These fractures are serious skeletal injuries and demand careful and expert care. If at all possible, displaced fractures and fracture-dislocations should be reduced. Depending on the injury and the circumstances, reduction could be closed or open. If the reduction is stable, immobilization could be effected in a cast or brace. If the reduction proves unstable, surgical fusion of the involved segment should be performed to insure spinal stability.

LOW BACK PAIN

Low back pain is one of the most frequent patient complaints heard by a physician. There are no accurate frequency figures available from the United States, but a study in Sweden concluded that 65 per cent of the adult Swedish population had, at one time or another, sought medical attention for back pain.

Low back pain is a symptom, not a diagnosis; hence it must be clearly understood that the causes are myriad and could be medical, obstetrical, gynecologic, urologic, metabolic, or psychosomatic, as well as musculoskeletal in origin. Disorders of the kidney, the pelvic viscera, retroperitoneal tumors, and abdominal aneurysms may all have the associated complaint of low back pain. Peripheral vascular disease causing intermittent claudication may on occasion mimic sciatic pain produced by spinal nerve root irritation.

Most low back pain, however, has a musculoskeletal basis. Some conditions of the spine that can cause low back pain have already been discussed in this chapter. The most frequent orthopaedic causes of low back pain are considered in this section and include acute lumbosacral strain, unstable lumbosacral mechanism, osteoarthritis of the lumbar spine, spinal stenosis, and problems involving the intervertebral disc.

General Considerations

Regardless of the underlying orthopaedic causes of low back pain, patients frequently have certain signs and symptoms in common. They may exhibit paravertebral muscle spasm of varying degree and severity. Their pain may be localized to the small of the back or may radiate up along the spinal column towards the neck and head or down into the pelvis, buttocks, or thighs. Low back pain may be associated with sciatica, which is a symptom of nerve root irritation and causes pain along the anatomic distribution of the sciatic nerve.

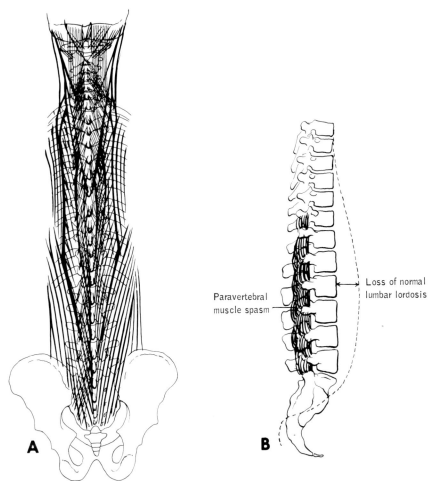

FIGURE 13–9. *A*, in normal health the paravertebral muscles act as guy wires to help hold the spine erect. *B*, following a painful stimulus, the paravertebral muscles may go into spasm as part of the body's defense mechanism.

PARAVERTEBRAL MUSCLE SPASM

The paravertebral muscles play a dual role in body mechanics (Fig. 13–9). Normally, they act as physiologic guy wires helping to hold the trunk erect. Their physiologic stimulus for postural tone is the upright position. These muscles are completely flaccid in the prone or supine position.

Their second role in body mechanics is that of a protective mechanism. A painful stimulus arising from the low back area may trigger paravertebral muscle spasm, which is defined as markedly exaggerated muscle tone, initiated by a stimulus of trauma or pain and maintained by the upright position. It is, in effect, a warning to the patient to protect the back from movement and from possible further damage. The occurrence and effects of paravertebral muscle spasm can be aborted by removing the stimulus of the upright position through absolute bed rest. If the patient is allowed to remain ambulatory, the low back area is progressively splinted by the muscle spasm. If unchecked, the clinical symptoms produced by paravertebral muscle spasm may cause extreme functional disability.

SCIATICA

Patients may present with low back pain and the additional complaint of posterior leg pain, representing an associated sciatica. This type of leg pain must be carefully differentiated from the diffuse muscular and ligamentous radiation pattern associated with tight hamstring muscles or accompanying some of the mechanical and degenerative lesions of the low back.

Sciatica attendant upon low back pain represents the peripheral manifestation of compression of the lumbosacral spinal nerve roots (Fig. 13–10). The most frequent causes of this compression are herniated intervertebral disc, compression of a spinal nerve root by an osteoarthritic spur, spinal stenosis, and intraspinal tumors. The symptoms and signs accompanying nerve root compression in this area, regardless of cause, are similar and constitute the so-called lumbosacral nerve root compression syndrome. A physician can uncover the presence of an associated nerve root compression syndrome by a thorough history and physical examination. Further

FIGURE 13–10. Relationship of lumbosacral nerve roots to lumbar vertebrae.

tests, however, are necessary to pinpoint the exact cause of the nerve root compression.

The predominant symptom of lumbosacral nerve root compression is leg pain that follows the sciatic distribution (buttock, posterior thigh, popliteal space, and calf) and which may then divide to involve either the medial or lateral part of the foot. The pain is aggravated by spinal movements and by anything that raises the intrathecal pressure, such as lifting, coughing, sneezing, or straining. The pain is characteristically sharp and severe and may be associated with tingling, a sensation of hot water running down the leg, or hypesthesia over the foot and toes. There is usually tenderness to palpation over the sciatic nerve trunk in the posterior thigh and buttock. If the pain is due to sciatica, it will be reproduced or aggravated by the straight leg raising test and the sitting root test.

The positive neurologic signs produced by lumbosacral spinal nerve root compression are those of a lower motor neuron lesion. The Achilles reflex and occasionally the patellar reflex, depending on the level of involvement, may be normal, depressed or absent, but never hyperactive. The muscles most frequently affected by compression at the lower lumbar levels are the anterior tibial and toe extensors. The motor power of these muscles may be normal, weak, or absent, but never increased or spastic. Sensation over the dermatome supplied by the compressed spinal nerve root may be normal, diminished, or absent, but not increased.

Examination of the Low Back

HISTORY

Once it has been ascertained that the patient's chief complaint is low back pain, the examiner should, by direct questioning, determine its specific location, duration, and character and whether or not it radiates to another part of the body. The location is best determined by asking the patient to point to the place that hurts.

The character of the pain is discovered by asking about its severity, constancy, and intensity. Acute low back pain is generally more severe and of shorter duration. Chronic low back pain is frequently described as an ache and tends to be present intermittently. Since most causes of musculoskeletal low back pain are mechanical in origin, it is important to discover if the pain is influenced by movement of the spine. Often, low back pain is aggravated by bending and lifting and relieved by resting the back. Frequently, particularly in degenerative lesions of the lumbar joints, an element of stiffness is noted by the patient following periods of relative immobility, as on arising from bed in the morning or after a long automobile trip.

It is important to determine whether the pain radiates to another part of the body. Frequently, the pain may radiate up the back toward the neck and head, down into the muscles of the buttocks and thighs, or down the posterior aspect of either leg. It is unusual for pain originating in the low back area to radiate to the abdominal or genital area.

PHYSICAL EXAMINATION

The patient should be undressed and draped so that the entire back, pelvis and legs are visible to the examiner. A satisfactory low back examination procedure is outlined in Table 13–1.

TABLE 13–1. Outline for Examination of the Low Back

HISTORY

1. Chief complaint and duration
2. Location of pain
3. Character of pain
   a. What aggravates pain?
   b. What relieves pain?
4. Radiation of pain
   a. Location
   b. Type

PHYSICAL EXAMINATION

1. Inspection—standing
   a. General contour of back
   b. Status of pelvis
   c. Status of paravertebral muscles
   d. Lumbar lordosis—present or absent
   e. Spinal motions
2. Palpation—standing
   a. General contour of back
   b. Status of iliac crests
   c. Status of paravertebral muscles
3. Palpation—lying
   a. General contour of back
   b. Status of paravertebral muscles
   c. Determination of areas of local tenderness
4. Hip joint range of motion
5. Leg length determination
6. Leg tests
7. Neurologic examination
8. Radiographic examination

FIGURE 13–11. Movements of the spine. (Courtesy American Academy of Ortho-paedic Surgeons.)

Inspection. The patient is first examined while standing erect with the back to the examiner. The general contour of the spine in the standing position is evaluated in terms of straightness, curvature, pelvic tilt, list, or other visible deformity (p. 334). The presence or absence of the normal lumbar lordotic curve is noted, since this finding is closely related to the presence or absence of paravertebral muscle spasm.

Movements of the low back are then examined and any pain or restriction of motion noted. The patient is asked to bend forward as far as possible *(flexion)* and then to bend backwards as far as possible *(hyperextension)*. Left lateral bend and right lateral bend complete the usual motions examined (Fig. 13–11).

Palpation (Standing). While the patient remains standing, the examiner palpates the back to assess the general contour and determine whether both iliac crests are level. The elevation of one iliac crest above the other indicates a pelvic tilt that could be related to curvature of the spine, paravertebral muscle spasm, or an inequality in leg lengths.

The tone of the paravertebral muscles is determined by palpation with the patient erect.

Palpation (Lying). The patient next lies completely prone on the examining table with the arms relaxed at the sides and the head comfortably turned.

The general contour of the back in this position is compared with that noted in the erect posture. The factors of spinal straightness, curvature, or pelvic tilt are compared between the erect and prone positions. All deformity directly related to paravertebral muscle spasm will disappear in the relaxed prone position. Deformity not directly related to paravertebral muscle spasm tends not to disappear in the prone position.

The paravertebral muscles should feel relaxed and flaccid when the patient is in the prone position. The examiner then notes the presence or absence of local tenderness about the lower lumbar spine and lumbosacral joint, sacroiliac joints, sciatic notch, and sciatic nerve trunk.

Hip Joints. Both hip joints should be put through a full range of passive motion and any restrictions noted. Degenerative diseases of the hip joint early in their course are associated with decrease in rotation motions of the hip that may cause pain radiating to the low back area.

Leg Length. The length of both lower extremities is measured with a tape measure from the anterior superior iliac spine to the medial malleolus with the patient lying supine and the pelvis straight. Unequal leg length may be related to pelvic tilt, curvature of the spine, or a prior condition associated with bone loss in the lower extremity and could be the cause of a gait abnormality and low back pain.

Leg Tests. Various tests involving passive bending of the low back or passive stretching of the legs have been popularized in the past to demonstrate mechanical abnormalities of the low back region and sciatica. These include the Gaenslen, Nacklas, Ober, Lasèque, and Patrick tests and are still performed routinely by some examiners.

Two leg tests should be done whenever lumbosacral nerve root compression is suspected. Both depend upon stretching the sciatic nerve and are positive if they reproduce or aggravate sciatica (Fig. 13–12).

1. *Straight leg raising test.* With the patient lying supine, the extended leg is flexed on the trunk at the hip by the examiner. If the patient has sciatica, the pain will be reproduced at some point before the examiner has completely raised the extended leg to the right angle. The examiner should document the approximate angle the leg has

FIGURE 13-12. A, straight leg raising test. B, sitting root test.

made with the examining table surface at the point pain is reproduced.

2. *Sitting root test.* The patient sits erect on the edge of an
examining table with the chin bent down on the chest. The examiner
fixes the thigh to the table with one hand while extending the leg on the
flexed thigh with the other. If sciatica is present, the pain will be
reproduced before the examiner has completed the extension of the
leg.

These tests are positive only if they reproduce or aggravate pain of
a sciatic distribution. They are considered negative if they produce
pure back pain or discomfort due to hamstring muscle tightness.

Neurologic Examination.   The neurologic examination should be
as complete as is warranted by the suspected condition. Routinely, the
Achilles and patellar reflexes should be tested. Examination is made of
the relative strength of the anterior tibial, long toe extensor, and
common toe extensor muscles. These muscles are routinely tested for
weakness because they are involved in the motor weakness pattern
most commonly associated with lumbosacral nerve root compression.
If present, the clinical findings associated with motor weakness of this
dorsiflexor muscle group may vary from simple impairment of toe
extension power to complete foot drop.

Tests for sensory deficit are made in the dermatome patterns of the
toes and foot. Part of the dermatome pattern of the first sacral nerve root
involves the fifth toe and lateral border of the foot. Nerve root compression at the lumbosacral interspace will implicate the first sacral nerve
root. Loss of sensation, if present, will therefore be found over the fifth
toe and lateral border of the foot.

Part of the dermatome pattern of the fifth lumbar nerve root
involves the great toe and medial border of the foot. Nerve root
compression at the L4–L5 interspace will implicate the fifth lumbar

nerve root. Loss of sensation, if present, will therefore be found over the great toe and medial border of the foot.

Radiographic Examination. Anteroposterior, lateral, and oblique views of the lumbar and lumbosacral spine area should be taken of every patient seeking attention because of low back pain.

Orthopaedic Causes of Low Back Pain

ACUTE LUMBOSACRAL STRAIN

Acute lumbosacral strain is the commonest cause of acute low back pain. The lumbosacral joint, because of its position in the skeleton, supports the body weight and acts as a fulcrum for this weight in activities involving bending and lifting. Mechanical stress to this joint is frequent because of the functional demands placed on the low back area by everyday activities. In this particular joint, the traumatic force is usually a lifting load applied to a forward flexed spine with the lumbosacral joint as fulcrum, or a load applied to the spine while it is twisted or rotated, or less often, a sudden force applied unexpectedly before the back muscles brace themselves to meet it.

The resulting pathologic change is a partial stretching or tearing of the overlying paravertebral muscles, lumbar fascia, and interspinous ligaments. If the injury results in more serious damage to the spine, by definition, it cannot be a lumbosacral strain. The injury to the soft parts initiates paravertebral muscle spasm, which accounts for the clinical picture seen with this entity.

Two facts are basic to the understanding of an acute lumbosacral strain. First, the stimulus for normal tone of the paravertebral muscles is the upright position. These muscles are in normal postural tone only in the standing or sitting positions and are completely flaccid in the prone or supine position. Spasm of the paravertebral muscles is markedly exaggerated tone initiated by the stimulus of overload and maintained by the stimulus of the upright position. It is this basic physiologic fact that accounts for the extreme duration of pain and disability in patients with paravertebral muscle spasm who are allowed to remain ambulatory. It also accounts for the rapid subsidence of symptoms that results from absolute bed rest. If the patient were put to bed rest immediately after sustaining the straining injury, it is doubtful whether the symptoms and signs associated with an acute lumbosacral strain could develop.

Secondly, in patients with acute lumbosacral strain, there is almost always a lag period between the time the low back damage was sustained and the onset of clinical symptoms. This lag period may vary from hours to days and is totally dependent upon the patient remaining upright. It is during this period that the paravertebral muscle spasm builds up to the point of clinical significance.

Clinical Features. The severity of the clinical features of acute lumbosacral strain depends directly upon the degree of paravertebral muscle spasm present. The patient gives a history of twisting or lifting injury to the low back area and states that the onset of symptoms occurred either immediately or, more commonly, following a lag period of hours or days. Walking is slow and guarded because movement of the spine is painful. The back may be held in a forward flexed attitude or may exhibit a list to one side, with a tilted pelvis (Fig. 13–13). The paravertebral muscles feel extremely taut and hard, and the normal lumbar lordotic curve is obliterated. Spinal movements are limited in direct proportion to the amount of spasm present and are associated with a sharp, diffuse "catching" type of pain in the low back area with possible radiation to the buttocks and thighs or up toward the neck.

It is painful for the patient to lie on the examining table and to turn from abdomen to back and vice versa. Once the patient is completely relaxed in the prone position, all the postural deformity caused by paravertebral muscle spasm seen in the upright position disappears

FIGURE 13–13. *A,* paravertebral muscle spasm with obliteration of lumbar lordosis, elevation of left side of pelvis, and list of spine to the right. *B,* the postural deformity disappears once the patient is relaxed in the prone position.

and the paravertebral muscles feel soft and flaccid. If the postural deformity of the spine noted in the upright position does not disappear in the prone position, the cause of the deformity is probably a structural disorder of the spine and not paravertebral muscle spasm.

Once the patient is able to lie flat and relax on the examining table, the physical findings are minimal because of the subsidence of muscle spasm. Palpation will reveal diffuse tenderness over the low back area, particularly at the lumbosacral joint and along the paravertebral muscle masses. Coughing, straining, or turning over on the examining table aggravates the low back pain. The straight leg raising and sitting root tests are negative in that they produce low back pain, not sciatic radiation. Passive movement of the hip joints does not produce pain, and the neurologic examination is negative. Radiographic examination of the spine is negative except for flattening of the normal lumbar curve noted on the lateral view, indicative of paravertebral muscle spasm.

Treatment. The basic principle of treatment is to remove the stimulus for paravertebral muscle tone by means of absolute bed rest. Only patients with minimal spasm can recover rapidly under treatment on an ambulatory basis. The most effective treatment for almost all patients is absolute bed rest, except for bathroom privileges, continued until the patient can turn from side to side in bed without pain. This usually takes from three to ten days. In addition to bed rest, local heat to the back, analgesics, and muscle relaxant drugs may be helpful. There is no rational reason to use traction in addition to bed rest for these patients.

Once the patient is able to move freely in bed without pain, ambulation can be allowed and gradually progressed to full activity.

Important Diagnostic Points. Some important considerations in arriving at a diagnosis are:

1. History of a lifting or twisting injury or sudden strain to the low back.

2. Usually a lag period between incident and onset of symptoms.

3. Severe paravertebral muscle spasm with all objective findings directly proportional to degree of spasm.

4. Degree of disability often out of proportion to severity of injury.

5. Negative radiographic examination; negative neurologic examination.

6. Rapid recovery with absolute bed rest and local heat.

UNSTABLE LUMBOSACRAL MECHANISM

The term unstable lumbosacral mechanism is used to describe a lumbosacral joint that is architecturally unable to meet the functional demands placed on it. As long as the functional demands do not exceed the strength of the joint, the patient remains asymptomatic. Factors allowing the functional demands to exceed the strength of the joint are called precipitating factors and include pregnancy, gradual loss of muscle tone due to overweight or increasing age, sedentary occupations, and local trauma to the back. When the strength of the joint is exceeded, the patient becomes symptomatic and presents with chronic low back pain or repeated episodes of acute low back pain.

Some of these patients complain of pain radiating to the buttock, anterior thigh, and groin or along the lateral aspect of the thigh to the knee, but this radiation is along a muscular and ligamentous distribution and not along nerve pathways. The patients with muscular leg radiation must be carefully differentiated from those with nerve root compression syndrome, in which the leg radiation is posterior and follows specific nerve root pathways.

Radiographic examination may be negative but usually will reveal some potential mechanical abnormality such as a congenital anomaly of the lumbosacral joint or the presence of an acute lumbosacral angle (Fig. 13–14).

FIGURE 13–14. Spina bifida occulta deformity involving the first sacral segments.

Treatment. Treatment consists of first relieving the paravertebral muscle spasm, if present, and then strengthening the unstable joint.

Each acute episode of low back pain sustained by the patient is treated exactly as an acute lumbosacral strain. Once the paravertebral muscle spasm has subsided, attention is directed to strengthening the low back area through spinal exercises.

Hyperextension spinal exercises can be used to increase the

FIGURE 13-15. An exercise program designed to strengthen the paravertebral muscles.

strength and tone of the paravertebral muscles until these muscles are strong enough to function as a physiologic brace for the spine (Fig. 13–15). In addition, many orthopaedists recommend mobilization by postural pelvic tilt and flexion exercises, which should be done regularly for at least a three-month period, then gradually decreased depending on symptoms. Between 50 and 75 per cent of patients can be maintained satisfactorily on exercises alone.

If exercises are not sufficient, or in patients who cannot exercise for one reason or another, the use of a firm lumbosacral belt or brace is indicated. It must be remembered that extrinsic support could further weaken the back muscles and everyone who wears a support should also exercise if at all feasible.

If symptoms are not adequately controlled by exercises or support, lumbosacral fusion is indicated. It has been estimated that no more than 10 per cent of patients ever progress to the point of requiring a fusion operation for pain relief.

OSTEOARTHRITIS OF THE LUMBAR SPINE

(See also p. 148)

The lumbar spine is a common site for osteoarthritis in patients past the fifth decade of life. The disorder may be either a part of a generalized disease process or localized to one spinal segment as a result of trauma or repeated occupational stresses over a long period of time. Patients may remain pain-free for long periods only to have symptoms triggered by trauma to the back. This is the condition usually referred to by the layman as "lumbago."

The disease attacks the articular hyaline cartilage and causes degeneration and thinning of the cartilage, which, along with thinning of the intervertebral discs, results in narrowing and irregularity of the joint space. With narrowing of the joint space, bone sclerosis gradually appears at the subchondral joint margins, giving the joint its characteristic dense appearance on the radiograph (Fig. 13–16). Spurs may form at both the anterior and posterior joint margins as a result of local pressure stresses and disease activity.

Clinical Features. The characteristic presenting complaint of patients with osteoarthritis of the lumbar spine is stiffness and ache in the low back area. Stiffness following periods of inactivity is typical. Patients note this stiffness particularly in the morning upon arising from bed or after prolonged periods of sitting or car-riding. The sensation of stiffness is relieved somewhat by motions of the spine and by activity, but prolonged activity will bring back the ache. Discomfort is usually aggravated by cold damp weather and is frequently relieved by

FIGURE 13–16. Osteoarthritis of the lumbar spine showing hypertrophic bone changes, spur formation, and narrowing of the intervertebral disc spaces. A, lateral view. B, AP view.

rest and local heat. Many patients have associated muscular and ligamentous radiation of pain into the buttocks, anterior thigh area, and pelvis, and along the tensor fascia lata to the lateral aspect of the knee. Often a trochanteric bursitis is associated with osteoarthritis of the lumbar spine.

If osteoarthritic spurs impinge on the lower spinal nerve roots in the root canals, the clinical picture will be complicated by sciatica associated with the signs of a lumbosacral nerve root compression syndrome.

The patient with this condition presents with a stiff, tight lumbar spine with spinal mobility decreased in proportion to the stiffness. There is usually little or no paravertebral muscle spasm but constant tenderness over the lumbar segment is noted on palpation. Radiographic examination reveals narrowing of the involved lumbar interspaces, dense sclerotic vertebral body margins, and the hypertrophic spur formation that is characteristic of the condition. In older patients and in patients with severe disabling pain, a degree of osteoporosis is usually noted in the affected segment.

Treatment. Effective relief of symptomatic pain and stiffness in these patients is dependent upon recognizing and treating the underlying osteoarthritis. Salicylates and several of the anti-inflammatory drugs seem to be beneficial when given in adequate doses. Oral steroid therapy seems to have little consistent effect in alleviating symptoms of osteoarthritis of the spine.

In addition to oral medication, treatment should include weight reduction if indicated, adequate rest, and the use of local heat in the form of hot tub baths. Exercises within toleration help to maintain muscle tone and joint mobility.

Brace and corset support should be avoided if at all possible. It will be remembered that these joints tend to stiffen with immobility and thus generally benefit if kept flexible by exercise while the symptoms are controlled by the systemic medication. Various physical therapeutic measures, such as diathermy and massage, may be helpful in relieving symptoms.

Surgery plays a very limited role in this condition. Unless the process is limited to the lumbosacral joint, a fusion operation would have to be quite extensive to control symptoms and the technical failure rate would be quite high. Surgical decompression of spinal nerve roots is occasionally necessary when osteoarthritic spurs impinge on the nerve roots to cause sciatica.

Important Diagnostic Points.   The following should be considered in making a diagnosis:

1. Most patients are in the older age group.

2. There is a characteristic history of low back pain and stiffness noted particularly after periods of relative inactivity.

3. There is little or no paravertebral muscle spasm.

4. The condition may be part of a generalized osteoarthritis.

5. There is a characteristic radiographic appearance.

6. Neurologic examination may show evidence of lumbosacral nerve root compression, and the myelogram may be positive if osteoarthritic spurs impinge on nerve roots.

Spinal Stenosis

Spinal stenosis is narrowing of any region or regions of the spinal canal or nerve foramina, usually with pressure on spinal nerves or on those vessels supplying the nerves. Spinal stenosis may have a congenital basis, such as might be encountered in a patient with achondroplasia. It may develop secondary to severe degenerative spinal changes or spondylolisthesis. It could develop following spinal surgery, such as laminectomy or spinal fusion, or it may develop following trauma to the spine or in association with such medical disorders as Paget's disease or fluorosis.

Pain may be chiefly in the back but is usually also present in one or both legs and is described as constant or intermittent in character. The pain is often aggravated by exercise, which might also increase sensory disturbances and motor weakness. The patient may have to rest after walking a short distance, because of increasing leg pain. The pain often resembles intermittent claudication. One distinguishing feature, however, is that in spinal stenosis, unlike intermittent claudication, the leg pain is not relieved by standing still.

Routine anteroposterior and lateral radiographic views, tomograms of the area, and transaxial tomography are all helpful in verifying the diagnosis of spinal stenosis. Myelography is an essential study in order to document both the location and extent of the stenosis, particularly if surgical treatment is planned.

If the patient is sufficiently disabled by symptoms produced by spinal stenosis, surgical laminectomy to decompress the spinal nerves and vessels should be considered.

The Intervertebral Disc

An intervertebral disc functions as a shock absorber between two vertebral bodies and consists of several parts (Fig. 13–17). The center is a semi-liquid, mucicartilaginous mass, the remnant of the embryonic notochord, called the *nucleus pulposus*. The nucleus is maintained in place by a thick fibrous band called the annulus fibrosus. The intervertebral disc is further stabilized by the superior and inferior cartilage end-plates that fix the structure to the vertebral bodies above and below. In addition, the anterior and posterior longitudinal spinal ligaments pass in front of and behind the disc thus also acting as limiting membranes. The normal intervertebral disc serves a definite purpose in the physiology of the human spine. It is the structurally abnormal intervertebral disc that alters the physiology of the spine and results in clinical symptoms.

Structurally, the normal intervertebral disc consists of collagen and mucopolysaccharides. The central part of the disc, the nucleus pulposus, is a gelatinous substance with a high water content in which the collagen network is masked by a rich layer of chondroitin sulfate. The collagen fibers form a fine network resembling a porous system. The annulus fibrosus has a considerably denser and more regular collagenous pattern. The fibrils are grouped in bundles of varying thickness that pass in a spiral course from one vertebra to the next. They are attached to the hyaline cartilage end-plate, which divides the bony structure of the vertebra from the intervertebral disc itself (Fig. 13–18). The normal shock-absorbing mechanism of the intervertebral disc depends upon the nucleus pulposus having the right amount of hydration and upon the annulus fibrosus and vertebral end-plates being intact.

In some individuals, a structural disintegration of the disc occurs that resembles premature aging. Chemically, the protein in the disc increases while the mucopolysaccharide decreases. The water content of this protein-polysaccharide complex gradually diminishes and the nucleus pulposus loses its gelatinous properties. Once the nucleus

FIGURE 13–17. Gross specimen illustrating a normal disc's role as an intervertebral shock absorber.

FIGURE 13–18. Cross section of normal intervertebral disc.

pulposus has undergone degeneration and has lost its gelatinous properties, it becomes converted into a fibrocartilaginous mass that no longer complies with the laws applicable to a fluid under a compressive force (Fig. 13–19). The forces once normally tolerated by an intact spine now place abnormal stress on the degenerated intervertebral disc, the apophyseal joints, and the annulus fibrosus. In a degenerated disc, the annulus fibrosus is subjected to a relatively higher stress than in a normal disc.

Once begun, degeneration of the intervertebral disc and annulus fibrosus is a progressive and irreversible process that may start as early as the second decade of life. This apparently natural biologic process, which has been observed in numerous other vertebrates, is probably a consequence of the special vascular conditions characterizing all adult cartilaginous tissue. Once growth has been completed, the intervertebral discs are totally avascular. Their normal metabolic balance presumably depends upon a nutrient diffusion mechanism from the vascular spaces of the cancellous bone through the hyaline cartilage end-plates and the nucleus pulposus gel to the notochordal cells. Interference with this nutrient diffusion mechanism may be the inciting factor in the onset of intervertebral disc degeneration.

The essential lesion, therefore, of intervertebral disc degeneration is a partial degradation of the protein-polysaccharide complex with a

FIGURE 13–19. Cross section of degenerated intervertebral disc.

loss of mechanical properties. Two clinical states may arise from the pathologic lesion of disc degeneration. If the annulus fibrosus remains intact, the abnormal mechanical stresses placed on the degenerated disc may cause chronic low back pain, and the condition is called degenerative disc disease. If the annulus fibrosus ruptures, fragments of degenerated nuclear material may bulge against the posterior longitudinal spinal ligament to compress the adjacent nerve root. This condition is called a herniated disc.

DEGENERATIVE DISC DISEASE

Degenerative disc disease involves the lumbosacral joint most frequently and is probably the most common cause of chronic low back pain. Advancing degeneration of the nucleus pulposus and annulus fibrosus means lessening of the mechanical efficiency of the disc to act as a shock absorber or insulator between two vertebral bodies. Under these circumstances, the anterior margins of the involved vertebrae soon begin to show wear and tear changes characterized by sclerosis and osteophyte formation. A degenerated disc loses height, allowing the vertebral bodies to move closer together. An additional pathologic finding secondary to the compromise of an intervertebral disc as a functioning entity is the change in the apophyseal joints. An intact disc not only keeps two vertebral bodies separate, but also serves as a center or axis for much of the spinal movement. With collapse of the intervertebral disc space, the axis of motion shifts posteriorly to the apophyseal joints. These joints cannot withstand the increased stress, and deteriorative changes soon follow to alter the smooth contour of the apophyseal joints.

Clinical Features. The clinical picture presented by these patients is chronic low back pain. Age may range from the second to the sixth decade of life. The pain is characteristically worse upon arising from bed in the morning and after long periods of sitting or car-riding. Prolonged standing, bending, lifting, coughing, and sneezing frequently aggravate the back pain. Many patients will have associated unilateral or bilateral leg pain. In all patients, the leg pain will be along muscular and ligamentous pathways and will not represent sciatica. In this condition, therefore, the objective neurologic examination will be negative. Paravertebral muscle spasm may develop if the patient overstresses the defective joint. Many of these patients also may develop symptomatic degenerative disc disease of the cervical spine.

Often the only positive physical finding will be tenderness on palpation of the lumbosacral joint.

Radiographic examination characteristically reveals narrowing of

FIGURE 13–20. Characteristic radiographic changes associated with degenerative disc disease involving the lumbosacral joint. *A*, AP view. Note degenerative changes involving the apophyseal joints. *B*, lateral view. Note narrowing of the height of the intervertebral disc space.

the height of the intervertebral disc space and frequently shows degenerative changes in the apophyseal joints (Fig. 13–20).

Treatment. The pain in degenerative disc disease is thought to arise from inflammation of the surrounding tissues induced by the chemical changes accompanying disc degeneration. Anti-inflammatory drugs if given in adequate doses are often quite useful in controlling the symptoms of low back pain and stiffness.

Once the pain is controlled, hyperextension spinal strengthening exercises should be started to increase the strength of the paravertebral muscles. The patient should be taught to bend and lift properly to protect the lumbosacral joint from stress. Many orthopaedists favor the use of back braces and supports in the treatment of degenerative disc disease. In some patients, however, the wearing of a back brace increases the sensation of low back stiffness.

For the few patients whose low back pain cannot be adequately relieved by nonoperative treatment methods, lumbosacral spine fusion is indicated.

HERNIATED INTERVERTEBRAL DISC

Abnormal physical stresses placed on a degenerated disc may exceed the mechanical strength of the degenerated disc and annulus fibrosus, with resulting rupture of the annulus. Herniation or prolapse of nuclear material, either wholly or in fragments, into the spinal canal to cause either compression of or tension on a lumbar or sacral spinal nerve root as it prepares to exit from the spinal canal is the essential pathologic lesion of the condition known as herniated intervertebral disc (Fig. 13–21). Lumbar discs, like cervical discs, usually herniate posteriorly rather than anteriorly and to one side rather than in the midline. The nuclear material may push the posterior longitudinal spinal ligament ahead of it like a hernial sac, or the material may rupture through the posterior longitudinal spinal ligament to extrude directly into the spinal canal.

The general process of intervertebral disc degeneration may extend over a period of years, but the clinical picture characteristic of herniated intervertebral disc does not arise until some of the nuclear material herniates or ruptures the posterior longitudinal spinal ligament to cause pressure on the adjacent spinal nerve root as it passes by on its way to exit from the spine. There is a special relationship between the nerve roots of the cauda equina and the disc space that needs to be appreciated. Before it exits through the neural foramen, a nerve root in the lumbar region turns at approximately a 45 degree

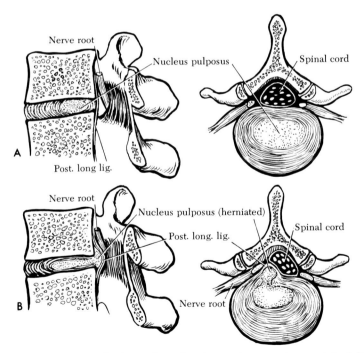

FIGURE 13–21. *A*, normal relationship of nucleus pulposus to intervertebral disc and spine. *B*, course taken by herniated nuclear material.

angle around the pedicle of its vertebra. Because of this anatomic arrangement, a nerve root is usually not involved in any herniation occurring at the disc space adjacent to its point of exit. A nerve root is commonly involved only in a herniation occurring at the disc space above its point of exit. Thus, disc herniation at the L4–L5 interspace will affect the fifth lumbar nerve root, and disc herniation at the lumbosacral joint will affect the first sacral nerve root (Fig. 13–22). The actual contact between disc material and nerve root may be quite sudden and commonly follows an acute rise in intrathecal pressure triggered, for instance, by sneezing, lifting, or straining at stool.

Clinical Features. Herniated intervertebral disc occurs most often between the ages of 20 and 45 years and is more common in males. Because the greatest motion in the lumbar spine occurs at the L4–L5 and L5–S1 joints, approximately 90 per cent of intervertebral disc herniations occur at either the L4–L5 interspace or lumbosacral interspace involving the fifth lumbar or first sacral nerve roots. Back pain is usually associated with the disc degeneration, but the predominant symptom is sciatic pain beginning when the nuclear material protrudes posterolaterally into the spinal canal and compresses a nerve root. In most instances, a diagnosis of herniated disc is untenable in the absence of sciatic leg pain. The point to remember is that although

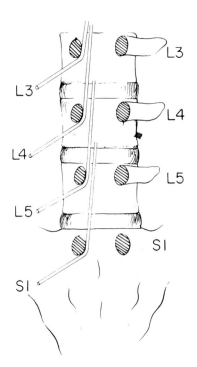

FIGURE 13–22. The anatomic basis for nerve root impingement by a herniated disc. (From Hoppenfeld, S.: Orthopaedic Neurology. A Diagnostic Guide to Neurologic Levels. Philadelphia: J. B. Lippincott Co., 1977.)

many back conditions may be associated with leg pain, only nerve root irritation at this level gives pain in the distribution of the sciatic nerve associated with signs of a lumbosacral nerve root compression syndrome.

The patient with herniated intervertebral disc presents with low back pain accompanied by radiation into the posterior buttock and leg or with just leg pain alone. When viewed standing, the patient may exhibit a list of the pelvis or the so-called "sciatic scoliosis." Anything that increases irritation of the affected nerve root (bending, lifting, coughing, sneezing) will aggravate the leg pain. There is usually tenderness to deep palpation over the affected vertebral interspace and over the course of the sciatic nerve. Straight leg raising and sitting root tests are positive if pain over the distribution of the sciatic nerve is reproduced. These tests do not indicate nerve root irritation if the pain produced occurs only in the low back area or if it is due to hamstring muscle tightness.

If the nerve pressure is severe enough, the Achilles reflex may be depressed or absent. The strength of the long toe extensors and anterior tibial muscle may be lessened, even to the point of a complete foot drop. The patient may complain of a sensation of numbness and tingling in the toes and feet associated with an objective sensory loss in the affected dermatome.

Routine radiographs are usually negative but may show narrowing of the affected interspace. Electromyographic examination and the myelogram are extremely helpful in localizing the site of the lesion, but the best guide to diagnosis is the clinical picture presented by the patient (Fig. 13–23).

Treatment.   Treatment is conservative for the most part, with some patients requiring surgery. Adequate conservative treatment should include a minimum of ten days of absolute bed rest combined with local heat and appropriate analgesics. Putting the patient to bed reduces intradiscal pressure. This frequently allows the disc "bulge" to subside and drop away from the irritated nerve root. Scar tissue may then form over the rent in the annulus fibrosus, thus accounting for the "cures" that follow successful conservative therapy.

Traction is often used although it has been shown to have no specific influence on a herniated disc and is probably justified only as a measure to keep the patient in bed.

The success of conservative therapy is measured by the gradual subsidence of the signs and symptoms of nerve root irritation. Once the nerve pressure subsides and symptoms disappear, the patient is started on back strengthening exercises. Some orthopaedists favor the use of a back brace after the acute symptoms have receded.

Bed rest or any form of conservative therapy will usually be

FIGURE 13–23. Myelogram showing positive filling defect at the lumbosacral joint on the right side.

unsuccessful if the nuclear material has ruptured through the posterior longitudinal spinal ligament to extrude directly into the spinal canal. Most of these patients require surgical decompression of the affected nerve root for relief of sciatic pain. Surgical treatment consists of excision of the protruding disc material. Most orthopaedists favor the combined operation of disc removal and fusion of the interspace if the protrusion is at the lumbosacral interspace. The indications for surgery are:

1. Failure of conservative treatment.

2. Repeated disabling attacks.

3. The presence of severe or progressive abnormal neurologic signs.

Important Diagnostic Points. The presence of a herniated intervertebral disc is suspected when:

1. The patient is between 20 and 45 years of age and has signs and symptoms of lumbosacral nerve root compression syndrome.

2. Leg pain follows the distribution of the sciatic nerve and is aggravated by raising the intrathecal pressure.

3. Paravertebral muscle spasm is not a predominant feature.

4. Straight leg raising and sitting root tests are positive.

5. Routine radiographs are not specifically helpful.

6. Neurologic examination, electromyographic examination, and myelogram are positive.

THE PELVIS

The term "pelvis" is derived from the Latin and means *basin*. The bony pelvis or pelvic ring is formed by the right and left ilium, ischium, and pubis, which articulate in front at the symphysis pubis and behind with the first three sacral vertebrae at the sacroiliac joints. The pelvic ring is built for the stability of the trunk and the protection of its contents. It is united to the vertebral column through the sacrum and lumbosacral joints. Contained within the pelvis are important visceral structures that may be torn or lacerated by pelvic trauma or secondarily compromised by diseases involving the pelvis.

Ankylosing spondylitis or Marie-Strumpell disease characteristically begins in the sacroiliac joints (see p. 146). Paget's disease is frequently found to involve the pelvis (see p. 129). Benign and malignant tumors may arise in the component bones of the pelvic girdle. Not infrequently metastatic deposits in the sacrum may involve the lumbosacral plexus to cause sciatic pain that might mimic the clinical picture of a herniated disc in the lower lumbar spine.

The pelvis is most often at risk from trauma. A high proportion of pelvic fractures are caused by vehicular accidents or falls from a height. Traffic accidents are responsible for about two-thirds of all pelvic fractures, and pedestrians are more frequently injured than are occupants of vehicles. A pelvic fracture may occur as an isolated injury or as an associated injury in a patient with multiple trauma. Fractures of the pelvis constitute about 3 per cent of all skeletal fractures and may be associated with a 5 to 20 per cent mortality rate (Fig. 13–24).

Pelvic fractures may be accompanied by severe intrapelvic hemorrhage, rupture of the membranous urethra or bladder and paralytic ileus. Published studies relating to this injury have pointed out that too frequently preoccupation with associated injuries has resulted in total neglect of the pelvic injury. Hypovolemic shock is combated by blood transfusion and volume expanders to restore blood volume. Valuable information about the integrity of the membranous urethra and bladder can be obtained by inserting an indwelling catheter to examine the urine for blood and as a means of performing a cystogram. Paralytic ileus should be treated by gastric suction.

Fractures of the pelvis can be identified by appropriate radio-

FIGURE 13-24. Extensive fracture of right side of pelvis.

graphic studies and can be classified as stable fractures of the pelvic ring and unstable fractures of the pelvic ring.

Stable fractures of the pelvis include fractures of one to three of the four pubic rami, fractures of the iliac ala, and fractures of the sacrum. Involvement of one to three of the four pubic rami is by far the most commonly encountered stable pelvic fracture. Visceral complications are rare with these injuries. Bed rest, from a few days up to six weeks, is the only treatment required for stable pelvic fractures.

Unstable pelvic fractures disrupt the pelvic ring and are frequently associated with severe intrapelvic hemorrhage or rupture of the urethra or bladder. Unstable fractures include hemipelvic displacement with dislocation of the sacroiliac joint, displaced fracture of all four pubic rami with involvement of the symphysis pubis, opening of the pelvic ring with disruption of the symphysis pubis and sacroiliac joints, and combinations of these injuries.

Depending on the particular fracture, treatment methods include bed rest, manipulation, pelvic slings, spica casts, and skeletal traction. Open reduction, with or without internal fixation, is occasionally employed in the treatment of unstable pelvic fractures.

References

DaRoza, A. C.: Primary intraspinal tumours: Their clinical presentation and diagnosis. J. Bone and Joint Surg., 46–B:8, 1964.

Hoppenfeld, S.: Orthopaedic Neurology. A Diagnostic Guide to Neurologic Levels. Philadelphia: J. B. Lippincott Co., 1977.

Macnab, I.: Backache. Baltimore: Williams and Wilkins Co., 1977.

Moe, J. H., Winter, R. B., Bradford, D. S., and Lonstein, J. E.: Scoliosis and Other Spinal Deformities. Philadelphia: W. B. Saunders Co., 1978.

Nachemsen, A., and Wiltse, L. L. (Co-Guest Eds.): Spondylolisthesis. Clin. Ortho. and Rel. Res., Vol. 117, 1976.

Rockwood, C. A., Jr., and Green, D. P.: Fractures, Vols. I and II. Philadelphia: J. B. Lippincott Co., 1975.

Rothman, R. R. (Ed.): Symposium on disease of the intervertebral disc. Ortho. Clin. North Am., 2:2, July, 1971.

Rothman, R. R., and Simeone, F. A.: The Spine, Vols. I and II. Philadelphia: W. B. Saunders Co., 1975.

Stauffer, E. S. (Guest Ed.): Spinal cord injuries. Clin. Ortho. and Rel. Res., Vol. 112, 1975.

Willis, T. A.: Lumbosacral anomalies. J. Bone and Joint Surg., 41–A:935, 1959.

CHAPTER 14

THE LOWER
EXTREMITY

GENERAL CONSIDERATIONS

Weight bearing and locomotion in the upright position are the principal activities required of the lower extremities in man. Proper performance of these functions requires strength and stability of the part, coupled with sufficient mobility to allow walking, running, climbing, and leaping. The stability demanded of the lower extremity is obtained at the price of mobility. As a consequence, the joints of the lower extremity do not have as great a range of mobility as those of the upper extremity.

As is also true in the upper extremity, the functions performed by the lower extremity influence to a great extent the type of musculoskeletal disorders encountered. The addition of weight bearing adds further stress to the joints and helps explain the higher incidence of degenerative joint disease in the lower extremity. All activities of daily living involve intermittent loading and oscillation of joints. Under normal circumstances articular cartilage is protected from the full effects of physiologic loading by the shock absorbing mechanism of joint motion combined with the lengthening of muscles under tension. Another shock absorbing mechanism that protects articular cartilage is the deformation of the subchondral bone. Subchondral bone normally has a compliance approximating that of soft wood and "gives" a little under physiologic load.

The ability to walk, run, climb, and jump carries with it the increased likelihood of injury by overloading of these protective shock absorbing mechanisms. It should not be surprising to learn, therefore, that trauma produces a great proportion of the musculo-skeletal problems involving the lower extremity.

Before discussing localized problems of the lower extremity, it should be appreciated that many general disorders exist that include deformities of the lower extremity in their clinical picture. As mentioned in Chapter 8, disorders of neuromuscular origin — such as cerebral palsy, anterior poliomyelitis, and Friedreich's ataxia — frequently are accompanied by lower extremity complaints and deformities. Rheumatoid arthritis, hemophilic arthritis, neuropathic joint disease, gout, and Paget's disease all may involve the lower extremity in the disease process. As mentioned in Chapter 9, the distal end of the femur and the proximal end of the tibia are sites commonly afflicted with benign and malignant bone tumors.

For descriptive purposes, local problems involving the lower extremity are presented in discussions of the hip joint, thigh, knee joint, leg, ankle joint, and foot.

THE HIP JOINT

The hip joint is the pivotal joint of the lower extremity, and its functional demands require great stability, coupled with a wide range of motion. To meet these demands the hip is built to be a close-fitting deeply set ball and socket arrangement between the femoral head and acetabulum. It is further supported by a strong capsule that extends circumferentially from the acetabular rim to the intertrochanteric line of the femur. The hip joint is inherently stable by virtue of its construction and, unlike the shoulder and knee joints, needs no particular supporting ligaments.

Normally, the femoral neck forms an angle with the shaft of the femur in the frontal plane that ranges between 120 and 135 degrees and is called the *angle of inclination*. If this angle is larger than 135 degrees, the resulting deformity is known as *coxa valga*. If this angle is less than 120 degrees, the resulting deformity is known as *coxa vara* (Fig. 14–1). The angle of inclination is not to be confused with the angle of anteversion (see Fig. 3–6).

The principal hip flexor muscle, the iliopsoas, is located anteriorly. Posteriorly, the gluteus maximus functions as the principal hip extensor. The gluteus minimus and medius abduct the thigh. They originate on the wing of the ilium and insert on the greater trochanter of the femur. The adductor muscles are grouped medially and consist of the adductors longus, brevis, and magnus and the

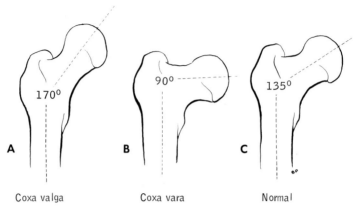

Coxa valga   Coxa vara   Normal

FIGURE 14-1. Angle of inclination of the femoral neck. A, coxa valga. B, coxa vara. C, normal.

gracilis. They originate largely from the inferior ramus of the pubis and insert on the inner side of the femur.

In ordinary activities, a great deal of pressure is applied to the hip joint as a result of the need of the hip abductor muscles to counterbalance body weight, with the hip joint acting as a fulcrum. Since the length of the lever arm from the fulcrum to the center of gravity of the body is two and one-half times the length of the lever arm from the fulcrum to the hip abductors, resulting total pressure on the hip joint surface during walking will be several times body weight.

Disorders affecting the hip joint in both children and adults are important and frequently serious clinical problems.

Clinical Aspects of Hip Disorders

The majority of patients presenting because of a hip joint problem may do so because of pain, stiffness, limp, or deformity.

Pain of hip joint origin may be localized to the groin and from there may radiate down the medial or anterior aspect of the thigh; pain may also arise in the region of the greater trochanter and radiate laterally along the course of the fascia lata toward the knee. Hip joint pain may present posteriorly in the region of the ischial tuberosity and must be carefully differentiated from the complaint of sciatica (see p. 350). Frequently the pain is referred to the low back area or knee and can be reproduced or accentuated by movements of the hip joint.

Subjective stiffness of the hip joint may be noted by the patient following periods of hip immobility, such as after prolonged sitting or upon arising from bed in the morning. In more advanced degenerative states affecting the hip joint, objective stiffness may be noted by the examiner. In degenerative arthritis of the hip joint, for example, the patient will lose hip joint motion sequentially, with the ability to rotate the hip being lost first, followed by abduction and adduction and hip flexion being maintained to the last. For this reason, many patients wih degenerative arthritis of the hip describe difficulty in putting a shoe and stocking on the affected leg since this action usually requires the ability to rotate the hip joint externally.

During normal gait the stance phase begins with heel-strike and ends with toe-off and constitutes two-thirds of the gait cycle. Swing phase begins with toe-off and ends at heel-strike and constitutes one-third of the gait cycle. Time in both stance and swing phase is bilaterally equal, giving normal gait its appearance of symmetry and rhythm.

Limp is a pathologic asymmetrical gait, and several mechanisms may be operating about a hip joint either singly or in combination to produce it. Shortening of the involved extremity and marked stiffness about the hip joint may be sufficient to alter gait patterns significantly. The limp may be protective as a reaction to weight bearing pain. This type of abnormal gait, called an *antalgic* gait, is characterized by a very short stance phase. The gait most characteristic of hip joint disease, however, is called a *gluteal lurch* and relates directly to a structural or functional weakness of the gluteus medius muscle on the affected side. Any abnormality of the pelvic-femoral lever arm may weaken the gluteus medius muscle. If this occurs, the muscle can no longer support the pelvis and trunk on the lower extremity. As a consequence, the patient's trunk lurches to the affected side with weight bearing (positive Trendelenburg test).

Visible deformity of the lower extremity is frequently associated with injuries or disease affecting the hip joint. A patient with a fracture of the hip joint usually presents with the lower extremity held in marked external rotation. A patient who has sustained a traumatic dislocation of the hip joint usually presents with the lower extremity held in internal rotation. Degenerative arthritis of the hip joint is frequently associated with contractures of flexion, adduction, and external rotation. Flexion and adduction contractures about the hip, external rotation position of the lower extremity, shortening of the leg, and limp are characteristic deformities that may be produced by hip joint disorders.

Examination of the Hip Joint

The patient must be suitably draped so that both lower extremities, the pelvis, and the spine are visible to the examiner.

INSPECTION

The examiner notes the appearance of the patient in the walking position, whether weight is borne equally on both feet with the legs in a normal position, and any increase in lumbar lordosis or pelvic tilt.

If the patient is able to walk, any limp or abnormal gait pattern is noted.

With patient lying supine, the legs are inspected for visible deformity.

PALPATION

The joint is palpated to detect evidence of swelling or local heat. The presence of tenderness over the joint anteriorly or posteriorly or over the greater trochanter is noted. The position of the greater trochanter relative to the anterior superior iliac spine is compared on both sides.

RANGE OF MOTION

With the patient lying supine on the examining table, the examiner puts both hip joints through a full range of passive motion, testing the motions of flexion, abduction, adduction, internal rotation and external rotation (Fig. 14–2). When testing abduction and adduction of the hip joint, the examiner steadies the pelvis by placing a hand on the iliac crest.

Extension of the hip joint is tested with the patient lying prone.

In the absence of joint stiffness, the range of active joint motion is tested to determine the presence or absence of muscle weakness about the hip joint.

SPECIAL MANEUVERS

Test for Hip Flexion Contracture. A hip flexion contracture can be hidden so well by an increased lumbar lordosis that its presence may be missed by the examiner unless it is revealed by a special maneuver.

With the patient lying supine, the normal hip is acutely flexed

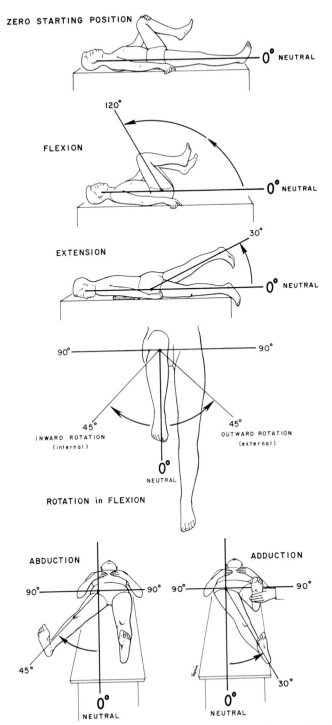

ZERO STARTING POSITION

0° NEUTRAL

120°

FLEXION

0° NEUTRAL

30°

EXTENSION

0° NEUTRAL

90°   90°

45°
INWARD ROTATION
(internal)

45°
OUTWARD ROTATION
(external)

0°
NEUTRAL

ROTATION in FLEXION

ABDUCTION

ADDUCTION

90°   90°   90°   90°

45°

30°

0°
NEUTRAL

0°
NEUTRAL

FIGURE 14–2. Motions of the hip. (Courtesy American Academy of Orthopaedic Surgeons.)

LIMITED MOTION in FLEXION

FIGURE 14-3. Test for hip flexion contracture. (Courtesy American Academy of Orthopaedic Surgeons.)

on the abdomen to flatten the lumbar spine and obliterate the lordosis permitting a hip flexion contracture to become apparent and its degree noted (Fig. 14–3).

Leg Length Measurement. Shortening of the leg may be caused by hip joint disorders. The amount of shortening is determined by accurate measurement with a tape measure. The patient lies supine on an examining table, with the body straight and both legs in the same position. The distance from the anterior superior iliac spine to the tip of the medial malleolus is measured on each leg and the results are compared.

Trendelenburg's Test. Normally, when all the body weight is borne on one foot and the opposite leg is raised from the ground, the pelvis on the raised side rises slightly with the leg. When the gluteal muscles on the affected side are unable to support the pelvis properly, the pelvis on the raised side does not rise but falls, and the test is said to be positive (Fig. 14–4).

A positive Trendelenburg test indicates some abnormality in the musculoskeletal mechanism between the pelvis and the femur. The test is positive in many deformities involving the femoral neck, dislocation of the hip joint, and weakness or paralysis of the gluteus medius muscle. This is the biomechanical mechanism operating to produce the so-called gluteal lurch in patients with various disorders of the hip joint.

RADIOGRAPHIC EXAMINATION

Proper evaluation of a problem affecting the hip joint cannot be made without radiographic examination. As a routine, an anteropos-

**DISTURBANCES OF
GLUTEUS MEDIUS
MECHANISM**

1. Bony
   a. Ankylosis (fibrous or bony)
   b. Deformity of the neck of the femur
      1) Coxa vara (congenital or acquired)
      2) Shortening of the neck of the femur
   c. Loss of continuity
      1) Fractures about the hip (intra- and extracapsular)
      2) Pseudoarthrosis
   d. Instability
      1) Dislocation of the hip
      2) Subluxation of the hip
2. Muscular
   a. Weakness or paralysis of the gluteus medius muscle
   b. Spasticity of the gluteus medius muscle

STANDING ERECT (Glut. med. relaxed)

LEFT LEG RAISED. PELVIS LIFTED ON LEFT (Rt. glut. med. contracts): Negative test

LEFT LEG RAISED. PELVIS "FALLS" ON LEFT (Rt. glut. med. mechanism disturbed): Positive test

FIGURE 14–4. Trendelenburg's test. (From Manual of Orthopaedic Surgery, American Orthopaedic Association.)

terior view of the pelvis and lateral view of both hip joints should be obtained of every patient with a problem of hip joint origin.

Disorders of the Hip Joint in Children

CONGENITAL DISLOCATION OF THE HIP

(See p. 64)

TRAUMATIC DISLOCATION OF THE HIP

Traumatic dislocation of the hip is an uncommon lesion in the child, but it has been seen following difficult deliveries, athletic injuries, and vehicular accidents. The majority of the patients are male. The femoral head is usually dislocated posteriorly so that the leg assumes the characteristic positional deformity of shortening and internal rotation.

The less common anterior dislocation of the femoral head carries with it the threat of impingement against the femoral artery.

Reduction of the dislocation should be carried out promptly, certainly within the first 24 hours following injury. The dislocation can usually be corrected by closed reduction, followed by a period of rest of the joint by means of traction or plaster cast. Weight bearing can be resumed three months following reduction. If there is no associated injury about the hip joint, the majority of patients make a full recovery from the injury.

The prognosis for future hip function is not good if the dislocation is associated with fracture about the femoral head or acetabulum, since this implies more severe violence to the joint at the time of injury. Open reduction of the fracture fragments may be required.

Some children sustaining fracture-dislocation of the hip joint may develop the complication of avascular necrosis of the femoral head (see p. 399) or of degenerative arthritis of the hip (see p. 394). Both of these complications may severely compromise the function of the involved hip joint for the remainder of the patient's life.

In general, however, traumatic dislocation of the hip in a child is a more benign injury in regard to future hip function than a similar hip injury in the adult.

SYNOVITIS OF THE HIP (OBSERVATION HIP)

A twisting strain applied to the hip joint may cause a traumatic irritation of the synovial membrane with the formation of a synovial effusion within the joint. Some authorities believe that an irritative synovitis may also be caused by a viral inflammation of the synovial membrane.

The child may develop a painful limp, muscle spasm about the hip, and limited joint motion. Radiographic examination is negative except for evidence of capsular distention.

The differential diagnosis between nonpyogenic synovitis of the hip and pyogenic arthritis, Legg-Calvé-Perthes disease, and tuberculosis of the hip is based upon an afebrile clinical course, negative radiographic examination, and the recovery of sterile fluid from the hip joint on needle aspiration.

Synovitis of the hip joint responds rapidly to rest, local heat, and close observation of the patient. Severe hip pain can be alleviated by traction applied to the leg in the form of Buck's extension.

An occasional patient originally believed to have a synovitis of the hip will eventually show radiographic changes in the capital femoral epiphysis characteristic of Legg-Calvé-Perthes disease. In these instances, it is believed that distention of the hip joint capsule by fluid produces pressure that exceeds the epiphyseal marrow pressure and thereby cuts off its circulation.

PYOGENIC ARTHRITIS OF THE HIP

(See p. 182)

TUBERCULOSIS OF THE HIP

(See p. 190)

LEGG-CALVÉ-PERTHES DISEASE

(See p. 97)

SLIPPED CAPITAL FEMORAL EPIPHYSIS

In the adolescent, it is not uncommon for the epiphysis of the femoral head to slip from the neck of the femur (Fig. 14–5). Unlike other epiphyses (Chapter 4), the capital femoral epiphysis may displace outward and backward from the femoral neck in the absence of specific trauma, for reasons that are still poorly understood. If this condition is not recognized early and treated rapidly, severe structural deformity of the head and neck of the femur may result. The problem assumes great functional significance because of the importance of the joint involved.

FIGURE 14–5. *A,* complete slip of capital femoral epiphysis of left hip. *B,* same patient after operative replacement of the epiphysis, bone pegging of the growth line, and fixation with metallic pins. (Courtesy Dr. John Dowling, Lankenau Hospital, Philadelphia, Pa.)

The condition occurs most frequently in boys 10 to 16 years of age and may be bilateral.

Etiology. The cause of slipping of the capital femoral epiphysis is unknown. Many authorities favor an underlying endocrine imbalance because the condition frequently occurs in two types of children: (1) the overweight child with underdeveloped genitalia (*Fröhlich's adiposogenital syndrome*) and (2) the tall thin child showing a rapid adolescent growth spurt. Proof for this hypothesis has not been forthcoming.

Other authorities have suggested trauma, low-grade infection, nutritional defects, and weakening of the periosteum as causes, but these too have not been proved.

Pathology. It has been reported that the basic pathologic change associated with slipped capital femoral epiphysis occurs in the cartilage of the growth plate. The growth plate, instead of producing enchondral bone, becomes transformed into fibrous tissue. This weakens the attachment of the capital epiphysis to the femoral neck and may allow it to slip off following minimal trauma.

The epiphysis gradually slips downward and backward on the neck of the femur, but because of periosteal attachment, the two structures never become completely separated. Callus tissue gradually forms in the angle between the head and neck of the femur, and, in time, the femoral neck becomes rounded.

The articular hyaline cartilage of the femoral head and acetabulum is unaffected.

Clinical Features. The onset of symptoms is gradual in the majority of patients and a history of some trauma may be obtained. The patient, frequently overweight, may complain of vague discomfort about the hip, with pain that radiates to the anterior thigh and knee. Often the pain will appear to be confined totally to the anterior aspect of the lower thigh and knee. An antalgic limp may be present, frequently associated with a sensation of stiffness. As the deformity progresses, the affected extremity may develop shortening and an externally rotated appearance and the limp becomes a gluteal lurch.

The telltale physical sign is the externally rotated position assumed by the thigh as the hip is flexed. Internal rotation of the hip is markedly limited.

In an occasional patient, acute and sudden displacement of the epiphysis may follow a specific trauma to the hip. In this instance, the physical signs produced will resemble those produced by fracture through the neck of the femur.

Radiographic Findings. The presence of this condition may be discovered on a radiograph before actual slipping of the epiphysis occurs. This is known as the preslipped phase and is characterized by an abnormally widened and irregular growth plate associated with some rarefaction in the metaphysis of the femur, but no actual displacement of the epiphysis.

Actual slipping of the capital epiphysis can be first detected on a lateral radiograph. The epiphysis tends to displace downward and backward in relation to the femoral neck. As the condition progresses, rounding of the femoral neck becomes apparent.

Treatment. To prevent further displacement, weight bearing should be prohibited as soon as the diagnosis is made. Active definitive treatment should be undertaken as soon as possible.

The goal of treatment is to correct whatever deformity exists between the head and neck of the femur and to bring about premature closure of the growth plate so that the capital epiphysis cannot slip again. The attainment of this goal is most often sought by surgical means.

No significant amount of deformity between the head and neck of the femur exists in the preslip stage or in those patients in whom the capital epiphysis has slipped less than one centimeter. In these instances, the surgeon proceeds directly to operative closure of the growth plate. This can be accomplished by driving a metal nail, or multiple metal pins, across the growth plate or by the use of bone graft. Weight bearing is prohibited until closure of the growth plate has occurred. Because this condition usually occurs towards the end of the growth cycle of the child, and because the proximal femoral growth plate contributes less than 30 per cent to the total length of the femoral shaft, no significant shortening of the leg follows premature closure of the growth plate in these patients.

In addition to inducing early premature closure of the growth plate, the surgeon may also have to correct structural deformity or malalignment between the femoral head and neck. Deformity between the head and neck can be corrected by careful surgical osteotomy through the neck of the femur or the subtrochanteric region. Bone fragments are held in the corrected position by some metallic internal fixation device.

Complications. If the diagnosis of slipped capital femoral epiphysis is made early before significant deformity occurs and if proper treatment is carried out promptly, the final result is excellent in the majority of patients. Delay in diagnosis and the presence of significant structural deformity increase proportionately the percentage of poor results.

A few patients, following surgical treatment, may develop acute cartilage necrosis of the femoral head or avascular necrosis of the femoral head because of damage to the blood supply (see p. 399). These complications usually result in a painful, stiff hip.

Residual deformity of the head and neck of the femur may cause mechanical malalignment of the hip joint. Weight bearing stresses on a mechanically imperfect joint may lead to the complication of secondary degenerative arthritis in later years (see p. 394).

Disorders of the Hip in Adults

FRACTURE OF THE HIP

Fracture of the hip refers specifically to fractures occurring through the neck of the femur or through the intertrochanteric region of the femur. This is a serious injury that occurs mostly in older patients. Fracture of the hip may occur in the child, but is a relatively rare occurrence. Management of the problem in the usual adult patient is complicated by the fact that about one-third of the injured patients have an associated medical disease of some significance, such as diabetes, renal deficiency, or a disorder of the cardiovascular system.

The fracture may occur following a twisting injury to the leg or a fall directly on the hip joint. In patients with osteoporosis, fracture of the hip may occur in the seeming absence of specific trauma. Metastatic tumors to the neck or intertrochanteric region of the femur may result in pathologic fractures. The patient may note severe pain and inability to move the leg or bear weight upon it. Following fracture of the hip, the affected leg assumes a characteristic position of shortening, adduction, and external rotation.

Fracture through the Neck of the Femur (Transcervical, Intracapsular). Fractures occurring through the neck of the femur are more difficult to treat and slower to heal than fractures occurring through the intertrochanteric region, mainly because the proximal fragment is small, contains a high proportion of cortical bone, and has a relatively poor blood supply. Even under optimal conditions, about 25 per cent of patients with transcervical fractures will develop nonunion.

The treatment of this fracture consists of accurate reduction of the two fragments by either closed or open methods, followed by operative insertion of some metallic internal fixation device, such as a compression screw or multiple threaded pins to fasten the broken fragments together until healing occurs. The use of an x-ray image

intensifier in the operating room greatly aids in the accurate placement of the metallic internal fixation device (Fig. 14–6). Effective
internal fixation allows the patient to be out of bed, but weight
bearing is prohibited until subsequent radiographic examination reveals complete healing of the fracture. This may take as long as six
months.

In selected frail or aged patients or in those few patients in
whom the head fragment cannot be reduced, the femoral head can
be removed and a metallic femoral head prosthesis inserted (Fig.
14–7). All things considered, however, it is better for the patient to
obtain healing of the fracture by means of internal fixation than to
have prosthetic replacement of the femoral head.

*Fracture through the Intertrochanteric Region of the Femur
(Extracapsular).* Intertrochanteric fracture of the femur occurs
most commonly in women. As a general rule, these patients are
older than those breaking the neck of the femur. Healing is more
favorable at this location, however, because of the blood-rich cancellous bone found here.

Treatment of this fracture is operative and consists of open reduction and internal fixation of the fragments in the reduced position by means of a metallic nail-plate device with or without a compression element (Fig. 14–8). Many of these fractures are
considered unstable, and rigid internal fixation may prove difficult
to achieve. Effective internal fixation, if achievable, allows early
ambulation for the patient, but weight bearing is prohibited until
subsequent radiographic examination reveals complete bone healing. This may take from four to six months.

Complications of Hip Fracture. It has been estimated that one
patient of every four sustaining a fracture through the neck of the
femur fails to obtain successful healing and develops nonunion of
the fracture. The main reasons for nonunion at this site are inadequate reduction of the fracture, inefficient internal fixation, and
damage to the blood supply to the femoral head fragment. Nonunion of the fracture is usually painful and functionally disabling
and requires another operation to correct. The choice at the second
operation would usually be between the insertion of a metallic femoral head prosthesis (see Fig. 14–7) or total hip replacement (see
Fig. 14–11).

Two complications of fracture through the neck of the femur
that may occur after the fracture has healed are avascular necrosis of
the femoral head (see p. 399) and degenerative arthritis of the hip
(see p. 394). Both complications are usually painful and may require
another operative procedure for correction.

Nonunion, avascular necrosis, and degenerative arthritis of the

FIGURE 14–6. *A*, displaced fracture through neck of right femur (transcervical). *B*, same patient after open reduction of fracture and multiple pin fixation.

FIGURE 14–7. Metallic femoral head prosthesis replacing head of femur.

FIGURE 14-8. *A*, intertrochanteric fracture of right hip. *B*, same patient after open reduction and nail-plate fixation of intertrochanteric fracture of right hip.

hip joint are rarely encountered following intertrochanteric fractures of the hip because of the relative abundance of the blood supply in this essentially cancellous segment of the femur. However, residual shortening of the leg is commonly encountered in these patients after the fracture has healed, because collapse of the fragments at the fracture site frequently occurs during the healing phase.

DISLOCATION OF THE HIP JOINT

Traumatic dislocation of the hip joint in the adult occurs most commonly as the result of an automobile accident in which the person's flexed knee strikes the dashboard and the transmitted force dislodges the femoral head posteriorly. The characteristic attitude assumed by the affected leg is shortening, flexion, and marked internal rotation (see Fig. 2–14).

Anterior dislocation of the hip joint in the adult is uncommon.

Other injuries that may accompany posterior dislocation of the hip, particularly as sustained in automobile trauma, are fractures of the patella, fractures of the posterior rim of the acetabulum, and stretch injury of the sciatic nerve sustained as the femoral head is displaced posteriorly.

Prompt reduction of the dislocation is essential to the preservation of good function in the hip joint, and, in the majority of patients, reduction can be achieved by closed manipulation. If this is unsuccessful, open reduction is carried out. Weight bearing is usually prohibited for three months following reduction. Large bone fragments broken from the rim of the acetabulum have to be replaced at operation and secured in position with metallic screws or the joint will be unstable and dislocation may recur (see Fig. 2–15).

Traumatic dislocation of the hip in the adult results from severe violence, since it takes a large force applied to the hip joint to effect dislocation. It takes much less force to effect traumatic dislocation of the hip in the child. For this reason, traumatic dislocation of the adult hip has more severe prognostic implications for future function than a similar lesion in a child.

It has been estimated that approximately 50 per cent of adult patients sustaining traumatic dislocation or fracture-dislocation of the hip develop secondary degenerative arthritis of the hip joint or avascular necrosis of the femoral head as later complications of the injury. Both of these complications may require major reconstructive hip surgery for their relief.

DEGENERATIVE ARTHRITIS OF THE HIP (OSTEOARTHRITIS)

Osteoarthritis involving the hip joint is a common, usually progressive disorder characterized pathologically by biochemical and enzymatic degeneration of articular hyaline cartilage and overgrowth of juxta-articular bone. The initiating cause of this sequence of events would seem to be increased stress on the cartilage. It is a disease mainly of middle and old age and affects females more frequently than males.

In general, osteoarthritis is a degenerative disease process of joints affecting mostly weight bearing joints. The hip joint, therefore, may become involved as part of the generalized disease process (see p. 148). Primary osteoarthritis of the hip may also occur in apparent absence of predisposing factors. In a third situation, the condition may be secondary, arising in a hip joint rendered abnormal by prior trauma or disease.

A long-standing mechanical malalignment within the hip joint may be a predisposing factor in osteoarthritis. In this instance, the stress of daily wear and tear gradually erodes the articular hyaline cartilage and induces the secondary effects characterized by the hypertrophic bone changes. Mechanical malalignment of the hip joint may be caused by primary hip disorders occurring in childhood, such as congenital dislocation of the hip, pyogenic arthritis of the hip, Legg-Calvé-Perthes disease, slipped capital femoral epiphysis, or traumatic dislocation of the hip.

Osteoarthritis of the hip may occur as a complication of other primary hip disorders in adults, such as fractures and fracture-dislocations involving the femoral neck, the femoral head, or acetabulum.

Clinical Features. Whether osteoarthritis of the hip develops as a primary disease process or as a secondary effect of long-standing mechanical malalignment, its clinical characteristics are the same. The problems of management are compounded if both hips are involved.

Osteoarthritis of the hip produces pain, limp, limited joint motion, and deformity of the affected leg. Pain is felt in the region of the groin and may be referred along the anterior surface of the thigh to the knee, along the lateral aspect of the thigh, or posteriorly to the buttock or low back area. Pain is invariably associated with a sensation of stiffness. In severe hip joint involvement, the affected leg tends to shorten and turn in the direction of external rotation. The leg is usually flexed and adducted at the hip joint.

Limp may be due to pain, stiffness, shortening of the leg, or disturbance in gluteus medius function. Often several of these factors operate to produce an abnormal gait in a patient with an externally rotated extremity.

Flexion contracture of the hip, if present, can be detected by performing the maneuver illustrated in Figure 14–3. The presence of limited joint motion is detected by comparing the passive range of motion obtained in both hips. As noted previously, patients with osteoarthritis involving the hip joint will lose hip joint motion sequentially. The ability to rotate the hip joint internally or externally is always lost first. The motions of abduction and adduction are lost next, with hip flexion being maintained to the last.

Radiographic Findings. Radiographic examination reveals the characteristic deformity of the hip joint (Fig. 14–9). Loss of articular hyaline cartilage results in a corresponding reduction in the joint space. Hypertrophic bone changes are evident about the femoral head and the acetabulum that reflect a dense appearance on the radiograph. Bone spurs appear as irregular projections extending outward from the joint margins around the femoral head and the edges of the acetabulum. Radiolucent cysts may be noted immediately beneath the joint surface in the subchondral bone of the femoral head and acetabulum. These cysts are probably caused by

FIGURE 14–9. Severe degenerative arthritis of the right hip.

joint fluid being forced into the subchondral bone through a defect in the articular cartilage. In the late stages of the disease, the cartilage space may appear totally obliterated with grossly deformed and irregular opposing joint surfaces.

Treatment. The symptoms in some patients with osteoarthritis of the hip may be controlled by nonoperative measures, such as the use of a cane in the opposite hand to "unload" the hip joint in order to relieve pain or the use of a heel lift on the affected side to compensate for shortening. The anti-inflammatory drugs may also be useful in relieving pain.

A great many patients with symptomatic degenerative arthritis of the hip, however, eventually require some type of operative treatment. The following four operative procedures would seem to have the greatest general usefulness:

DISPLACEMENT OSTEOTOMY. Osteotomy means the surgical cutting of a bone. When applied to osteoarthritis, displacement osteotomy refers to cutting through the shaft of the femur at the trochanteric level, displacing the fragments to change the line of weight bearing thrust on the hip joint, and rolling the femoral head up or down to bring a normal area of articular cartilage in contact with the acetabulum. This operation is designed for those patients who are early in the course of their disease and exhibit minimal deformity and loss of motion. Its chief benefit is pain relief. It usually does not result in any increase in hip joint motion.

ARTHRODESIS. This term refers to the operative procedure designed to stiffen a joint permanently by fusing the apposing joint surfaces together, usually with a bone graft (Fig. 14–10). This results in a painless and stable hip joint. The obvious disadvantage is that there is no motion in the joint. The use of this operative procedure would have to be considered very carefully in a patient with involvement of both hip joints.

Many patients refuse to consider arthrodesis at the present time in light of the interest in joint replacement with the retention of joint motion. Nevertheless, arthrodesis appears to continue to have a place in treatment for the patient with prior or present hip joint infection. The young male planning to do heavy work in his career and with only one hip severely involved would be well advised to accept hip arthrodesis.

TOTAL HIP REPLACEMENT. Since 1961 in Europe and 1971 in the United States, a new surgical procedure has become available for the surgical reconstruction of the arthritic hip that produces excellent results more frequently, more readily, and more routinely in more difficult problems than any other method. The operation is called total hip replacement. In this procedure, the femoral head

FIGURE 14–10. Arthrodesis of right hip by a technique that involved use of a large iliac bone graft fixed with screws, bone chips along superior margin of the joint, and subtrochanteric osteotomy.

and neck are replaced by a metallic prosthesis and the acetabulum is replaced by a plastic cup, both components being fixed to bone by methyl methacrylate or "bone cement" (Fig. 14–11).

Polymerization of the methyl methacrylate commences when the methacrylate powder and the liquid methacrylate monomer are mixed together. When doughy in consistency, the "cement" can be applied to the prepared bone surfaces. Although it does not adhere to bone in the nature of a glue or cement, it gains fixation by extruding into the ramifications of the bone trabeculae and into special holes made in the bone to receive projections of the methacrylate bolus as anchoring sites. Once polymerized (a process usually taking from eight to twelve minutes), the methacrylate holds the components rigidly in place.

Because of the procedure's relative newness, many long-term end result studies are not yet available. The United States Food and Drug Administration did not release methacrylate for general use in the hip joint until 1971. Short-term studies indicate an expected excellent result in about 85 per cent of patients in whom total hip replacement was performed for osteoarthritis of the hip. However, as the surgical follow-up period approaches 10 years for

FIGURE 14–11. Total hip replacement unit in right hip. Opaque material represents methacrylate "cement."

many patients, a relatively small but disturbing incidence of delayed deep wound infection and loosening of the components is being reported. Although in most instances of component loosening it is possible to operate again and cement in a new total hip unit, deep infection usually requires complete removal of the total hip unit and the cement for its control. This will leave the patient with an unstable and shortened lower extremity.

Total hip replacement has gradually replaced other forms of arthroplasty of the hip, such as cup arthroplasty and metallic femoral head prosthesis, as the surgical procedure of choice for osteoarthritis of the hip. Cup arthroplasty is still a valuable procedure in the patient 50 years of age or younger with rheumatoid arthritis of the hip (see Fig. 1–17). Until total hip replacement can be evaluated over a long period of time, it is considered wise to limit its use in unilateral hip disease to patients 60 years of age and older and in bilateral hip disease to patients 50 years of age and older. An absolute contraindication to total hip replacement is a history of prior hip joint infection.

TOTAL JOINT SURFACE REPLACEMENT. This is a recent variation of total hip replacement designed to save bone stock and believed to have an indication in patients generally considered too young to undergo total joint replacement. Designed in Europe, the procedure is just beginning to be evaluated in the United States.

In this operation, only the joint surfaces are replaced, not the joint itself. The joint surface of the femoral head is capped by a metallic shell held in place by methyl methacrylate. The acetabular cavity receives a plastic cup, also anchored by "bone cement." The main advantage of this technique is that the femoral head and neck are preserved rather than resected. This allows the retention of adequate bone stock for further reconstructive hip surgery should these implants fail.

AVASCULAR NECROSIS OF THE FEMORAL HEAD (OSTEONECROSIS)

The term "avascular necrosis" is used to describe the changes that occur in bone tissue after interruption of its blood supply by trauma or disease. This condition may affect any living bone, but it is encountered most frequently in the head of the femur.

When avascular necrosis of the femoral head complicates fractures or dislocations about the hip joint, the mechanism of physical interference with the extraosseous and intraosseous blood supply is usually obvious; but when avascular necrosis of the femoral head occurs in systemic conditions without associated trauma, such as decompression syndromes, hypercortisonism, and alcoholism, the mechanism is less well understood. It has generally been assumed that some degree of vascular insufficiency is common to all of these conditions, but the precise mechanism of osseous ischemia resulting in infarction remains obscure.

Avascular necrosis of the femoral head may complicate the treatment of a congenital dislocated hip or a slipped capital femoral epiphysis in a child or a fracture or fracture-dislocation of a hip in an adult. Avascular necrosis is the underlying pathologic process encountered in the osteochondroses (see p. 96). Osteochondritis dissecans is thought to represent localized bone necrosis (see p. 419).

The known systemic conditions associated with nontraumatic avascular necrosis of the femoral head in adults include decompression syndromes (caisson disease), sickle cell hemoglobinopathies, hypercortisonism, alcoholism, pancreatitis, and Gaucher's disease.

In a large group of patients the cause of the femoral head avascular necrosis cannot be positively identified. The condition is then termed idiopathic *femoral head necrosis* or *Chandler's disease*.

Pathologic Features. Interruption of the circulation to an area of bone results in death for that segment of bone tissue. The affected bone softens and dies. The pathogenesis of the necrosis produced by systemic nontraumatic causes is a matter of considerable controversy. There seems little doubt, however, that the bone end-stage following both traumatic and nontraumatic causes is remarkably similar. Necrotic bone is removed and replaced by viable bone through a process called "creeping substitution." This is the method bone tissue uses to repair the effects of avascular necrosis.

Highly vascularized fibrous tissue from the adjacent viable bone tissue invades the interstices of the dead bone, generates osteoblasts to resurface the dead trabeculae, and resorbs necrotic bone and marrow debris with the aid of osteoclasts and histiocytes.

The final stage of avascular necrosis is that of reossification. Areas where dead bone has been resorbed are filled with new bone; other areas have appositional new bone deposited on the surfaces of dead bone trabeculae. Cellular death, removal of dead bone, and reossification occur simultaneously in different parts of the affected bone.

Radiographic Findings. Radiographic examination of an area of avascular necrosis in bone reveals intermingled irregular areas of decreased bone density and increased bone density (Fig. 14–12). The areas of decreased bone density represent living bone that has undergone atrophy with decalcification; those of increased density represent zones of hypertrophic living bone, necrotic bone with reactive bone around it, and dead bone. The resorptive activity of the granulation tissue is usually focal, resulting in a radiographic appearance of irregular islands of mottled radiolucent spaces in the dead bone.

Necrotic bone is unable to stand the stress of weight bearing, and secondary subchondral fractures may occur through the necrotic segment. The necrotic segment may thus appear flattened and depressed on the radiographs because of compaction of dead cancellous bone fragments into a smaller volume (Fig. 14–13).

Treatment. In the child, treatment of avascular necrosis of the femoral head is the prevention of weight bearing for a period long enough to allow "creeping substitution" to revitalize the affected

FIGURE 14–12. Avascular necrosis of both femoral heads.

FIGURE 14–13. Section through femoral head with avascular necrosis secondary to sickle cell disease. Arrows point to necrotic segments showing collapse and fragmentation.

portion of the head. Weight bearing must be prohibited to prevent the soft necrotic femoral head from becoming flattened and deformed.

In the adult, "creeping substitution" does not appear to be the effective repair mechanism that it is in the child, possibly because weight bearing is rarely prohibited early. Flattening and collapse of the necrotic segment are seen more frequently in the adult patient. Fragmentation and collapse represent an advanced and probably irreversible stage of avascular necrosis. For this reason, most adult patients with avascular necrosis of the femoral head require reconstructive surgery of the hip joint for pain relief. Depending upon the stage of hip joint destruction, osteotomy, cup arthroplasty, metallic femoral head prosthesis, or total hip replacement would be considered in choosing the proper surgical procedure.

THE THIGH

FRACTURE OF THE FEMORAL SHAFT

Fracture through the femoral shaft is a relatively common injury that may occur in children or adults. It is usually produced by severe trauma. The line of pull and the great strength of the muscles of the hip and thigh produce, as a rule, marked displacement of the bone fragments (Fig. 14–14). This fracture is typically accompanied by extensive hemorrhage into the soft parts of the thigh, sometimes severe enough to precipitate shock. Generally, in civilian medical practice, this fracture is closed rather than open.

The affected leg appears shortened and the thigh may present an anterior and lateral angulation. The lower part of the limb usually lies in abnormal rotation. The patient is unable to move the leg, and attempts to do so cause severe pain. Damage to the sciatic nerve may accompany this fracture.

In children, fractures of the femoral shaft may be treated by closed reduction followed by immobilization in a plaster hip spica cast or by the use of traction. It is generally agreed that open reduction of these fractures is rarely required in children.

Fractures of the femoral shaft in adults are often treated in skeletal traction initially, followed by the use of an ambulatory cast brace. If the fracture is treated surgically, the choices would include open reduction and compression plate fixation or the use of an intramedullary nail introduced across the fracture fragments at the time of open reduction or introduced by a closed technique aided by use of an x-ray image intensifier.

FIGURE 14-14. *A*, transverse fracture through the lower shaft of the femur in an adult. *B*, same patient after open reduction of fracture and fixation with intramedullary rod.

MYOSITIS OSSIFICANS

Myositis ossificans has been discussed previously in relation to the elbow joint (see p. 274).

The condition may also occur in the anterior aspect of the thigh in response to hemorrhage in the quadriceps muscle. The cause is trauma to the front of the thigh. Contusion and tearing of muscle fibers with resulting hematoma in the muscle, a common sports injury, is called a "charley horse." If this muscle hematoma becomes converted to bone, the condition is called myositis ossificans.

OSTEOMYELITIS OF THE FEMUR

Open fracture involving the femur may be complicated by the development of infection that may progress to osteomyelitis. Closed fractures treated by open reduction with internal fixation may develop wound sepsis that also may progress to osteomyelitis.

The treatment of this disease in the femur follows the general principles outlined in Chapter 7 (see p. 170).

THE KNEE

General Considerations

The knee is the largest joint in the body, but it is far from the strongest. Because of its exposed position in the limb and the great functional demands imposed by weight bearing stresses, such as walking, running and jumping, the knee suffers derangement of its function and stability more frequently than any other joint.

The knee is basically a hinge joint between the femur and tibia; it permits the motions of flexion and extension. A slight amount of rotation and lateral motion is allowed when the kneee is flexed. Since the knee lacks the inherent bony stability of the hip joint, it must depend upon muscles and strong ligaments to bind the component bones together (Fig. 14–15).

The hinge effect of the knee joint is formed between the rounded femoral condyles and the shallow depressions on the tibial plateaus. The tibial spine is a twin-peaked projection that lies between and separates the tibial plateaus. Lying on top of the tibia are two semilunar shaped pieces of fibrocartilage known as the medial and lateral menisci. The menisci move forward and backward with the tibia and act to promote a snugger fit between the femur and tibia when the knee joint is in extension.

The patella, the largest sesamoid bone in the body, lies within the substance of the quadriceps tendon. A thin layer of quadriceps tendon passes over the anterior surface of the patella to join the patellar tendon, which inserts distally into the tibial tubercle. The function of the patella, in addition to protecting the femoral condyles from injury, is to increase the mechanical advantage of the quadriceps tendon.

Active knee extension is achieved by the quadriceps muscles. The muscle forces are transmitted to the patella through the quadriceps tendon, then to the patellar tendon, and finally to the tibia at the tibial tubercle. When the knee is extended, the force required of the quadriceps muscles is influenced by the patella, because this bone causes an increase in the length of the moment arm through which the quadriceps muscles work. If the patella is removed, the moment arm is shortened and the muscular force required to extend the knee is

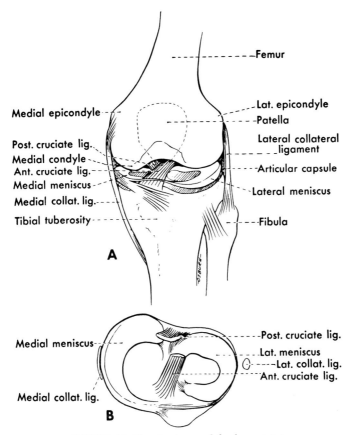

Medial epicondyle

Post. cruciate lig.
Medial condyle
Ant. cruciate lig.
Medial meniscus
Medial collat. lig.
Tibial tuberosity

Femur

Lat. epicondyle
Patella
Lateral collateral
ligament
Articular capsule
Lateral meniscus
Fibula

A

Medial meniscus

Medial collat. lig.

Post. cruciate lig.
Lat. meniscus
Lat. collat. lig.
Ant. cruciate lig.

B

FIGURE 14-15. Anatomy of the knee joint.

increased. Without a patella, the quadriceps muscles cannot provide this additional force and the knee cannot be extended fully.

Medial stability of the knee joint is provided by the joint capsule and the medial collateral ligament which runs from the medial femoral condyle to the medial tibial condyle. The deeper layer of the medial collateral ligament is attached to the outer border of the medial meniscus.

Lateral stability of the knee joint is provided by the joint capsule, the iliotibial band, and the lateral collateral ligament, which runs from the lateral femoral condyle to the fibular head but has no attachment to the lateral meniscus.

Within the joint itself are found the cruciate ligaments, two binding ligaments so named because they run in a criss-cross fashion. The anterior cruciate ligament runs from the anterior surface of the tibia to the posterior aspect of the femur and acts to prevent forward displacement of the tibia on the femur. The posterior cruciate ligament runs from the posterior surface of the tibia to the anterior aspect of the femur and acts to prevent backward displacement of the tibia on the femur.

The knee joint is lined with a relatively thick synovial membrane containing many folds and villi that secrete lubricating fluid. The synovial membrane of the knee joint is continuous with the suprapatellar pouch, which extends about four inches above the upper pole of the patella on the anterior aspect of the thigh.

The knee joint is braced and stabilized to a great extent by the quadriceps muscles in order to support the body weight. It is generally accepted that the action of the quadriceps muscles and extensor apparatus is the most important factor in maintaining the erect position in man.

Normal knee function is possible, therefore, only in the presence of muscular control, intact supporting ligaments, and smooth well-aligned joint surfaces.

Clinical Aspects of Knee Disorders

The majority of patients presenting with a knee joint problem do so because of pain, joint swelling, limited joint motion, or joint instability.

PAIN

Pain of knee joint origin may be noted anteriorly or posteriorly, or it may be localized to either the medial or lateral side of the knee. The pain is characteristically aggravated by the use of the joint and may be referred to the muscles of the thigh or calf.

SWELLING

Joint swelling may indicate synovial effusion or hemarthrosis. Synovial effusion is an outpouring of essentially normal-appearing synovial fluid in response to irritation of the synovial membrane. Synovial irritation may arise as a result of trauma, mechanical disorder, or disease. The excess fluid distends and swells the joint and suprapatellar pouch resulting in pain and limitation of joint motion.

Hemarthrosis is extravasation of blood within the joint, where it is mixed with synovial fluid. The presence of blood within the joint may occur with hemophilia or it may follow major injury to the knee.

JOINT MOTION

In reference to the knee, limited joint motion means a decrease in the arc of motion between complete flexion and full extension. Motion may be limited because of pain, stiffness, fluid, muscular weakness, or joint locking.

Following trauma to the knee, the joint may be held firmly in the position of semiflexion by hamstring muscle spasm, and the patient may voluntarily resist all efforts to extend the knee because of pain.

Stiffness is synonymous with limited joint motion and may indicate degenerative or mechanical malalignment of the articular surfaces or flexion contracture of the joint.

Fluid within the joint limits motion because of the pain of capsular distention and the hydraulic effect of intra-articular liquid.

Locking is the situation that arises when a loose piece of tissue interposes itself between the femur and the tibia and effectively blocks full extension of the joint. A joint that is locked presents in flexion and cannot be extended until the lock is released. True mechanical locking must be differentiated from other causes that limit knee extension, such as knee pain with hamstring muscle spasm, joint effusion, quadriceps muscle weakness, and flexion contracture of the joint.

INSTABILITY

Joint instability may occur with rupture of one or more of the supporting ligaments of the knee. The sensation of the joint "giving way" may be associated with quadriceps muscle weakness or a torn meniscus.

Examination of the Knee Joint

The patient must be draped so that both lower extremities are visible for examination. Patients must remove their slacks or trousers. Both knee joints are examined for comparison purposes.

VISUAL EXAMINATION

The physical appearance of both knee joints is compared and any deformity, swelling, or malalignment is noted.

PALPATION

The knees are palpated for evidence of swelling or deformity. The patellae are compared for contour and mobility, and areas of palpable tenderness over the lower femur, upper tibia, articular margins, or in relation to the patella are noted. The presence of quadriceps muscle wasting can be confirmed by comparing the circumference measurement of both thighs. The measurement is taken at corresponding locations three inches above each patella.

RANGE OF MOTION

The average range of motion in the normal knee joint begins at the zero starting position in full extension and moves through a 135 degree arc of motion in the direction of flexion (Fig. 14–16).

SPECIAL MANEUVERS

Test for Collateral Ligament Rupture. Abnormal opening of the medial aspect of the knee joint noted when the medial collateral ligament is stretched with the knee partially flexed indicates damage to the medial collateral ligament. When opening is noted on the

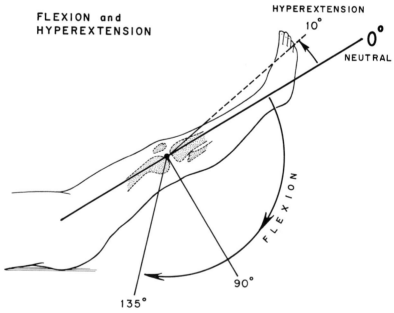

FIGURE 14–16. Range of motion allowed by knee joint. (Courtesy American Academy of Orthopaedic Surgeons.)

lateral aspect of the knee joint, the lateral collateral ligament has been damaged (see Fig. 14–20).

Test for Cruciate Ligament Rupture. With the patient's knee flexed, the examiner grasps the leg just below the knee with both hands and pulls the tibia forward. Abnormal forward mobility of the tibia on the femur suggests rupture of the anterior cruciate ligament (drawer forward test). Abnormal backward mobility of the tibia on the femur suggests rupture of the posterior cruciate ligament (drawer backward test).

McMurray's Test for Torn Meniscus. With the patient lying supine, the knee is fully flexed and the foot is forcibly rotated outward to its full capability. With the foot held in the outwardly rotated position, the knee is slowly extended. A painful "click" indicates tear of the medial meniscus. If the painful "click" is felt when the foot is rotated inward, the tear is in the lateral meniscus.

ASPIRATION OF THE KNEE JOINT

The knee joint may be aspirated of fluid, blood, or pus as an aid to diagnosis, for the purpose of treatment, or to relieve the pain of joint distention. For this procedure, aseptic precautions and local anesthesia are recommended. Aspiration can be carried out through the suprapatellar pouch or through the anterior approach to the joint (see p. 17).

RADIOGRAPHIC EXAMINATION

Routine radiographs of the knee joints include anteroposterior and lateral views. Special views may be taken as indicated.

ARTHROGRAM OF THE KNEE

An arthrogram of the knee is a special radiographic study performed after a mixture of air and radiopaque dye has been injected into the knee joint cavity (Fig. 14–17). This allows roentgenographic visualization of some of the structures inside the knee joint, such as the menisci and the cruciate ligaments which ordinarily are not visualized on x-ray examination. Depending upon the contour of the dye on the x-ray film, it is possible to get useful information about the menisci, many of the ligamentous structures, the integrity of the capsule, and the presence or absence of cysts arising from the knee joint.

FIGURE 14–17. Arthrogram of knee. Arrow points to dark cleft indicating transverse tear in meniscus.

ARTHROSCOPIC EXAMINATION

It is possible to examine the inside of the knee joint by direct vision using a special instrument called an arthroscope. With the arthroscope, it is possible to visualize the synovia, the menisci, the cruciate ligaments, the articular cartilage of the joint, and the under-surface of the patella. This allows the trained observer to make an accurate assessment of the state of health of the visualized tissues.

Disorders of the Knee Joint

PREPATELLAR BURSITIS

(See p. 164)

TRAUMATIC SYNOVITIS

A jarring or twisting injury to the knee joint may irritate the synovial membrane and cause, some hours later, an outpouring of normal-appearing synovial fluid. Fluid distention of the joint and suprapatellar pouch may cause pain, limitation of motion, and a limping gait.

A diagnosis of traumatic synovitis may be entertained if injury to the joint surfaces, supporting ligaments, or menisci has been ruled out. Radiographic examination of the knee joint will be negative except for possible capsular swelling due to the accumulation of fluid.

Treatment of traumatic synovitis consists of rest and support to the joint. Joint distention may be relieved by aspiration of the excess joint fluid.

HEMARTHROSIS

Extravasation of blood within the knee joint is rarely produced by trivial injury. It may be seen following severe sprain of the joint accompanied by a tear in the synovial membrane and joint capsule, rupture of the anterior cruciate ligament, fracture through the articular surface of the tibia, or fracture of the patella. Swelling of the knee joint appears much more rapidly with hemarthrosis than with traumatic synovitis.

Blood should be aspirated from the joint because its continued presence may cause irritation of the joint and may contribute to the formation of adhesions. The presence of fat globules in the aspirated blood should alert the examiner to the possibility of an intra-articular fracture.

FRACTURE OF THE PATELLA

The patella may be broken by a direct blow, such as a fall on the knee, or a dashboard injury, or it may be broken in two by a sudden and violent contraction of the quadriceps muscles.

Direct blows and sudden violent contraction of the quadriceps muscles, such as may occur when a person tries to keep from slipping or falling, may snap the patella in two. Usually, tears of the quadriceps expansion to the medial and lateral side of the fracture site accompany this injury and allow marked displacement of the fragments. When this occurs, the patient loses the ability to extend the knee actively (Fig. 14–18).

If there is little or no displacement of the two fragments, the fracture may be treated by immobilizing the knee in a plaster cast in the position of extension. If the fragments are displaced, operative

FIGURE 14–18. Lateral view of knee, showing displaced fracture of patella.

intervention is required. Two techniques are in popular usage. The fragments may be wired together and the torn quadriceps expansion repaired. Alternatively, the smaller fragment may be simply excised and the quadriceps tear and patellar tendon repaired. After healing, the remaining patellar fragment functions as a smaller patella.

A direct blow to the patella may cause a crushing injury resulting in a severely comminuted fracture. If immobilized and allowed to heal, a severely comminuted patellar fracture may heal with a deformed and irregular articular surface, and the patient may have a painful knee because of grating between the irregular undersurface of the patella and the underlying distal femur. For this reason, severely comminuted fractures of the patella may be treated by total excision of the knee cap with repair of the quadriceps expansion. It must be borne in mind that the patella functions as the fulcrum for the quadriceps extensor apparatus. For this reason, some patients are unable to achieve full active knee extension after removal of the patella.

RUPTURE OF THE QUADRICEPS EXTENSOR APPARATUS

In an older person, a sudden violent contraction of the quadriceps muscles may cause the extensor apparatus to rupture instead of causing the patella to snap in two. If this occurs, a sulcus may be palpated in the thigh just above the knee, and if rupture is complete, the patient will lose the ability to extend the knee actively.

Treatment is operative repair of the defect.

CHONDROMALACIA PATELLAE

The word "chondromalacia" means softening of cartilage and is applied most frequently to a poorly understood disorder affecting the undersurface of the patella. This condition is seen most commonly in young adults and is associated with softening and degeneration of the articular hyaline cartilage lining the undersurface of the patella. The biochemical changes causing the softening are believed to be similar to the articular cartilage changes seen in osteoarthritis. The earliest biochemical change in both conditions is loss of chondroitin sulfate from the matrix. Chondromalacia may follow trauma to the knee cap, but in many patients the cause is not apparent. When examined grossly, the cartilage surface of the patella may appear yellowish and opaque and may be soft and pitted. The remainder of the knee joint is usually normal. The patient may complain of pain in the region of the patella, usually aggravated by bending the knee or stair climbing. Motions of the knee are often accompanied by a grating sensation beneath the patella that is caused by rubbing of the irregular articular surfaces. The patient may complain of a "giving away" sensation. There may be an associated irritation of the synovial membrane, with a synovial effusion.

The grating sensation beneath the patella can usually be felt by the examiner when the knee is flexed and extended. Tenderness may be elicited by pressing the undersurface of the patella.

Radiographic examination frequently shows a normal knee, since articular cartilage casts no shadow. Occasionally, an irregularity of the undersurface of the patella may be noted on the lateral radiograph.

In later life, some of these patients progress to develop all the signs and symptoms of osteoarthritis of the knee and some do not. Symptoms of chondromalacia of the patella may be relieved by use of the anti-inflammatory drugs, combined with support to the knee. Frequently, quadriceps exercises are helpful. More severe cases may require operation in which the soft cartilage is scraped from the undersurface of the bone to aid in restoring a smooth articular surface. If all else fails and the symptoms are severe enough, patellectomy may be performed.

RECURRENT DISLOCATION OF THE PATELLA

The patella may be dislocated forcibly by an injury or repeatedly as a result of congenital and postural factors. The second situation is more common and is known as recurrent dislocation of the patella. This condition occurs most frequently in adolescent girls who often have an accompanying knock-knee deformity and a congenitally flattened and small lateral femoral condyle. It is thought that the insertion of the patellar tendon is more laterally placed in these children. Contraction of the quadriceps muscles allows the patella to be pulled to the outside, where it slips over the flattened lateral femoral condyle and dislocates to the lateral side of the knee.

Children so afflicted may suffer frequent or infrequent dislocations accompanied by pain, joint swelling, and marked disability. Dislocations may become so frequent that they seriously curtail the child's physical activity.

Reduction of the dislocated patella is usually accomplished quite easily by fully extending the knee and manipulating the bone back into location. However, this does not cure the underlying defect, which requires more extensive treatment. In some instances, increasing the strength of the quadriceps muscles by resistance exercises may be sufficient to stabilize the patella. If this procedure is not successful, surgical repair is carried out. Muscle pull on the patella can be realigned surgically by releasing the soft tissues laterally and reefing the quadriceps muscles medially.

INTERNAL DERANGEMENTS OF THE KNEE JOINT

The term "internal derangement" is used to group together a variety of joint conditions — usually of traumatic origin — in which the internal structure of the joint is affected to such an extent that its function and mechanics are compromised.

Meniscus Lesions. A rotatory force applied to the knee joint may trap a meniscus between the femur and tibia to produce the familiar "torn cartilage" lesion. A meniscus cannot be torn while the knee is in extension. To produce a tear, the knee joint must be first rotated in a flexed position to trap the meniscus and then extended to produce the tearing force on the tissue. This combination of motions is frequently encountered on the football field or basketball court.

MEDIAL MENISCUS. Tears of the medial meniscus are encountered about nine times more frequently than tears of the lateral meniscus. This is believed to be so because the medial meniscus has less mobility being attached to the deep layer of the medial collateral ligament, and because the mechanisms that cause tearing are more frequently applied to the medial aspect of the joint. Usually, the patient sustaining this injury is a healthy young male who is hurt while engaging in some athletic activity.

Tear of the medial meniscus is associated with pain referred to the medial side of the joint and with synovial effusion. The pain caused by a torn meniscus is frequently aggravated by forced rotation of the foot and leg. Pain or a "click" may be produced by the McMurray test. Locking of the joint may or may not be present, depending upon the location of the tear.

Two types of tears occur most frequently:

1. The punch-press effect of the femoral condyle on the trapped meniscus may cause *splitting of the meniscus along its longitudinal axis* producing the so-called "bucket handle" tear (Fig. 14–19). In this instance, the inner portion of the torn cartilage may displace into the joint to cause locking. The joint may be unlocked by manipulation, but healing of the tear does not occur since the avascular meniscus lacks the capacity for total regeneration. This type of tear causes repeated locking of the joint and is the lesion usually present in the athlete with a "trick knee."

Treatment of a longitudinally torn meniscus is operative removal of the meniscus.

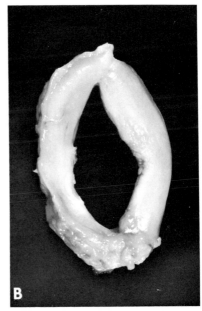

FIGURE 14–19. *A*, excised medial meniscus exhibiting tear along longitudinal axis. *B*, the bucket handle is opened when the inner portion of the meniscus is displaced into the joint. This may cause the knee to lock.

2. Under certain circumstances, the *meniscus may be torn along its transverse axis*. This type of tearing usually does not cause locking of the joint. Pain is produced by momentary impingement of the irregular meniscus between the femur and the tibia on motions of the joint.

The symptoms caused by a transverse tear of the meniscus can frequently be relieved by the use of the anti-inflammatory drugs combined with rest of the joint. If symptoms persist, operative excision of the meniscus is indicated.

LATERAL MENISCUS. Lesions of the lateral meniscus include tears, cystic degeneration, and discoid menisci.

Tears similar to those seen in the medial meniscus may involve the lateral meniscus, but they are less common.

Cystic degeneration, on the other hand, is much more common in the lateral meniscus than in the medial meniscus. In this condition, multiple cysts containing gelatinous material appear within the peripheral border of the meniscus. It is thought that repeated trauma causes their appearance. Once developed, cartilage cysts may cause pain and often can be seen and palpated along the lateral border of the knee joint.

Treatment consists of operative removal of the entire cystic meniscus.

A discoid meniscus is a congenitally abnormal lateral meniscus in which the structure assumes a thickened and rounded shape. Because of its thickness, the meniscus does not glide smoothly between the femur and the tibia, but must force its way through. As a result, a loud clicking noise is heard when the knee flexes or extends, but locking does not occur. The patient is usually a child who is brought for an examination because of the loud snap. If symptoms are present, the entire meniscus should be surgically excised.

In the absence of locking, a tear of a meniscus can be difficult to diagnose. Before surgical treatment is undertaken, confirmatory evidence should be sought by careful evaluation of radiographic changes, by the performance of McMurray's test, and by an arthrogram or arthroscopic examination of the knee joint.

Injury to Knee Ligaments. The medial and collateral ligaments, the anterior and posterior cruciate ligaments, and the joint capsule all work together to maintain the integrity of the stability of the knee joint. Twisting injuries, particularly those sustained in athletics, may sprain or rupture these ligaments to produce painful and often disabling conditions of the joint.

MEDIAL COLLATERAL LIGAMENT. A rotatory twist of the leg with the knee in flexion, such as may occur in skiing or football, may sprain or stress the medial collateral ligament. Pain and tenderness are noted along the course of the ligament, but there is no instability since the continuity of the ligament remains intact. Radiographic examination is negative in the presence of sprain of a collateral ligament. This injury usually responds rapidly to rest and support to the joint.

Much more serious and disabling to the patient is complete rupture of the medial collateral ligament. The mechanism for this fairly common injury is usually a force applied to the lateral aspect of the knee joint when it is partially flexed or extended as might be produced by a football block or "clip."

The ligament may be torn loose from its femoral or tibial attachment or it may rupture through its midportion. Tears of the anterior cruciate ligament frequently accompany rupture of the medial collateral ligament. Severe trauma may cause simultaneous tearing of the medial collateral ligament, anterior cruciate ligament, and medial meniscus. This combination is known as the "terrible triad."

Rupture of the medial collateral ligament produces instability of the medial side of the joint. The diagnosis may be confirmed by taking an anteroposterior radiograph of the partially flexed knee while an abduction force is being applied to the joint. This is known as a *stress x-ray* (Fig. 14–20). Opening of the medial side of the joint indicates rupture of the medial collateral ligament.

FIGURE 14–20. Positive stress x-ray indicating rupture of medial collateral ligament of right knee.

Treatment is immediate operative repair of the torn ligament.

LATERAL COLLATERAL LIGAMENT. Rupture of the lateral collateral ligament is relatively uncommon, but may be produced by a force applied to the medial aspect of a partially flexed knee joint. The diagnosis may be confirmed by taking an anteroposterior radiograph of the partially flexed knee while an adduction force is being applied to the joint. An opening in the lateral side of the joint indicates rupture of the lateral collateral ligament (stress x-ray).

Treatment is immediate operative repair of the torn ligament.

ANTERIOR CRUCIATE LIGAMENT. The anterior cruciate ligament is frequently ruptured in association with tears of the medial meniscus or rupture of the medial collateral ligament. Isolated ruptures of this ligament may occur if the femur is forcibly driven backward when the knee is flexed. This may cause an avulsion fracture of the tibial spine, which pulls off and carries with it the inferior insertion of the anterior cruciate ligament.

The patient with a torn anterior cruciate ligament may exhibit a positive drawer forward test (see p. 409).

Treatment is operative repair of the torn ligament.

If the patient sustains a fracture of the tibial spine, reduction of the fracture may be carried out successfully by immobilizing the knee in the extended position. If this proves unsuccessful, open reduction of the tibial spine fragment is indicated.

POSTERIOR CRUCIATE LIGAMENT. Rupture of the posterior cruciate ligament is relatively uncommon. It may occur with an injury that forces the tibia backward when the knee is flexed.

The patient with a torn posterior cruciate ligament may exhibit a positive drawer backward test (see p. 409).

Treatment is operative repair of the torn ligament.

Loose Bodies. Loose bodies are fragments of cartilage, bone, or calcified tissue that lie free within the joints causing pain, joint irritation, and locking (see p. 407). Loose bodies have been discovered in practically every joint in the body, but occur most frequently in the knee. Locking occurs if the loose body becomes wedged between the bones, thereby forming a mechanical obstruction to complete extension.

The fragments may be pieces of bone broken from the articular surface, such as a piece of tibial spine, a detached bone spur in an osteoarthritic knee joint, or a torn portion of a meniscus, or they may result from osteochondritis dissecans or osteochondromatosis.

Loose bodies containing bone or calcified cartilage are visible on radiographic examination (Fig. 14–21). Loose bodies that are fragments of cartilage are not visible on routine radiographs, but may be visualized by arthrography. They are removed from the joint by opera-

FIGURE 14-21. Loose bodies within the knee joint.

tion to relieve the symptoms produced and to protect the joint surfaces from further damage.

OSTEOCHONDRITIS DISSECANS. Osteochondritis dissecans is a relatively uncommon joint condition, primarily affecting children and young adults. The process consists of a localized segmental area of avascular necrosis in the end of a long bone. This ultimately results in formation of a button-shaped piece of dead subchondral bone covered with articular hyaline cartilage. If the overlying cartilage degenerates around the edges of the defect, the entire piece may separate from the rest of the bone and drop into the joint as a "loose body."

The exact cause of the localized avascular necrosis is unknown, but trauma, thrombosis of an end-artery, or an underlying metabolic defect have all been suggested. The condition occurs most commonly in the knee joint, but may also be seen in the elbow, ankle, and hip joint.

The usual area of involvement in the knee joint is the medial femoral condyle close to the intercondylar notch. The presence of the

FIGURE 14-22. Osteochondritis dissecans of medial femoral condyle.

defect may cause pain and joint irritation with synovial effusion and a "giving away" sensation. If the involved piece of condyle becomes detached, it may drop into the joint cavity to act as a loose body and cause locking.

The area of involvement on the medial femoral condyle may be visible on the radiograph (Fig. 14-22).

If the diagnosis of osteochondritis dissecans of the knee joint is made before the fragment completely separates, healing of the defect by "creeping substitution" may occur if the joint is put at rest and protected from weight bearing. This process may take months. If healing does not occur, or if the fragment becomes detached, the knee joint should be operated upon and the lesion excised.

OSTEOCHONDROMATOSIS. Osteochondromatosis is an unusual condition in which the synovial villi within the joint undergo metaplasia into bone and cartilage masses. The disorder may arise in any joint, but it is most often seen in the knee joint. When these small hard masses become detached from the synovial membrane, they may drop into the joint cavity to act as loose bodies.

Radiographic examination may be quite dramatic in that the joint may be flooded with literally hundreds of these small calcified bodies.

Treatment is excision of the synovial membrane and all the loose bodies.

BAKER'S CYST (POPLITEAL CYST)

Baker's cyst is the name given to a firm, tense cystic mass occasionally found along the medial border of the popliteal space in children. Although the condition may represent herniation through the posterior capsule of the knee joint, most popliteal cysts are believed to represent fluid distention of the bursal sac that is associated with the gastrocnemius and semimembranosus muscles.

The patient is usually a child, but popliteal cysts may also be seen in adults, particularly in patients with rheumatoid arthritis. Some cysts communicate directly with the joint cavity. No symptoms other than swelling may be noted. In some patients, however, the cyst may cause vague pain and discomfort associated with a sensation of weakness and "giving away."

Because a Baker's cyst consists of soft tissue, no particular abnormal findings are noted on a routine radiographic examination. However, the cyst can frequently be outlined by arthrogram.

If the cyst produces symptoms, it may be removed surgically.

KNOCK KNEE (GENU VALGUM)

A knock knee deformity is one in which the legs deviate outward from the long axis of the femur with the apex at the knee joint. When normally straight legs are placed together in the extended position, the medial femoral condyles and the medial malleoli touch. In knock-knee deformity, the medial malleoli are separated (Fig. 14–23A).

Knock knee may be caused by strain placed on the knee by severely pronated feet or may arise secondarily to growth plate injury at the knee. Knock knee may also be produced by rickets in the child or unicompartmental arthritis of the knee joint in the adult.

Shoe corrections for pronation may relieve the valgus strain on the knee. Leg braces may be helpful, particularly in children with remaining growth potential at the knee. Severe deformity may require surgical osteotomy through the femur or tibia in order to realign the leg.

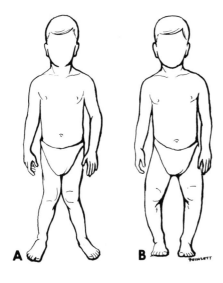

FIGURE 14–23. *A*, knock knee deformity. *B*, bowleg deformity.

BOWLEG (GENU VARUM)

Bowleg deformity is a lateral curvature at the knee joint involving either one bone or both. In bowleg deformity, the medial femoral condyles are widely separated when the legs are placed together in the extended position (Fig. 14–23*B*).

The causes of bowleg are essentially the same as those of knock knee except that the deforming force affects the opposite side of the knee joint. Bowleg may be treated with shoe corrections, bracing, or surgical osteotomy.

DEGENERATIVE ARTHRITIS OF THE KNEE JOINT (OSTEOARTHRITIS)

Osteoarthritis involving the knee joint is a common and frequently progressive disorder seen mainly in middle aged and older patients. As discussed in Chapter 6, osteoarthritis is characterized by deterioration of articular cartilage with narrowing of the joint space and overgrowth of the juxta-articular bone. The disease tends to strike females more frequently than males and affects mainly weight bearing joints.

The knee joint, as a major weight bearing joint, may become involved as part of the generalized disease process. It is not uncommon to see both knees involved. Quite frequently, osteoarthritis may affect one side of the knee joint more severely than the opposite side, resulting in the development of an angular deformity at the knee. Narrowing of the medial side of the joint may cause a genu varum deformity. A genu valgum deformity may result from narrowing of the lateral side of the joint. Long-standing or severe angular deformity may cause knee joint instability (see Fig. 6–2).

Osteoarthritis of the knee may follow as a later complication of an intra-articular fracture of the joint. Removal of a torn meniscus may be followed in later life by the development of osteoarthritis in that compartment of the joint, associated with an angular deformity (Fig. 14–24). This very common condition will cause the patient to complain of pain, grating, and stiffness in the joint, and, on occasion, joint deformity with instability. Pain may be referred to the thigh and calf muscles. Synovial effusion is frequently present, and the patient may complain of a tightness in the back of the joint. The joint outlines may be distorted by the effusion or by thickening of the synovial mem-

FIGURE 14–24. Narrowing of the medial joint space seen 10 years after excision of medial meniscus.

brane. Some limitation of the joint motion usually occurs and a flexion contracture may develop.

Radiographic examination of the knee joint may disclose narrowing of the joint space associated with sclerotic changes in the subchondral bone. Bone spurs may arise along the joint margins and at the pole of the patella. Changes may be more marked on one side of the joint than the other. In advanced disease, the tibia may appear subluxed on the femur.

Treatment. Symptoms produced by degenerative arthritis in the knee joint frequently may be relieved by the use of intra-articular hydrocortisone following aspiration of the effusion if present. The systemic use of anti-inflammatory drugs is usually helpful in relieving symptoms of pain and stiffness. Locally applied moist heat, mild support to the joint, and the occasional use of a cane to unload the joint may also be helpful in relieving painful symptoms.

Some of these patients may require surgical treatment in order to relieve pain, correct deformity, or restore joint motion. The choice of

FIGURE 14–25. *A,* AP radiograph of knee showing degenerative arthritis of medial joint space and angular deformity. *B,* same knee after correction of angular deformity by proximal tibial osteotomy. Metal staple used for internal fixation.

surgical treatment clearly will depend on the specific findings and aims of surgery in the individual patient.

1. *Proximal Tibial Osteotomy*. In a patient with disease confined primarily to one side of the joint, the development of an angular deformity, varus or valgus, usually aggravates the pain because of the abnormal distribution of weight bearing forces on the joint. This angular deformity can be corrected by an osteotomy through the proximal tibia, which realigns the abnormal weight bearing stresses on the osteoarthritic joint and relieves pain (Fig. 14–25). Healing is rapid because the surgery is performed through cancellous bone just proximal to the tibial tubercle. The deformity is corrected at its origin, and there is relief of pain together with retardation of progressive deformity and further damage to the joint in the usual patient.

2. *Total Knee Replacement*. Recent biomechanical and biomaterial advances have made possible the design of satisfactory units for total knee replacement. The component parts are metal and plastic implants fixed to bone with methyl methacrylate (see p. 397). In general, two types of total knee replacements are commercially available, the nonconstrained type and the constrained type. The nonconstrained type consists of two separate components that simply cover the surfaces of the articulating bones. Stability of the unit is totally dependent upon good musculature and intact ligaments. The constrained type is articulated or hinged, thus supplying its own stability. This type is used for unstable knees.

Total knee replacement is indicated more frequently in rheumatoid arthritis than osteoarthritis because joint destruction is usually more advanced. In osteoarthritis, it is considered advisable to restrict total knee replacement to those patients with severe functional disability and for whom nothing else can be offered (Fig. 14–26).

3. *Arthrodesis*. Severe painful osteoarthritic changes in one knee, usually associated with joint instability, can be treated by fusion of the joint provided the patient has a normal knee on the opposite side (see Fig. 1–16). Arthrodesis of the knee is the choice of last resort and is generally performed when only a single knee requires surgical correction.

PYOGENIC ARTHRITIS OF THE KNEE JOINT

(See p. 183.)

TUBERCULOSIS OF THE KNEE JOINT

(See p. 191.)

FIGURE 14–26. *A*, lateral radiograph of knee, showing advanced degenerative arthritis. *B*, same knee after insertion of total knee unit. Femoral component is metal and tibial component is plastic. Opaque material represents methacrylate "cement." (Courtesy Dr. Jerome Cotler, Thomas Jefferson University Hospital, Philadelphia, Pa.)

FRACTURES INVOLVING THE KNEE JOINT

Tibia. Fracture through one of the tibial condyles is the most common fracture involving the knee joint. This injury may be produced by direct compression, such as might occur when one jumps from a high place, or by a force applied to the outer or inner side of the leg, producing abduction or adduction at the knee joint.

Fracture of the lateral tibial condyle occurs more frequently than fracture of the medial condyle, because the outer side of the knee is unprotected and more exposed to trauma. All degrees of displacement and comminution may be seen on the radiographs.

A force applied to the outer side of the leg to produce an abduction strain on the knee joint may cause a fracture through the lateral tibial condyle and simultaneously a rupture of the medial collateral ligament.

Some displaced tibial condyle fractures may be reduced by closed methods and held in a long leg lcast. Others are best treated by skeletal traction. If these methods are not feasible, open reduction may be carried out and the fragments held in position by some form of internal fixation.

Femur

IN CHILDREN.   A hyperextension force applied to a child's knee may cause traumatic separation of the distal femoral epiphysis from the femoral shaft. The small distal epiphyseal fragment typically displaces to the front of the shaft and is tilted backward by pull of the gastrocnemius muscle.

The separated distal femoral epiphysis is usually reduced by closed manipulation and held in position by a plaster cast applied with the knee joint in a flexed position.

This is considered a serious joint injury in children. Complications are common and include residual shortening of the affected leg and subsequent development of angular deformity at the knee.

IN ADULTS.   Direct trauma of the knee in the adult may produce a fracture through the supracondylar region of the femur. The small distal bone fragment usually displaces to the front of the shaft and is tilted backward by pull of the gastrocnemius muscle. The popliteal artery may be damaged by projecting bone spikes on the end of the large femoral shaft fragment.

Theoretically, this fracture may be reduced by manipulation and immobilization in a hip spica cast or treated by skeletal traction. However, because the majority of adult patients sustaining supracondylar fractures of the femur are in the older age group, many orthopaedists elect open reduction and internal fixation in order to obtain early ambulation for the patient.

DISLOCATION OF THE KNEE

Traumatic dislocation of the knee joint is a relatively rare lesion in children. The forces that would result in dislocation of the knee in the adult usually cause displacement of the distal femoral epiphysis in the child.

Dislocation of the knee joint in the adult is caused by severe direct or indirect violence. Classification of the dislocation depends upon the position of the tibia relative to the femur. Anterior, posterior, medial, or lateral dislocation may occur, with anterior being the most common.

Successful treatment of complete dislocation of the knee joint depends upon prompt reduction of deformity, but there is no uniformity of opinion about the method used to achieve this result. It is generally accepted that closed reduction under general anesthesia is indicated. The decision whether surgical repair of the torn soft tissue structures is necessary remains unsettled. Fractures of the tibia or fibula occurring with knee joint dislocation are usually minor and usually can be treated by simple immobilization.

The complications of knee joint dislocation may be disastrous and must be carefully anticipated. Injury to the popliteal artery is the most devastating complication, because it may result in amputation of the extremity at the level of the knee joint or higher. Because of the relatively fixed position of the popliteal artery as it leaves the adductor hiatus and enters the soleus arch, it is extremely vulnerable to damage, particularly in a hyperextension injury. Because of the anatomically poor arterial anastomoses around the knee, interruption of the popliteal artery usually results in gangrene of the leg unless continuity of the artery is restored. Obvious initial signs of vascular insufficiency or severe and increasing pain after reduction should alert the physician to the possibility of vascular injury. Early arteriography is mandatory if vascular injury is suspected. Repair of the damaged popliteal vessel should take precedence over all other injuries once reduction of the dislocation has been accomplished.

THE LEG

TIBIAL TORSION

The term "tibial torsion" refers to a deformity of the tibia seen in infancy in which the bone is twisted on its longitudinal axis in an inward or outward direction. With the patella pointing straight forward, the foot turns inward or outward depending on the direction of the torsional deformity.

Tibial torsion is usually congenital and may be aggravated by allowing the baby to sleep on the abdomen. Internal tibial torsion is more common than external tibial torsion, and if not corrected, will produce an in-toe or pigeon-toe gait. Internal tibial torsion may accompany clubfoot deformity or may be associated with knock knee or bowleg.

During infancy, tibial torsion may be corrected by manipulative exercises or by the use of plaster casts. More severe cases may require a corrective Denis Browne splint. Older children may need surgical osteotomy to straighten the leg, but this is rare.

Congenital Pseudarthrosis of the Tibia

(See p. 77.)

Fracture of the Tibia and Fibula

The exposed human shin is often the recipient of trauma sufficient to simultaneously break both bones of the lower leg. Industrial, highway, and athletic accidents all contribute to the incidence of severe lower leg trauma that fractures both the tibia and fibula. Open fractures are common since the entire medial surface of the tibia is subcutaneous.

A direct blow to the shin delivered, for example, by the bumper of an automobile may cause a transverse fracture through the proximal midshaft or distal portions of the bones. The fracture frequently is comminuted. A torsional injury to the leg incurred, for example, while skiing may result in a spiral or long oblique fracture. In either instance, immediate pain and disability are noted by the patient. Usually the foot and ankle are rotated outward in relation to the knee.

Treatment is directed towards restoring alignment and obtaining union of the tibial fracture, since this is the weight bearing bone of the leg. Reduction of the fibula usually accompanies reduction of the tibia.

Many of these fractures can be reduced by closed methods and held in alignment by a long leg cast (Fig. 14–27). Early weight bearing in a specially designed cast has been shown to be associated with rapid healing of the fracture in a high percentage of patients.

A severely comminuted fracture of the tibia and fibula may require treatment in skeletal traction with the traction pin inserted through the os calcis.

A few fractures may require open reduction with the bone fragments held in alignment by means of an intramedullary nail or a compression plate.

Nonunion of fractures located in the middle or lower third of the shaft of the tibia is not uncommon. In a high proportion of patients, nonunion characterizes either open fracture or fractures associated with a high degree of soft tissue trauma. This complication requires a bone graft for its correction.

FIGURE 14-27. AP (*A*) and lateral (*B*) radiographs of patient with fracture of tibia and fibula, after closed reduction and application of cast.

Osteomyelitis of the Tibia

Open fractures involving the tibia may be complicated by the development of infection that may progress to osteomyelitis. Closed fractures treated by open reduction with internal fixation may also develop wound sepsis that may progress to an osteomyelitis.

The treatment of osteomyelitis in the tibia follows the general principles outlined in Chapter 7.

Rupture of the Achilles Tendon

Traumatic rupture of the Achilles tendon is not an uncommon occurrence, particularly in men during the prime of life. Sudden contraction of the calf muscle with the foot fixed to the floor may cause the Achilles tendon to pull suddenly apart. The tendon usually pulls apart within the sheath, leaving the sheath intact.

A patient so afflicted will immediately note sharp pain in the area associated with inability to plantar flex the foot. On examination, a gap in the continuity of the tendon can be palpated.

Immediate operative repair of the Achilles tendon is recommended. Meticulous surgical technique is required because the skin overlying the area does not possess a copious blood supply. The operation may be complicated by skin necrosis during the healing phase.

It is possible to treat this injury by the application of a walking cast with the foot held in marked plantar flexion. This position allows the ruptured tendon fragments to glide closer together within the intact sheath and ultimately heal. Healing by use of the plantar flexed cast usually takes between six and eight weeks, but recurrence of the rupture has been reported following cast removal.

RUPTURE OF THE PLANTARIS TENDON

The plantaris is a thin, inconstant muscle that lies between the gastrocnemius and soleus muscles. Rupture may occur with vigorous use of the legs, causing the patient to experience a sharp, stinging pain in the calf. Plantar flexion is unaffected.

Surgical treatment is not required. Rest, support to the calf, and the use of a heel lift are the only supportive measures needed.

THE ANKLE JOINT

The ankle joint is the hinge between the long lever arm of the leg and the presenting weight bearing surface of the foot. Because the body weight, poised over this hinge joint, may transmit abnormal forces along the tibial lever arm by means of running, jumping, twisting, or sliding motions, the ankle is one of the most frequently injured joints in the body.

General Considerations

Anatomically, the ankle is a hinge joint formed by the lower end of the tibia and the talus. The distal tibia contributes the medial malleolus and the distal fibula contributes the lateral malleolus. The malleoli grasp the sides of the talus to form the ankle joint mortise. The bones are enclosed in a capsule, the anterior and posterior parts

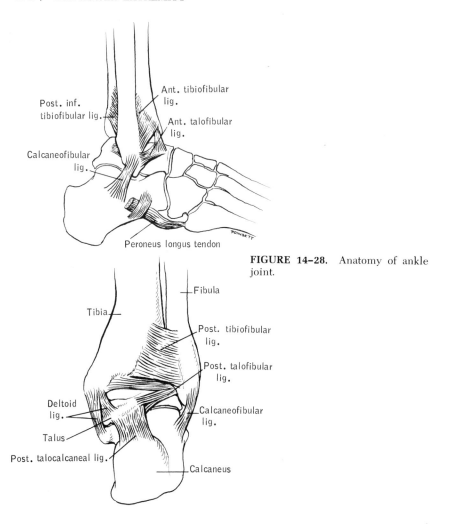

Post. inf. tibiofibular lig.

Ant. tibiofibular lig.

Ant. talofibular lig.

Calcaneofibular lig.

Peroneus longus tendon

FIGURE 14–28. Anatomy of ankle joint.

Fibula

Tibia

Post. tibiofibular lig.

Post. talofibular lig.

Deltoid lig.

Calcaneofibular lig.

Talus

Post. talocalcaneal lig.

Calcaneus

of which are loose to allow the hinge motions to occur. Strong ligaments add support to the medial and lateral joint margins (Fig. 14–28).

As in all hinge joints, the muscles that move the hinge are grouped in front and behind. The anterior tibial and toe extensor muscles lie in front of the joint and act as dorsiflexors of the ankle. The gastrocnemius and soleus muscles lie posteriorly and perform the motion of plantar flexion of the ankle joint.

The motions of eversion and inversion of the foot do not occur in the ankle joint proper, but rather through the joints below or distal to the ankle joint. These joints, frequently referred to as the "subtalar joints," consist of the talocalcaneal joint, the talonavicular joint, and the calcaneocuboid joint. The posterior tibial muscle acting through these joints is the chief inverter muscle of the foot; the peroneals are the everters.

Disorders of the Ankle Joint

A force applied to the ankle joint may cause a sprain, ligamentous rupture, fracture, or dislocation or a combination of injuries, depending on the amount of force applied, the duration of its application, and its direction. In all patients, details concerning the mechanism of injury, careful physical examination, and radiographic studies made in anteroposterior and lateral planes are prerequisites for correct diagnosis and proper treatment. Treatment should be carried out promptly because of the great tendency for the ankle joint area to swell rapidly following trauma.

SPRAIN

A sprain of the ankle joint is a stretch injury applied to the joint capsule and supporting ligaments by a twisting force. Rapid swelling and stiffness of the joint and increased pain with walking are characteristic of joint sprain.

Examination frequently reveals the maximum swelling and tenderness to be localized to the tissues immediately below the lateral malleolus. Radiographic examination is negative.

Ankle sprains respond favorably to rest and support. This may be obtained by strapping the joint, or by supporting it in a plaster splint or cast. Crutches may be required. Immediate swelling may be controlled by ice packs. Later, soaking the ankle in hot water relieves residual edema and tenderness.

RUPTURED LIGAMENTS

Ruptures of the supporting ankle ligaments may occur as isolated injuries, but they more frequently occur in association with certain ankle fractures.

In the absence of joint fracture, radiographic evidence of displacement of the talus in relation to the tibia or fibula indicates rupture of supporting ligaments. In the absence of talar displacement, the diagnosis of ligament rupture is made by a stress x-ray examination. Tilting of the talus on an anteroposterior radiograph with the foot forcibly inverted or everted confirms the diagnosis of ligament rupture. Confirmed rupture of supporting ankle ligaments should be treated by surgical repair and immobilization.

FRACTURES

Ankle fractures, although relatively common in occurrence, are often quite complicated injuries that pose difficult treatment problems. Many complex mechanisms of injury may be applied to the ankle joint by vehicular, pedestrian, or athletic trauma producing a variety of fracture combinations. The physician who undertakes the treatment of these often complicated and difficult fractures must be well versed in the biomechanical and biological concepts of ankle injuries in order to consistently produce satisfactory treatment results.

In order to understand the fracture, it is essential to know something of the mechanism by which it is produced. The mechanism of injury to an ankle is usually delivered in the direction of external rotation, abduction, adduction, vertical compression or various combinations of these forces. The combination of external rotation and abduction is the most common mechanism by which ankle fractures are produced. In addition to this, the fracture produced by the injuring mechanism is modified somewhat by the position of the foot at the time of injury. For example, external rotation with the foot supinated first injures the lateral side of the ankle, but external rotation with the foot pronated first injures the medial structures.

Since the principle underlying successful reduction of ankle fractures is reversal of the injuring forces, knowledge of the mechanism of injury is necessary to carry out successful reduction. For example, fractures produced by external rotation and abduction should be reduced by internal rotation and adduction of the foot.

Specific details concerning the ankle fracture are identified by the radiographic examination. Routinely, anteroposterior, lateral, and mortise views should be obtained. Stress x-rays and examination of the joint by arthrogram are obtained as indicated.

Ankle fractures require accurate repositioning of the fragments to restore normal weight bearing joint surfaces. This can frequently be accomplished by closed manipulative reduction. If closed reduction is not successful or feasible, open reduction is carried out with the fragments held in the reduced position by internal fixation (see Fig. 2–9). The goals of treatment should include anatomic positioning of the talus in the ankle mortise, a joint line that is parallel to the ground, and a smooth articular surface. Acceptance of lesser goals frequently results in a poor clinical outcome.

A description of the varied types of ankle fractures encountered in clinical practice is beyond the scope of this book, and the interested reader is referred to authoritative fracture texts. Suffice it to say, ankle fractures include fractures of the lateral malleolus (distal fibula), fractures of the medial malleolus (distal tibia), fractures of both malleoli, and, if a vertical compression force is part of the mechanism, fracture of the posterior lip of the tibia. These fractures may occur singly or in various combinations depending on the mechanism of injury. In addition to the fracture or fractures, one or more of the ankle's supporting ligaments may be ruptured (Fig. 14–29).

With displacement of either malleolus, the talus may shift either medially or laterally depending on the location of the fracture. A shift of the talus toward the side containing a fractured malleolus, in the face of an intact malleolus on the opposite side, indicates rupture of the supporting ligaments on the side of the intact malleolus.

Fracture-Dislocation of the Ankle Joint. A severe twisting force applied to the ankle may, in addition to causing fracture of the malleoli, dislocate the talus from its position beneath the tibia. Fracture-dislocation of the ankle joint is often an open injury because the malleoli lie just beneath the skin. The open wound is usually made when the tibia or fibula burst through the skin as the foot is forcibly displaced to one side.

Radiographic examination will disclose the fracture-dislocation and the position of the fragment.

Many fracture-dislocations of the ankle joint can be accurately placed into normal alignment by closed reduction. Any accompanying wound must be surgically debrided and closed.

FIGURE 14–29. Common types of ankle fractures. *A*, fracture of lateral malleolus. *B*, fracture of medial malleolus. *C*, bimalleolar fracture (Pott's fracture). *D*, fracture of posterior lip of tibia.

Isolated dislocation of the ankle joint without accompanying malleolar fracture is a rare injury.

RECURRENT SPRAINS OF THE ANKLE JOINT

Occasionally, a patient will complain of a weak ankle or an ankle that "gives way" or is repeatedly sprained. The condition can usually be traced to a specific injury in which the fibular collateral ligament ruptured and the proper diagnosis was not made. Invariably, the patient will tell of being treated for a bad ankle sprain in the past. When weight bearing is resumed, the talus may rock inward and forward on certain motions of the foot and give the sensation of instability.

The diagnosis may be confirmed by demonstrating tilt of the talus on a stress radiograph taken with the foot forcibly inverted.

Treatment is surgical reconstruction of the fibular collateral ligament.

RECURRENT DISLOCATION OF THE PERONEAL TENDONS

The peroneal tendons run through a bony groove behind the lateral malleolus at the ankle. In some patients, these tendons may be loosely attached in a shallow groove allowing them to slip forward over the malleolus on active dorsiflexion of the foot. This abnormality may be associated with pain, weakness, and a "giving way" sensation about the ankle joint.

If symptoms warrant, the condition may be alleviated by surgical deepening of the peroneal groove.

OSTEOCHONDRITIS DISSECANS

An area of osteochondritis dissecans may occasionally involve the weight bearing surface of the talus (see p. 419).

The defect should be visible on anteroposterior and lateral radiographs. The lesion may heal following a period of prolonged non–weight bearing. If this is unsuccessful, the fragment should be excised.

DEGENERATIVE ARTHRITIS OF THE ANKLE JOINT

Degenerative arthritis may involve the ankle joint as part of a generalized disease process but, more commonly, involves the joint as a complication following ankle joint trauma. In this situation, the patient frequently gives a history of sustaining a fracture or fracture-dislocation of the ankle joint some years previously. Treatment of the original injury is typically followed by a period of relative calm, finally disturbed by the onset of symptoms of pain and stiffness in the ankle.

Radiographic examination may disclose evidence of degenerative arthritis in the joint, usually superimposed on bone showing residual effects of trauma (Fig. 14–30).

Symptoms may be relieved by support to the joint in the form of an elastic bandage, Gibney boot, arch support, or brace. Intra-articular injections of corticosteroid may be helpful. If pain and disability are severe, the operation of joint fusion may be performed for joint relief. Some work is being performed on the development of a total ankle replacement unit using the same metal, plastic, and methyl methacrylate combination used for total hip and total knee replacement. It is not at all clear at the present time whether total ankle replacement will prove satisfactory in the long view.

FIGURE 14–30. Degenerative arthritis in ankle joint nine years after reduction and internal fixation of ankle joint fracture.

PYOGENIC ARTHRITIS OF THE ANKLE JOINT

(See p. 181.)

TUBERCULOSIS OF THE ANKLE JOINT

(See p. 184.)

THE FOOT

The foot is the platform that supports the body weight during standing and moves the body during walking, running, and jumping. To bear this load most efficiently in the erect position, the foot has to be constructed from a number of small bones aligned in the form of resilient arches (Fig. 14–31). The bones are lashed together by ligaments supported to a certain extent by the surrounding musculature. Structural weakness in the foot, imbalance between the bones and supporting musculature, or abnormal demands placed on the part may contribute to the production of symptoms referable to the feet.

The longitudinal arch of the foot spans the distance between the

FIGURE 14–31. Skeletal anatomy of the foot. (From Hauser, E. D. W.: Diseases of the Foot.)

os calcis and the metatarsal heads. Its longer medial segment contains the os calcis, talus, navicular, three cuneiform bones, and first three metatarsal bones. Its shorter lateral border contains the os calcis, cuboid, and fourth and fifth metatarsal bones.

The anterior or metatarsal arch is formed by the heads of the five metatarsal bones. The presence of this arch can be appreciated only with the foot in a non–weight bearing position. In this position it can be noted that the first and fifth metatarsal heads are more prominent than the others. This arch flattens and disappears on weight bearing, as each of the five metatarsal heads bears a proportionate amount of weight.

Examination of the Feet

The feet are examined in both the non–weight bearing and standing positions and are observed with the patient walking.

During the visual examination, notice is taken of any visible deformities of the feet or toes, including positional or structural abnormalities, edema, corns, calluses, or ulcerations. The status of the longitudinal arch is observed in the resting and standing positions.

The various motions allowed by the foot are checked by the examiner and any decrease in flexibility is noted. Plantar flexion and dorsiflexion occur through the ankle joint. Eversion (outward rotation of the foot and heel) and inversion (inward rotation of the foot and heel) occur through the "subtalar" joints.

It is also possible to swing the forepart of the foot inward or outward in relation to the heel part of the foot, provided the heel part is firmly held by the examiner. This motion occurs through the talonavicular and calcaneocuboid joints. Outward swinging of the forepart of the foot is called forefoot abduction; inward swing is forefoot adduction.

The muscles supplying activity of the foot are tested for strength and ability to perform. These include the anterior tibial, posterior tibial, peroneals, calf muscles, and the flexors and extensors of the toes.

The presence of any areas tender to palpation is noted. These areas are most likely to be found on the sole of the foot, in the region of the sinus tarsi, and between the metatarsal heads and the dorsum of the foot.

The toes are examined for evidence of structural deformity, joint stiffness, or callus formation.

An assessment of the circulation of the foot can be made by noting the dorsalis pedis and posterior tibial pulsations and by evaluating the efficiency of the venous circulation.

Congenital Disorders of the Foot

CONGENITAL CLUBFOOT

(See p. 58.)

CONGENITAL METATARSUS VARUS

(See p. 62.)

Disorders of the Arches

The arches of the foot may fail to function with full efficiency in children and adults for a variety of reasons. Breakdown of these important weight-supporting structures may give rise to gait abnormalities, symptoms of pain and ache in the feet or legs, or pain referred to some distant segment of the body.

Abnormalities involving the longitudinal arch may be seen in children and adults and are often lumped together under the descriptive term "flatfoot." Breakdown of the metatarsal arch occurs primarily in adults and, as a rule, poses no particular difficulty in diagnosis or treatment.

The descriptive term "flatfoot" is misleading and confusing when used to classify disorders associated with depression of the longitudinal arch. It is true that the foot assumes an appearance of flatness with weight bearing in all of these disorders, but the causes and frequently the treatment will vary. For that reason, "flatfoot," from an orthopaedic standpoint, can stand a more detailed dissection. The three most important types of flatfoot are *pronation, structural flatfoot,* and *spastic flatfoot.*

DISORDERS OF THE LONGITUDINAL ARCH IN CHILDREN

Pronation. Pronation refers to the position assumed by some feet on weight bearing. Most feet called flat in children fall into this category. In this condition, the bone structure is normal and the longitudinal arch appears unaffected in the non–weight bearing position. However, with weight bearing, congenital ligamentous laxity about the small bones of the feet allows the heel to evert and the forefoot to abduct, causing the foot to roll into a position of pronation (Fig. 14–32). The clinical impression received on viewing such feet is that of flatness of the arch.

FIGURE 14-32.   Child with pronated feet.

As a rule, pronated feet are quite loose and flexible. The heel cord is usually slack, permitting extreme passive dorsiflexion of the foot. The synonym for this type of flatfoot is *weak foot*.

CLINICAL PICTURE.   Pronation may vary in degree and in the secondary effects produced. The most extreme degree of pronation may be noted shortly after birth in an infant whose feet are held in a markedly everted and dorsiflexed position. This deformity is frequently called congenital calcaneovalgus but, in reality, represents the extreme degree of pronation.

At the other end of the scale is the child whose feet appear normal in the non–weight bearing attitude, but roll into slight pronation with standing. Moderate or severe pronation may delay the onset of standing or walking in an infant for several months, presumably because of the unsteadiness of the platform presented for weight bearing.

After walking begins, pronation may cause abnormalities. Parents may complain of an in-toe or out-toe gait in the child or may simply describe the gait as awkward. Pronation may be a frequent cause of knock knee deformity (see p. 421).

In later childhood, pronation may cause aching legs because of muscle fatigue due to positional strain of the leg muscles. The ache

FIGURE 14–33. Shoe deformity caused by severely pronated feet.

characteristically comes on at night while the child is in bed and may be relieved by massaging the affected leg.

A a rule, pronation in a child does not cause pain in the feet; however, it does cause a typical deformity of their shoes (Fig. 14–33).

TREATMENT. The child is placed in regular shank, hard-soled, high-top shoes with ⅛-inch inner heel wedges as soon as a standing position is assumed. The purpose of the wedge is to prevent the heel from everting in the standing position. The wear of the shoes is carefully watched. If treatment is effective, the shoe wear will appear balanced.

As the child's activity increases, the initial wedge usually loses its effectiveness and the shoe may appear "undercorrected." This usually occurs between 14 and 18 months of age. At this time the correction in the shoe may be raised to a ³/₁₆-inch inner heel wedge and a ⅛-inch outer sole wedge.

At two years of age the child may be placed in regular shank low oxfords with a ³/₁₆-inch rubber longitudinal arch pad or scaphoid pad. Corrections continue until the arch tightens and tends to hold itself in the balanced position. When this occurs, the presence of the arch pad may cause a previously balanced shoe to appear "overcorrected."

Structural Flatfoot. Structural flatfoot is caused by skeletal deformities that allow depression of the longitudinal arch. Although much less common than pronation, structural flatfoot is a more serious and disabling condition.

The skeletal deformities usually found include congenital sagging or opening of the talonavicular joint or the presence of a talus that is tilted down in a fixed plantar flexed position.

A structural flatfoot soon assumes a flat appearance with or without weight bearing, but maintains good flexibility except for possible limitation of dorsiflexion. This type of flatfoot is frequently associated with pain in the feet.

Radiographic examination confirms the diagnosis.

Treatment depends on the type of skeletal abnormality present. Some feet may be adequately supported by molded metal arch supports; others may require operative intervention for their correction.

Spastic Flatfoot.   Spastic flatfoot is associated with a constant tightness or spasm of the peroneal tendon that pulls the foot into an everted or flat position. The peroneal spasm is usually associated with a tarsal abnormality, frequently a congenital bony bridge that locks the os calcis and navicular bones together.

A spastic flatfoot is usually very painful because of the peroneal spasm. The foot is held in rigid eversion by the tight peroneal tendons thus maintaining a constant flat appearance. The presence of tarsal abnormalities may be demonstrated on oblique radiographs of the foot.

Some patients with spastic flatfoot may obtain relief of pain by the use of molded metal arch supports. A few patients may obtain pain relief by manipulation of the foot under anesthesia. Most patients, however, require surgical intervention for relief. If the diagnosis is made before secondary joint changes occur, resection of the bony bridge may be curative.

DISORDERS OF THE LONGITUDINAL ARCH IN ADULTS

Flatfoot in the adult is associated with painful feet and legs and has, as a rule, the same causes as flatfoot in children.

The most common cause of flatfoot in the adult is residual pronation. Some of these patients give a history of wearing shoe corrections in childhood. Others may deny having problems with their feet until the onset of foot pain. Some patients with pronation escape trouble during childhood only to develop painful feet as adults. In these instances, arch breakdown is usually aided by occupational demands for prolonged standing or walking, by obesity, by poor muscle tone, or by the use of shoes that do not give adequate support.

In some instances, severe pronation in the adult may be associated with excessive sweating of the feet, edema about the foot and ankle, and varicose veins.

The symptoms produced by pronated feet in the adult can usually be relieved by the use of resilient longitudinal arch supports.

Painful feet in the adult caused by structural or spastic flatfoot

FIGURE 14–34. AP radiograph of foot with bunion.

may require operative fusion of the "subtalar joints" for pain relief (triple arthrodesis).

DISORDERS OF THE METATARSAL ARCH

If the bones forming the metatarsal arch are asked to bear a disproportionate amount of weight, thick calluses may form on the ball of the foot and the patient may experience a painful burning sensation in this area with weight bearing. This condition is known as metatarsalgia.

Metatarsalgia occurs primarily in adults and is more common in the female. It may occur alone, but it is frequently seen in association with pronation. In addition to the burning pain in the front of the foot and the callus formation, tenderness to palpation is usually noted between the metatarsal heads on the dorsum of the foot. Severe cases may be associated with clawing of the toes.

Symptoms can usually be relieved by the use of rubber metatarsal arch supports. These come in various sizes and are placed in the shoe to lie just behind the metatarsal heads.

Disorders of the Toes

HALLUX VALGUS (BUNION)

In general usage, the term "hallux valgus" or "bunion" refers to a deformity of the large toe consisting of three elements: lateral angulation of the large toe towards the second toe, bony enlargement of the medial side of the head of the first metatarsal bone at the metatarsophalangeal joint, and formation of a bursal sac over the point of the bony enlargement. In addition to being laterally deviated, the large toe frequently rotates medially on its longitudinal axis (Fig. 14–34). As the large toe progresses in a lateral direction, the long toe extensor tendon becomes displaced laterally and aids in maintaining the abnormal position. The deformity is frequently bilateral. It has been stated that a first metatarsal bone that is congenitally short or one that is deviated medially is a factor in causing bunion. It is also believed that the wearing of pointed and poor-fitting shoes or high heels is a contributing factor.

Bunions are found most frequently in women at or just past middle age. They may be painless and may give concern only because of a shoe fitting problem. Pressure of the shoe against the bursa may cause painful inflammation of the bursal sac. Extreme lateral deviation of the large toe may cause an overlapping of the second toe on the large toe. Bunion formation may be associated with hammer toe deformity of some of the remaining toes (Fig. 14–35).

Conservative treatment of bunion consists of wearing shoes that provide a wide forefoot or "bunion pocket" and the use of bunion pads to relieve shoe pressure on the bursal sac.

If the deformity is painful or extreme enough to make shoe fitting a problem, operative correction may be carried out. There are many operative techniques for removing the bursal sac and bony enlargement of the medial side of the first metatarsal head and correcting the lateral angulation of the large toe.

FIGURE 14–35. Bilateral bunions with overlapped second toes.

HALLUX RIGIDUS

The term "hallux rigidus" refers to a painful stiffness of the first metatarsophalangeal joint that is due to degenerative arthritis. The arthritic changes may accompany generalized degenerative arthritis or may follow local trauma to this joint.

Pain is usually first noted with walking when the joint stiffness prevents normal dorsiflexion of the large toe. The first metatarsophalangeal joint, in addition to being stiff, becomes enlarged and tender. Radiographic examination reveals narrowing of the joint space, with subchondral bone sclerosis and spur formation at the joint margins.

Conservative treatment consists of passive manual stretching of the first metatarsophalangeal joint combined with the use of intraarticular corticosteroid. The sole of the shoe may be stiffened to decrease pain in the joint on walking.

If symptoms warrant, operation can be carried out and a joint fusion or an arthroplasty performed.

HAMMER TOE

The term "hammer toe" refers to a positional deformity of the toe consisting of a flexion contracture of the proximal interphalangeal joint and an extension of the metatarsophalangeal joint. The end of the toe tends to point straight downward into the shoe, and painful calluses may develop on the tip of the toe and on the dorsum of the flexed interphalangeal joint (Fig. 14–36).

The deformity may be congenital in origin or may follow depression of the metatarsal arch with imbalance between the flexors and extensors of the toe.

Conservative treatment consists of passive manual stretching of the tight proximal interphalangeal joint and the use of a metatarsal arch support. If symptoms warrant, operation can be carried out and the flexed proximal interphalangeal joint fused in a straight position.

BUNIONETTE

Bunionette, or little bunion, is a bony enlargment of the lateral side of the head of the fifth metatarsal bone at the metatarsophalangeal

FIGURE 14–36. Hammer toe deformity of second and third toes.

joint. It is usually associated with an overlying bursal sac and a medial deviation of the fifth toe.

As in the case of bunion, treatment of a bunionette may be conservative or surgical.

INGROWN TOENAIL

The term "ingrown toenail" refers to a common and painful ailment usually affecting the outer margin of the large toenail. The nail margin grows into the soft lateral nail groove and surrounding skin. This is usually caused by the pressure of tight shoes or socks on a nail that has been cut too short. As a rule, the violated skin fold becomes infected and hypertrophied with granulation tissue.

Mild cases may respond to soaking the toe in hot water and tucking a small piece of cotton beneath the corners of the nail to raise it from the skin fold. If this is not successful, the involved margin of nail and a portion of the hypertrophied skin fold may be excised under local anesthesia.

PLANTAR NEUROMA (MORTON'S TOE)

The most lateral branch of the medial plantar nerve lies in the third webspace of the foot between the third and fourth metatarsal heads and supplies sensation to the third and fourth toes. Chronic impingement of this nerve between the metatarsal heads may lead to the formation of a neuroma or thickening of this branch of the nerve. Pressure on the neuroma with weight bearing may produce rather characteristic painful symptoms known as plantar neuroma or Morton's toe.

The condition is more common in women. The pain is usually localized to the metatarsal area of the foot, with radiation into the third and fourth toes. Most patients state they can relieve the pain by removing the shoe and massaging the ball of the foot. Occasionally, numbness and tingling are noted in the affected toes. A similar neuroma formation may appear in the other webspaces of the foot.

The pain can usually be reproduced by exerting downward pressure on the third webspace with a small object, such as the eraser end of a lead pencil, while maintaining upward pressure with the thumb on the sole of the foot between the third and fourth metatarsal heads.

The symptoms arising from pressure on a plantar neuroma are often relieved by the use of a metatarsal arch support. If this is not successful, the enlarged segment of nerve may be excised at operation.

Local Foot Problems

CORNS

Corns are localized painful hard thickenings of skin due to continuous shoe pressure on bony prominences. They may be found associated with bunions and bunionettes, beneath the metatarsal heads on the sole of the foot, and on the dorsal surface of hammer toes at the flexed interphalangeal joint.

A corn may be softened with hot water or preparations containing salicylic acid and then trimmed with a scalpel or razor blade. Steps must also be taken to relieve continuous shoe pressure on bony prominences.

SOFT CORNS

Soft corns are found between the toes and are produced when a small projecting bone spur on one toe presses into the skin of the adjacent toe. They are moist and painful.

A piece of cotton placed between the toes may separate them sufficiently to relieve pain. If symptoms warrant, surgical excision of the projecting bone spur may be carried out.

CALLUS

Callus is a circumscribed thickening of the skin similar to a corn, but generally larger in extent. Callus is found most frequently on the sole of the foot at the points bearing an abnormal amount of weight. Callus formation on the ball of the foot commonly accompanies depression of the metatarsal arch.

PLANTAR WART

A plantar wart is an extremely painful vascular papillomatous growth that may occur in any part of the skin on the sole of the foot. The surface of the wart is flat and continuous with the adjacent skin and is pressed inward by weight bearing. Callus may form over the surface of the wart, increasing the degree of local tenderness.

A plantar wart may be removed by local excision with electrocoagulation or by surgical excision. Recurrence is not uncommon.

Traumatic Disorders

PAINFUL HEELS

The complaint of pain in the heel with weight bearing is frequently heard from children and adults. The most common cause in children is calcaneal apophysitis or Sever's disease (see p. 103). The most common cause in adults is plantar bursitis (see p. 166).

MARCH FRACTURE (STRESS FRACTURE)

Fracture of a metatarsal shaft, usually the second or third, may result from the stress associated with weight bearing after prolonged walking has exhausted the muscular and tendinous support of the foot. This type of stress or fatigue fracture is especially common in army recruits during their basic training.

Pain is usually noticed by the patient, not at the moment of fracture as in traumatic fractures, but a week or so later after callus begins to appear. Radiographic examination at that time typically reveals the fracture line surrounded by exuberant callus formation.

March fractures are treated by immobilization, which may be supplied by adhesive strapping or plaster cast.

FRACTURES OF THE FOOT

Toe. Fracture of a toe may be caused by a weight falling on the toe or by stubbing the toe while barefoot. As a rule, these are painful, but not serious injuries. The objective of treatment is to maintain the alignment of the toes so that overlapping or hammer toe does not result. This frequently can be accomplished by strapping the broken toe to its neighbor. If multiple toe fractures are present, a walking cast may be applied for immobilization.

Metatarsal. Fractures of the metatarsal bones are common and may be caused by twisting injuries of the forefoot or by heavy objects dropping on the foot. The objective of treatment of metatarsal shaft fractures is to maintain the alignment of the longitudinal arch.

A fracture through the neck of the metatarsal may allow the metatarsal head to displace towards the sole of the foot. Normal alignment must be restored to prevent the subsequent development of a painful plantar callus.

Many displaced metatarsal fractures can be treated by closed reduction and immobilization in a plaster cast. If this is unsuccessful, skeletal traction, percutaneous pinning, or open reduction with internal metallic fixation may be elected.

Heel.   The os calcis is the most frequently fractured of the tarsal bones. The injury may be relatively insignificant or very complex. The fracture may be caused by a powerful contraction of the gastrocnemius and soleus muscles or by direct trauma to the heel. As a rule, two general types of fractures are seen: an avulsion fracture through the posterior portion of the bone, and comminuted or crush fractures of the bone involving the talocalcaneal joint. The objective of treatment is to restore contour of the bone, particularly the plantar surface and the talocalcaneal joint if possible, and yet, at the same time, maintain as much joint motion as is practical.

Many os calcis fractures are best managed by no active attempted reduction, but by compression dressings, non–weight bearing and early joint motion. Fractures that result in widening of the os calcis often can be reduced by manual compression and immobilized in a short leg cast. Depending on the location of the fracture and the degree of comminution, a few fractures may require skeletal traction, pin fixation, or open reduction with bone graft.

The major complication after os calcis fracture is the development of traumatic arthritis at the talocalcaneal joint. If this occurs, the patient will have pain on weight bearing, particularly with motions requiring eversion and inversion of the foot. If the pain arising from traumatic arthritis of the talocalcaneal joint cannot be controlled by nonoperative treatment methods, the operation of triple arthrodesis is carried out.

References

Adams, J. A.: Transient synovitis of the hip joint in children. J. Bone and Joint Surg., 45-B:471, 1963.

Barnes, R., Brown, J. T., Garden, R. S., and Nicoll, E. A.: Subcapital fractures of the femur. A prospective review. J. Bone Joint Surg., 58-B:2, 1976.

Bianco, A. J.: Slipped capital femoral epiphysis. J. Bone and Joint Surg., 47-A:432, 1965.

Bianco, A. J.: Treatment of mild slipping of the capital femoral epiphysis. J. Bone and Joint Surg., 47-A:387, 1965.

Chung, S. M. K., and Ralson, E. L.: Necrosis of the femoral head associated with sickle-cell anemia and its genetic variant. J. Bone and Joint Surg., 51-A:33, 1969.

Cracchiolo, A. (Guest Ed.): Statistics of total knee replacement. Clin. Ortho. and Rel. Res., No. 120, October 1976.

D'Aubigne, R. M., et al.: Idiopathic necrosis of the femoral head in adults. J. Bone and Joint Surg., 47-B:612, 1965.

Epstein, H. C.: Posterior fracture-dislocation of the hip: Long-term follow-up. J. Bone and Joint Surg., 56-A:1103, 1974.

Freeman, M. A. R. (Guest Ed.): Total surface replacement hip arthroplasty. Clin. Ortho. and Rel. Res., No. 132, August 1978.

Gartland, J. J., and Benner, J. H.: Traumatic dislocations in the lower extremity in children. Ortho. Clin. of North Am., Vol. 7, No. 3, July 1976.

Giannestras, N. J.: Foot Disorders: Medical and Surgical Management, 2nd Edition. Philadelphia: Lea and Febiger, 1973.

Helfet, A. J.: Diagnosis and management of internal derangement of the knee joint. Am.

Academy of Orthopaedic Surgeons Instructional Course Lectures, Vol. XIX. St. Louis: C. V. Mosby Co., 1970.

Inglis, A. E., Scott, W. M., Sculco, T. P., and Patterson, A. H.: Ruptures of the tendo-achillis. An objective assessment of surgical and nonsurgical treatment. J. Bone and Joint Surg., 58-A:990, 1976.

Jones, J. P., Jr., and Engelman, E. P.: Osseous avascular necrosis associated with systemic abnormalities. Arthritis Rheum., 9,5:728, 1966.

Lauge-Hansen, N.: Fractures of the ankle. II. Combined experimental-surgical and experimental-roentgenologic investigations. Arch. Surg., 60:957, 1950.

Radin, E. L., Simon, S. R., Rose, R. M., and Paul, I. L.: Practical Biomechanics for the Orthopaedic Surgeon. New York: John Wiley & Sons, Inc., 1978.

Robert, N.: Osteochondritis dissecans. J. Bone and Joint Surg., 39-B:219, 1957.

Sarmiento, A. (Guest Ed.): Fractures of the tibia. Clin. Ortho. and Rel. Res., No. 105, December 1974.

Smillie, I. S.: Injuries of the Knee Joint. Edinburgh and London: E. & S. Livingstone, 1970.

Urist, M. (Editor-in-Chief): Current practice in hip joint surgery. Clin. Ortho. and Rel. Res., No. 106, February 1975.

Urist, M. (Editor-in-Chief): Newer knowledge of total hip arthroplasty. Clin. Ortho. and Rel. Res., No. 120, December 1976.

Urist, M. (Editor-in-Chief): Hip and knee joint surgery. Clin. Ortho. and Rel. Res., No. 132, May 1978.

CHAPTER 15

ORTHOPAEDIC REHABILITATION

Phillip J. Marone, M.D. *

The reader is reminded that the definition of orthopaedics given in Chapter 1 contained the admonition that this discipline is concerned also with the restoration of the function of the skeletal system, its articulations, and associated structures. This means, of course, that the treating physician has a responsibility to restore patients to normal living after illness or injury. Persons born with afflictions of the musculoskeletal system grow and develop with compensatory mechanisms that enable them to function within the scope of their disability. However, if a person is sound and then becomes disabled because of injury or disease, the return to full function frequently becomes a major effort.

The purpose of this chapter is to bring to your attention some of the methods utilized to return these patients to the point of being able to care for themselves.

*Chief of Orthopaedic Surgery and Physical Medicine, Methodist Hospital, Philadelphia, Pa.; Clinical Associate Professor of Orthopaedic Surgery, Clinical Associate Professor of Rehabilitation Medicine, Jefferson Medical College of Thomas Jefferson University, Philadelphia, Pa.

453

TERMINOLOGY

It is essential to define some of the terms used in orthopaedic rehabilitation before the principles of orthopaedic rehabilitation can be discussed.

RANGE OF MOTION (R.O.M.)

The term "range of motion" refers to joint motion or the ability to move a part through its arc of motion at a joint. Many diseases of the musculoskeletal system cause, or are associated with, impaired joint motion. In testing joint range, the physician must be aware of the normal range of motion for each specific joint (see Fig. 14–2).

The instrument used for these determinations is called a *goniometer*, and the R.O.M. is conveniently expressed in degrees.

MUSCLE TESTING (M.T.)

Muscle testing is used to determine the degree of impairment in affected muscles. The usual method of testing is manual and subjective. Various degrees of resistance are applied to the muscles, which are graded accordingly. The patient is placed in a test position that varies for each muscle or muscle group to be tested. The patient is then asked to move the muscles being tested through their full R.O.M. The muscle or muscle group is graded according to the response elicited. Three methods of recording these actions are in general use: (1) grade 0 through 5; (2) percentage of normal, 0 per cent to 100 per cent; (3) the Lovett scale, zero to normal. Although these methods of recording are interchangeable, an examiner should master and stick to one method. The Lovett scale is a convenient method of recording muscle strength. The terms used in the Lovett scale are defined as follows:

Zero — no contraction felt or seen.

Trace — muscle is felt to tighten, but cannot produce movement.

Poor — motion with the force of gravity eliminated, but muscle cannot function against gravity.

Fair — patient can raise the part against gravity, but not with any outside resistance added.

Good — patient can raise the part as in fair, but with resistance added.

Normal — muscle overcomes a greater resistance than a "good" muscle and, in actuality, possesses the same strength as its contralateral muscle when it is tested.

Muscle testing and its accompanying R.O.M. are fundamental in the diagnosis, evaluation, and programming of the disabled orthopaedic patient.

ACTIVITIES OF DAILY LIVING (A.D.L.)

The A.D.L. are the basic activities essential to carrying on daily life, including transportation and working where applicable. The goal to be reached in A.D.L. is to make the patient self-sufficient. A very close interrelationship exists between A.D.L. and exercise. The goals to be achieved depend upon whether one is dealing with bed patients, wheelchair patients, or ambulatory patients. Orthopaedics deals mostly with ambulatory patients, and the goal should be to return these patients to their environment as efficiently as possible.

OCCUPATIONAL THERAPY (O.T.)

Occupational therapy is the art and science of directing man's response to selected action to promote and maintain health, to prevent disability, and to treat or train patients with physical dysfunctions.

The occupational therapist, therefore, instructs and actively involves patients in a wide variety of purposeful activities common to their immediate environment or culture. They are thus stimulated to develop what is necessary to be productive and independent.

While it is usually the most seriously disabled patient who requires occupational therapy, it is necessary to be aware of its availability, as many times patients will achieve their goals more quickly with this service.

GAIT

Gait is defined as the manner or style of walking. No physical examination of the locomotor system is complete unless the gait pattern is analyzed. Limp is defined as a pathologic gait (p. 379). To recognize a pathologic gait, one must be familiar with the normal gait pattern.

The gait cycle consists of two phases: *stance phase* and *swing phase*. These phases repetitiously and rhythmically alternate to produce normal locomotion. When these motions become asymmetric, they are considered pathologic.

The stance or support phase starts with the foot in the forward position and the heel down. It ends with the toe pushing off and the foot leaving the ground, and measures longer than the swing phase. The swing phase, shorter in duration than the stance phase, begins when the foot leaves the ground and lasts through the next heel strike. There is a brief period when both legs are on the ground simultaneously. This is called the *period of double support.*

Gait is a three-dimensional activity. When one moves forward or backward, several forces work to produce three-dimensional displacement of the body. Even though the legs play the most conspicuous role in ambulation, other body elements, such as pelvis, trunk, and even the upper extremities, also play important parts. All of these elements, consequently, must be carefully observed in a gait analysis.

ORTHOTICS

Orthotics deals with the application of exoskeletal devices to limit or to assist motion of any given segment of the human body. These exoskeletal devices are called *orthoses* when applied to patients suffering from neuromuscular or skeletal disorders. This, therefore, is a more inclusive term for devices than the old terms such as brace or splint.

PROSTHETICS

Prosthetics is the addition or application to the body of an artificial device, called a *prosthesis,* to replace partially or totally missing extremities or organs.

The terms quadriplegia, paraplegia, and hemiplegia have already been defined in the chapter on neuromuscular disorders (p. 194).

PRINCIPLES OF PHYSICAL MEDICINE

THERMAL THERAPY

Heat is one of the measures most commonly employed in orthopaedic rehabilitation. It is frequently utilized before massage and exercise because it enhances the effects of the subsequent treatment measures. The physiologic effects of heat are to bring about an increase in tissue temperature, to produce vasodilatation, and to increase local circulation. These changes cause an increase in tissue metabolic activity, which leads to a further increase in tissue temperature and further vasodilatation, thus increasing transduction of tissue fluids. Excessive basal heat is controlled by blood flow away from the heated area to other parts of the body. Another well-known effect of heat therapy is mild sedation, with relief of pain and muscular tension.

The methods of heat application are classified as *radiant, conductive,* or *conversive.* Each form has certain effects and indications for use. Radiant heat is infrared. Conductive heating is the direct application of heat to the body in the form of hot water packs or bottles, towels, paraffin baths, or electrically heated pads. Conversive heating is an indirect form of heat resulting from the conversion of various forms of primary energies to heat in the body tissues. Radiant and conductive heating are superficial and readily available.

Superficial heating can be supplied by the infrared lamp, whirlpool bath, Hubbard tanks, hot packs, contrast baths (hot and cold), and paraffin baths. Any form of superficial heating takes between 20 and 30 minutes to produce the desired effect; the temperature increase is greatest in the skin and less in the deeper tissues. There is no significant rise in temperature beyond 1 to 2 cm. beneath the skin surface. The most commonly utilized means of applying superficial heat are the infrared lamp and the forms of hydrotherapy. Little danger of overdosage exists with superficial heating if local circulation and skin sensation are intact. The main contraindications to the use of superficial heat are the absence of skin sensation and a decrease in local blood supply. Superficial heat should never be applied to a part during the first 24 hours following an acute injury.

Deep, or conversive, heating is the result of high frequency alternating currents, and its margin of safety is lower than that of the superficial forms of heating. The deep heating devices in general use are short-wave diathermy, microwave, and ultrasound.

Short-wave diathermy has a maximum penetration of 2 to 3 cm. beneath the skin surface over a period of 30 minutes. The high frequency currents tend to spread as they enter the body and tend to heat a fairly large area. The large area heated and the margin of safety in its usage are advantages of short-wave diathermy over microwave and ultrasound. Although short-wave diathermy gives more equal heating than infrared, it possesses no other advantage over the superficial forms of heating.

Microwave is applied by means of radiated electromagnetic waves, which must go through a director, or head, focused several inches away from the skin surface. A layer of subcutaneous fat one-half inch thick will absorb 30 per cent of microwave energy, and part of microwave energy is lost by reflection from the body surface.

Ultrasound is energy that comes from a series of mechanical vibrations. Direct contact with skin is necessary for ultrasound treatment, since these waves do not travel through air. A coupling medium, such as mineral oil, is a necessary part of its use. The subcutaneous fat must be at least 2 inches thick before 30 per cent of ultrasound energy is absorbed. No ultrasound energy is lost by reflection from the body surface.

In deep tissues of high water content, such as muscle, ultrasound has a greater penetration than microwave. The reverse is true in tissue of low water content, such as bone. Adequate deep heating effects can be obtained with either source of heat to a tissue depth of 5 to 6 cm. With proper application, an effective rise in temperature will occur within 15 to 20 minutes with microwave and within 3 to 10 minutes with ultrasound. The area that may be treated with either modality is small. The use of these modalities must be discontinued if unpleasant sensations of heat occur.

Ultrasound or microwave may be indicated to supply deep heat in the treatment of bursitis, myositis, tenosynovitis, and tendinitis. Neither should be used in the presence of infection, malignant disease, peripheral vascular disease, acute hemorrhage, or a metallic implant, or over a fracture site before callus has formed. Both should be used with caution over growing bone or over any bony surface that lies superficially beneath the skin surface. They should also be used with caution in the region of the eyes, over the testes, or over larger nerve structures. Deep heating modalities should never be used in the presence of an acute injury.

COLD THERAPY

Cold therapy has a more limited use than heat therapy, but it is occasionally of value because it causes vasoconstriction, with consequent decreases in local tissue blood flow, local metabolic activity, and local tissue temperature. These effects, in turn, produce a decrease in edema or local swelling of the part. Ice bags and cold compresses are used extensively to minimize the local reaction that results from acute trauma such as sprain, fracture, or dislocation. If edema or local swelling can be minimized in an injured part by the use of cold therapy, the patient will respond more favorably to the range of motion and exercise program needed to restore the preinjury state of function. The local use of ice also seems to decrease muscle spasm and pain in chronic joint problems such as strains. It has been theorized that cold anesthetizes the skin and reflexly causes muscles to become relaxed and less painful. Most often, ice packs are utilized as the means of cold therapy. A machine is available that combines a 40° F temperature circulating through a sleeve for the affected extremity with intermittent pressure. This method of cold combined with alternating increase and release of pressure reduces edema more quickly than the older, time-tested method of ice bags. Following this treatment, a patient is usually able to carry the joint involved through a range of motion and therefore decrease the amount of time that is necessary to return the joint to function. The use of cold therapy is contraindicated in the presence of peripheral vascular disease.

Contrast baths (hot and cold) have some beneficial effect in the relief of local pain and the reduction of tissue edema. They are thought to produce alternating contraction and relaxation of blood vessels, with a significant increase in local blood flow. Contrast baths are used as follows: hot (110° F to 115° F) for 10 minutes, cold for one minute; hot for four minutes, cold for one minute; hot for four minutes, cold for one minute; hot for four minutes, cold for one minute; the baths finish with four minutes of hot water. The Cryotemp machine described above can be an effective way of using contrast baths if it is used following the use of the intermittent pressurized cold method.

MASSAGE

Massage is a therapeutic measure performed by a trained therapist. Its use should always be preceded by some form of heating.

Many physiologic effects are attributed to massage. Its use seems to be followed by an increase in blood flow, which increases the interchange of substances between the cells and the bloodstream. External mechanical pressure increases the flow of lymph from tissue spaces into the venous circulation. The mechanical pressure of massage removes excess tissue fluid and decreases the likelihood of fibrosis. Connective tissue fibrosis responds to massage by the mechanical stretching and disruption of fibers by friction. Muscle nutrition improves following massage because the mechanical stimulation aids in removal of the extravascular fluids.

Two types of massage are generally utilized. Stroking (*effleurage*) is superficial and light. Compression (*petrussage*) consists of kneading a portion of a muscle or a group of muscles between the thumb, its eminence, and the fingers. The muscle is then compressed from side to side as the hand moves up the muscle in the direction of the venous flow.

Massage is indicated for the relief of pain, relaxation of muscle tension, improvement in local circulation, reduction of induration or edema, and the stretching of adhesions. Massage is contraindicated in the presence of acute inflammation, malignant tumors, and acute peripheral vascular disorders, such as phlebitis or thrombosis.

As mentioned, massage should be preceded by the use of local heat, as this will enhance the desired effects of the massage. Both heat and massage should be followed by an active or passive exercise program so that the maximum benefits of exercise can be obtained.

THERAPEUTIC EXERCISE

Therapeutic exercise is utilized to improve the balance and stability of the body. Its objectives are to improve coordination, to increase endurance and power, and to increase joint range of motion. Once an indication for therapeutic exercise has been identified and a purposeful goal established, the therapeutic exercise program must be carefully planned or the goal will not be reached. The exercise program should be on a graduated basis, tailored to the patient's needs as identified by periodic re-evaluation. A therapeutic exercise program can be successful only with a cooperative patient and an adequate prescription designed to improve what can be improved and to stabilize what cannot be improved.

The following types of exercises are available:

Passive exercise is accomplished by a therapist, with no effort by the patient. This form of exercise prevents joint contractures and maintains a normal joint range of motion and is usually used with a patient whose muscles are paralyzed or very weak.

Active assistive exercise is usually the first step in a muscle re-education program. Strength can be obtained only by active contraction of the muscle by the patient; the therapist assists by supporting the weight of the extremity so that gravity is eliminated or resistance overcome. This form of exercise not only helps to strengthen muscles but also aids range of motion and muscle coordination.

Active exercise is performed actively by the patient, who contracts the muscle with resistance and against the pull of gravity. Active exercise increases strength and improves function of the part. It may be started when a muscle is rated in the fair range.

Resistive exercise is an active exercise program with resistance added. It is usually carried out by applying manual resistance throughout the range of joint motion. Resistive exercise is used only when the muscle is rated good to normal. Its major purpose is to develop muscle strength.

Progressive resistive exercise (P.R.E.) is essentially the same as resistive exercise, except that progressive resistance is added by means of weight varying from a light load to a load maximal for a muscle. The aim of this type of exercise is to increase the strength and endurance of the exercised muscle as quickly as possible.

Isokinetic exercise is a relatively new method designed as a concept of accommodating resistance at a constant angular velocity throughout the range of motion. While isometric strength testing measures the maximum force exerted at one position, therefore determining static strength, isotonic testing measures dynamic strength typically by the one repetition maximum method.

Isokinetic exercise is a form of isotonic exercise with one major difference. This is continuous exercise throughout a range of motion, which is caused by accommodating resistance against a lever moving at a fixed speed. This can therefore document maximum dynamic strength throughout the range of motion.

AMBULATION

There are many devices available to help a disabled patient become ambulatory. The goal of rehabilitation is to enable the patient to become as independent as possible, either with or without the aid of a device. The type of device chosen and the length of time it will have to be used by the patient depend greatly upon the medical reason for disability. A patient with a fracture of a bone in the lower extremity is usually considered to have a temporary problem and is not as difficult to ambulate as a patient with paraplegia, which is a permanent problem. However, before an effort is made to ambulate a patient who has either a temporarily or permanently disabling medical problem, it first must be determined that the patient has sufficient muscle strength and coordination to handle an ambulation program. If not, an extensive exercise and conditioning program must be undertaken before ambulation can be realistically attempted.

The standard ambulation aids are as follows:
1. Crutches (metal or wood)
   a. Conventional
   b. Adjustable
   c. Lofstrand
2. Canes (metal or wood)
   a. Conventional (C curve or T top)
   b. Tripod
   c. Quadriped
3. Walkers (metal)

There are two methods in general use to measure a patient for crutches. One method is to measure from the patient's anterior axillary fold to the bottom of the shoe or heel and add an additional 2 inches to the measurement. The second method is to measure the patient from the anterior axillary fold to a point 6 inches lateral to the side of his foot. The handpiece of the crutch should be adjusted so that the elbow assumes a 30 degree flexion attitude with the wrist in extension. Lofstrand crutches, canes, and walkers can also be measured with the patient's elbow in a 30 degree flexion attitude with the wrist in extension.

Occasionally special adaptations become necessary because of problems in the upper extremities. Such adaptations can be made by an orthotist in accordance with the individual patient problem.

There are seven different aided gait patterns; choosing one depends on the patient's ability to take steps with either one or both of the lower extremities.

1. Four-Point Alternate Crutch Gait. This gait has the following sequence: right crutch, left foot; left crutch, right foot. This is a simple gait that is used if weight bearing is allowed and if the patient can place one foot in front of the other. It is a safe gait pattern, as there are always three points of support on the floor.

2. Two-Point Alternate Crutch Gait. This gait has the following sequence: right crutch and left foot simultaneously, followed by left crutch and right foot. This is a speeding up of the four-point gait, but it is not as safe, as only two points are supporting the body at one time.

3. Three-Point Crutch Gait. In this gait pattern, both crutches and the weaker lower extremity start out, followed by the stronger lower extremity. This gait is used when one lower extremity cannot take full weight bearing and the other one can support the entire body weight. Orthopaedists frequently prescribe this gait for patients who have suffered lower extremity or pelvic trauma. The amount of weight borne on the affected extremity can be modified by allowing weight bearing to vary from simple touching down of the toes of the extremity to full weight bearing. The amount of weight borne on the extremity is usually monitored by the pain tolerance of the patient.

4. and 5. Tripod Crutch Gait. This gait is used when a patient has no active means of placing one extremity ahead of the other, as would occur in paraplegia. There are two tripod gaits in use: the tripod alternate (drag-to) is first mastered, and then the tripod simultaneous (a faster, but not as safe, gait) is taught.

6. and 7. Swing Crutch Gait. There are two variations of this type of gait, the swing-to gait and the swing-through gait. Both are speedier modifications of the tripod gaits, but they require more energy output to balance safely.

In summary, walking aids, whether they be crutches, canes, or walkers, are utilized to assist the patient in becoming ambulatory. Each patient will have an aided gait tailored to fit the individual problem. Whenever possible, at least two gaits should be taught, one to be used for speed and the other for safety. It must be remembered that the use of walking aids greatly adds to the energy requirements of the patient. Older patients and patients with medically debilitating illnesses must be instructed with walking aids and gait patterns that are the least fatiguing.

REHABILITATION OF THE AMPUTEE

LOWER EXTREMITY AMPUTATION

The majority of amputations performed in civilian medical practice are of the lower extremities. The chief medical reasons for amputation in a civilian practice are peripheral vascular diseases, diabetes, and severe trauma. If amputation becomes necessary, the surgeon must make every effort to save as much limb length as possible for prosthetic fitting. It is difficult for a patient with a short stump to ambulate satisfactorily in a prosthesis, and the gait pattern developed is less cosmetically acceptable than the pattern developed by the patient with a long stump. An amputee will require a good stump and a comfortable, cosmetically acceptable prosthetic device to be rehabilitated satisfactorily. If at all possible, the surgeon should endeavor to save the knee joint. If an amputation is carried out above the knee, the prosthetic device must contain a mechanical knee joint, which adds another dimension to the prosthesis and is energy consuming and awkward for the patient.

Today, when amputation is performed for peripheral vascular disease or diabetes, it is more usual to be able to save the knee joint than not. This is a decided reversal of the earlier trend and has only become true over the past two decades. One of the chief reasons for the reversal is the use of the rigid dressing technique of amputation surgery. With this technique, the surgeon applies a cast in the nature of a patellar tendon bearing socket immediately after closing the amputation stump. The added resistance to swelling and the "mechanical pump set-up" combat edema and result in more rapid tissue healing.

The type of amputation performed and the prosthetic component required vary according to the amputation site, which is dictated essentially by the underlying disease or trauma.

Patients undergoing *toe amputation* need no special prosthetic device for ambulation. If amputation is required through the metatarsal or tarsal area of the foot, either a filling device or a special prosthesis will be necessary for the shoe.

Amputation through the ankle joint is called a Syme amputation. Its chief advantage is that the stump is end bearing, but the stump has a tendency to a bulbous shape that is cosmetically objectionable to most female patients. The prosthetic device used for a patient who has undergone a Syme amputation is called the Syme prosthesis. Along with most of the other lower extremity prosthetic devices, the Syme prosthesis has an S.A.C.H. foot (solid ankle, cushioned heel).

A *below knee amputation* level may vary from anywhere above the malleoli to 5 cm. below the tibial plateau. The actual site of amputation below the knee will have to depend upon the level of available good skin and muscle. Ideally, a 15 cm. length stump should be sought in a below knee amputation. The prosthesis used for a patient with a below knee amputation is of the patellar tendon bearing, below knee type, with or without an added thigh lacer. The thigh lacer is necessary for patients with short or tender stumps, as it helps distribute the pressures about the stump and adds to stump comfort. It also serves as an added suspensory mechanism in a patient with a very short stump. The old conventional type of prosthesis (open ended) is still occasionally utilized, especially for those patients with distal stump pain, skin problems in the stump, or recurrent edema of the stump. One of the newest modifications to eliminate distal stump pain or skin problems within the stump is a special socket called a slip socket. This simply is one socket within another, which allows room for pistoning and therefore avoids some of the abrasiveness that occurs with the rigid patellar tendon bearing socket.

An *above knee amputation* should be performed anywhere from 10 cm. above the knee joint to 10 cm. below the hip joint. The distance of 10 cm. above the knee joint is required for the mechanical knee that is added to the prosthesis. Many types of knee mechanisms are available for the patient with an above knee amputation. The one most commonly used is called the single axis constant friction knee. The socket of the prosthesis is of the total contact design, and the top is quadrilateral in shape. This tends to shift most of the weight to the ischial tuberosity, with the remainder distributed peripherally about the stump. The prosthesis can be suspended by either suction or by a suctionless arrangement. A suction socket should not be used in conditions associated with skin changes, local edema, or skin ulceration. The patient with an above knee amputation cannot develop a gait as cosmetically acceptable as that of the patient with a below knee amputation. The energy required to propel an above knee prosthesis is much greater than the energy necessary to propel a below knee prosthesis. This is another reason for saving the knee if at all possible so that a below knee prosthesis can be utilized.

Occasionally a patient will be seen who requires a *hip disarticulation, hemipelvectomy,* or *hemicorporectomy.* Prosthetic devices have been designed for these patients, and they consist of modifications of the Canadian hip prostheses and other types of pelvic support prosthetic devices. The energy necessary to propel these devices is even greater than the energy needed for the above knee prosthesis. It is for this reason that it is rare to see someone who has had an amputation at these levels learn to ambulate in a prosthesis. These patients usually prefer to get about with the aid of crutches because the energy requirement is less than that expended using a prosthetic device.

Upper Extremity Amputation

The objectives of upper extremity prosthetics are to give the patient prehension and to restore body image. As in lower extremity surgery, as much length as possible must be maintained for better prosthetic fit. A patient with a below elbow amputation will generally function better than a patient with an above elbow amputation.

Prehension and cosmesis are difficult tasks to accomplish in the same terminal device. In most instances, a patient must have two devices — one for function (the hook) and the other for cosmesis (the hand).

As in the lower extremity, the prosthetic device for an upper extremity amputee will depend upon the level of amputation.

Patients with a *partial hand amputation* cannot be fitted with a prosthesis.

Patients with a *wrist disarticulation* can become quite functional in a prosthesis, as they retain nearly full supination and pronation power in the prosthetic device. The terminal devices for this prosthesis, and for almost all other upper extremity prostheses, are either voluntary opening or voluntary closing devices, which are controlled by scapular abduction, shoulder flexion, or a combination of both. These motions are transmitted to the terminal device by a shoulder harness and a cable. Once the device is opened on a voluntary basis, terminal closing is supplied by rubber bands or spring loads. Voluntary closing devices allow the terminal devices to be locked at any angle of opening. However, a second motion is required to unlock the terminal device. The two terminal devices, the hook and the hand, are interchangeable, but most upper extremity amputee patients prefer the hook to the hand, as it is lighter, more durable, and more suitable for manual labor. The hand is really for cosmetic purposes and is not designed for work.

Below elbow amputees with longer stumps can be fitted with the same prosthesis as patients with wrist disarticulations. The Muenster prosthesis seems to work well for the patient with a short below elbow amputation stump. In this prosthesis, the socket extends posteriorly about the olecranon and fits closely about the biceps muscle. This arrangement suspends the prosthesis and eliminates the need for the elbow hinge and triceps cuff. It does limit elbow flexion and extension, but this proves to be of little significance in a patient with a unilateral amputation.

An *elbow disarticulation* maintains desirable function, as these patients retain full internal and external rotation in the prosthesis. However, the prosthesis required is cosmetically objectionable to most female patients because of the bulk produced about the elbow by the addition of outside lock hinges. The elbow unit contains an alternating locking mechanism, with one controlled motion locking the elbow and the other motion unlocking the elbow. Terminal device control and elbow flexion are supplied by the same motions as occur in the wrist disarticulation prosthesis. In this instance, the housing is split so that when the elbow is unlocked, elbow flexion occurs. When the elbow is locked, the same control motion will produce terminal device operation.

The patient with an *above elbow amputation* can be fitted with the same prosthesis as is used by the patient with an elbow disarticulation, the prosthesis being modified only at the elbow unit and in its socket configuration. These patients will need a device to assist in rotation.

The patient who has undergone *shoulder disarticulation* may be fitted with a prosthesis that has the same basic units as those required by the patient with an above elbow amputation, but the socket must cover the scapular and pectoral muscles.

A patient undergoing *forequarter amputation* currently has no way of being fitted with a functional prosthesis. However, testing is now underway on a prosthesis for these patients, fitted with an externally powered device. At the present time, most patients undergoing forequarter amputation may use a lightweight shoulder cup with a passive cosmetic arm if they desire.

REHABILITATION OF THE INJURED ATHLETE

Participation in sports activities is extremely popular and encompasses all age groups and all levels of competence, ranging from the professional to the sandlot athlete. A physician who elects to treat patients with sports-related injuries, whether it be on the professional, college, high school, or sandlot level, must possess the necessary skills not only to treat the injury properly but also return the patient to full function and full sports participation as quickly as possible.

Rehabilitation of the athlete begins with first aid on the athletic field and continues until the athlete has returned to full participation. The first step in rehabilitation is to make an accurate diagnosis of the extent of the injury. If the injury is such that surgical intervention is necessary, the operation should be performed as quickly as possible.

If the injury is such that surgery is not required, cold packs, pain medication, and splinting where appropriate are good initial measures. It is important to remember that splinting may be associated with muscle atrophy which should be avoided in the athlete if possible. It is important that exercise begin as quickly as possible even if it has to be performed intermittently during the day with the protective splint removed. The injured part should be mobilized as quickly as possible. The remainder of the body, including the other extremities, must be involved in an exercise program which combines work for endurance and strength. All exercises and movements should be controlled and guided by pain, which is a good indicator and should never be provoked.

It is important to relieve swelling in and about a joint as quickly as possible. Hematomas and joint effusions should be aspirated. If localized fluid collections are not present, ice packs are used. After the first day of cold therapy the various means to promote reparative processes and decrease edema, previously mentioned, are begun. Active mobilization of the injured part is begun as soon as practical, to stimulate venous and lymph return and prevent joint adhesions. Massage may be performed during this period but must be done by someone trained in its application. Gradual weight bearing and walking should begin as soon as the physician determines the activity would not be detrimental to the well-being of the injured athlete.

The injured athlete has a justifiable concern about loss of muscular capacity in relation to the particular characteristics of the sport involved. The rehabilitation team should immediately test these characteristics and follow them through the treatment and rehabilitation period. A diary can be kept with the active participation of the athlete so that all involved in the rehabilitation process can review the progress or regression. All extremities should be tested and compared, assuming that the injured part had the same qualities as the noninjured part before the injury. Extremity circumferences are measured with a tape. Range of joint motion is recorded with a goniometer, and standard muscle tests should be performed and recorded.

There has been some controversy in the past over the best type of exercise for the injured athlete. Studies have shown that isometric exercises promote more rapid rehabilitation of the injured knee than do isotonic exercises. Presently, isometric exercises are favored as the first step in reconditioning. High-resistance, low-repetition exercises develop strength, whereas low-resistance, high-repetition exercises promote endurance. Although both qualities need to be developed, strength should be emphasized first. After the affected extremity reaches its normal strength, the athlete is ready to start specific athletic training and competition. Specific athletic training commences by setting a goal and a period within which to attain that goal. A program is then set up to return the athlete to the prior performance level attained in whatever sport is involved.

References

Barnes, G. H.: Skin health and stump hygiene. Artif. Limbs, 3:4, 1956.

Block, M. A., and Whitehouse, F. W.: Below knee amputation in patients with diabetes mellitus. Arch. Surg., 87:682, 1963.

Bloomberg, M. H.: Orthopaedic Braces. Philadelphia: J. B. Lippincott Co., 1964.

Burgess, E. M., and Romano, R. L.: The management of lower extremity amputees using immediate post surgical prosthesis. Clin. Orth. and Rel. Res., 57:137, 1968.

Ducroquet, R., Ducroquet, J., and Ducroquet, P.: Walking and Limping, A Study of Pathological Walking. Philadelphia: J. B. Lippincott Co., 1968.

Elftman, H.: Biomechanics of muscles with particular application to studies of gait. J. Bone and Joint Surg., 48-A:363, 1966.

Hoover, R. M.: Problems and complications of amputees. Clin. Orth. and Rel. Res., 37:47, 1964.

Klopsteg, P. E., and Wilson, T. D. (Eds.): Human Limbs and Their Substitutes. New York: McGraw-Hill, 1950.

Marmor, L. (Ed.): Amputations and prosthesis. Clin. Orth. and Rel. Res., No. 37, 1964.

Rusk, H. A.: Rehabilitation Medicine, 3rd Edition, St. Louis: C. V. Mosby Co., 1971.

Ryan, A. J., and Allman, F. L.: Sports Medicine. New York: Academic Press, 1974.

Sarmiento, A., Bella, J. N., Sinclair, W. F., McCollough, N. C., and Williams, E. M.: Lower extremity amputations: The impact of immediate post-surgical prosthetic fitting. Clin. Orth. and Rel. Res., No. 68, 1970.

Saunders, J. B. deC.M., Inman, V. T., and Eberhart, H. D.: The major determinant in normal and pathological gait. J. Bone and Joint Surgery, 35-A:543, 1953.

Scott, M. G.: Analysis of Human Motion — A Textbook in Kinesiology. New York: F. S. Crofts and Co., 1942.

Smodlaka, V.: Rehabilitating the injured athlete. The Physician and Sports Medicine. November 1977, pp. 43–52.

Swinyard, C. A., Deaver, G. G., and Greenspan, L.: Gradients of functional ability of importance in rehabilitation of patients with progressive muscular and neuromuscular diseases. Arch. Phys. Med., 38:574, 1957.

Syllabus on Heat in Physical Therapy, 7th Edition. Milton, Wis.: Burdick Co., 1969.

Thompson, R. G., et al.: Above-the-knee amputation and prosthetics. J. Bone and Joint Surg., 47-A:619, 1965.

Williams, M., and Lissner, H. R.: Biomechanics of Human Motion. Philadelphia: W. B. Saunders Co., 1962.

Zohn, D. A., Leach, R. E.: Stryker laws: A comparison of isometric and isotonic exercises of the quadriceps after injuries of the knee. Arch. Phys. Med. 45:571–574, 1964.

Glossary

Abduction: a movement by which a part of the body is drawn away from the mid-line of the body.

Active motion: movement occurring as a result of the patient's own muscular activity.

Adduction: a movement by which a part of the body is drawn toward the mid-line of the body.

Amputation: the removal of part or all of a limb by cutting through the bone.

Ankylosis: abnormal immobility or stiffness of the joint caused by fibrous or bony tissue bridging the joint space.

Antalgic gait: a self-protective limp due to pain and characterized by a short stance phase.

Arthrodesis: the operation by which fusion is obtained between the bony parts of the joint. This term may be used interchangeably with the words *fusion* and *ankylosis*.

Arthrography: x-ray examination of a joint performed after injection of a contrast material, usually either air or a radiopaque dye, for the purpose of visualizing an internal derangement.

Arthropathy: general term used to refer to any joint disease.

Arthroplasty: a reconstructive operation performed on a joint previously damaged by trauma or disease, designed to restore, as far as possible, the integrity and functional power of the joint.

Arthroscopy: the technique of looking inside a joint through an arthroscope.

Arthrotomy: the operation of cutting into a joint.

Aspiration: the act of withdrawing fluid material from a joint through a needle.

Bone grafting: the operation by which bone tissue is transplanted from one site in the body to another bone in order to give added strength to the recipient bone or to induce healing of a fracture nonunion.

471

Calcaneus: a deformity in which the foot is maintained in a position of dorsiflexion, so that with walking only the heel touches the floor (opposite of *equinus*).

Capsulotomy: the surgical cutting of a joint capsule.

Cavus: exaggeration of the longitudinal arch of the foot due to contraction of the plantar fascia or bony deformity of the arch.

Congenital: existing at or before birth.

Coxa: pertaining to the hip or hip joint.

Coxa valga: an increase in the femoral neck-shaft angle.

Coxa vara: a decrease in the femoral neck-shaft angle.

Crepitus: the crackling or grating sound or sensation produced by bone fragments or joint surfaces rubbing together.

Cubitus valgus: an increase in the normal carrying angle at the elbow.

Cubitus varus: a decrease in the normal carrying angle at the elbow.

Curettage: the surgical scraping of bone with a sharp cup-shaped instrument called a *curette*.

Debridement: the surgical cleansing of a wound to remove dead, devitalized, infected, or soiled tissue.

Disarticulation: the removal of a limb by cutting through a joint.

Dislocation: complete displacement of the bones forming a joint.

Displacement osteotomy: the operation of cutting a bone and shifting the fragments to change the alignment of the bone or to alter the weight bearing stresses applied to the associated joint.

Dorsiflexion: the movement of backward flexion or bending. When used in reference to wrist or ankle joints, it means extension of the joint.

Effusion: formation of abnormal amounts of synovial fluid within a joint cavity, resulting in distension of the joint.

Epiphysiodesis: the operation creating permanent premature closure of a growth plate.

Equinus: a physical deformity of the foot and ankle, in which the heel is elevated and the foot dropped forward into a plantar flexed position (opposite of *calcaneus*).

Eversion: turning the plantar surface of the foot outward in relation to the leg.

External rotation: turning the anterior surface of the limb outward or laterally.

Forefoot: the front part of the foot, consisting of the toes and metatarsal bones.

Fusion: has the same orthopaedic significance as the term *arthrodesis*.

Genu valgum: the orthopaedic term for "knock knee."

Genu varum: the orthopaedic term for "bowleg."

Hanging cast: a plaster cast designed and applied not only to immobilize a fracture but also to deliver a traction force through the "hanging effect" of its own weight. Used frequently for the treatment of fractures through the lower half of the humerus.

Hemarthrosis: the distension of a joint by blood lying free within the joint cavity.

Hemilaminectomy: the operation of removing a portion of the vertebral lamina in order to gain exposure to an underlying nerve root or intervertebral disc.

Hindfoot: the rear part of the foot, consisting of the talus and calcaneus.

Internal rotation: turning the anterior surface of the limb inward or medially.

Inversion: turning the plantar surface of the foot inward in relation to the leg.

Limp: an asymmetrical pathologic gait.

Midfoot: the middle part of the foot, consisting of the navicular, cuboid, and cuneiform bones.

Myopathy: a general term used to refer to any disease of muscles.

Neurectomy: the surgical excision of a part of a nerve.

Neuropathy: a general term used to refer to a degenerative or noninflammatory disease of a nerve or nerves.

Orthosis: any device applied externally to assist or support a segment of the body.

Osteotomy: the surgical cutting of a bone.

Palmar flexion: a term used to denote the motion of flexion at the wrist causing the hand to be bent downward.

Passive motion: movement occurring by means of an external force, such as might be applied by an examiner.

Plantar flexion: a term used to denote the motion of flexion at the ankle joint causing the foot to be bent downward.

Pronation: when applied to the arm, the active turning of the forearm so that the palm of the hand faces downward; when applied to the foot, the combination of eversion and abduction, movements taking place in the tarsal and metatarsal joints and resulting in a "rolling over" of the longitudinal arch and an apparent "flat" foot.

Prosthesis: an artificial replacement for a part of the body that is diseased, damaged, or deficient. The term prosthesis also means an artificial limb.

Pseudarthrosis: a false joint formed when bone tissue does not successfully bridge a gap following an arthrodesis or fusion operation.

Recurvatum: a backward bending of a part or a joint.

Spica: a plaster cast applied in a figure-of-eight fashion, used to immobilize the trunk and an extremity, e.g., shoulder spica or hip spica.

Spinal fusion: the operation of fusing together two or more vertebral segments in order to eliminate motion between them.

Subluxation: partial displacement of the bones forming a joint.

Sugar-tong splint: a form of plaster immobilization useful in fractures of the wrist, forearm, humerus, ankle, and tibia. To immobilize the wrist or forearm, a continuous plaster splint is applied that begins just behind the metacarpal heads dorsally and extends along the dorsal aspect of the forearm, around the flexed elbow, and along the volar aspect of the forearm to end at the distal palmar flexion crease.

Supination: a turning of the forearm so that the palm of the hand faces upward.

Synovectomy: the operation of excision of the synovial membrane of the joint.

Tendon lengthening: the operation of lengthening a tightened or contracted tendon.

Tendon transplantation: the surgical relocation of the tendon of a normal muscle to another site to take over the function of a muscle permanently inactivated by trauma or disease.

Tenotomy: the surgical cutting of a tendon.

Total joint replacement: a special type of arthroplasty in which both sides of the joint are replaced by metal or plastic implants anchored to the bone by methyl methacrylate bone cement.

Valgus: in reference to a joint, the position assumed by the joint when the apex of the angle formed by the longitudinal axes of the component bones points toward the mid-line of the body; in reference to the foot, the term is usually applied to the heel and means that the heel is rotated outward on its longitudinal axis or everted.

Varus: in reference to a joint, the position assumed by the joint when the apex of the angle formed by the longitudinal axes of the component bones points away from the mid-line of the body; in reference to the foot, the term is usually applied to the heel and means that the heel is rotated inward on its longitudinal axis or inverted.

Index

Note: Page numbers in *italics* refer to illustrations. Page numbers followed by the letter t refer to tables.